AF776156

Updates in Anesthesia - The Operating Room and Beyond

Edited by Anna Ng-Pellegrino and Stanislaw P. Stawicki

Published in London, United Kingdom

Updates in Anesthesia - The Operating Room and Beyond
http://dx.doi.org/10.5772/intechopen.100964
Edited by Anna Ng-Pellegrino and Stanislaw P. Stawicki

Contributors
Akram M. Zaaqoq, Heidi J. Dalton, Mariam Gabrial, Kathryn Foster, Steven S Silvonek, Franzes Anne Z. Liongson, Rina Bhalodi, Christopher McCarthy, Sanjay V. Menghani, Ajaz Siddiqui, Wayne B. Bauerle, Jennifer Hwang, Anthony P. Allsbrook, Vanessa Reese, Prabhdeep Hehar, Suresh Kumar Singhal, Manisha Manohar, Judith Adrianne Deutsch, Kata Šakić, Tomica Bagatin, Johann Nemrava, Dinko Bagatin, Sadhana S Kulkarni, Savani S. Futane, Ellen Louise McHugh, Samina Khatib, Syed S.N. Razvi, Mudassir M. Shaikh, Mohammed Moizuddin Khan, James Pellechi, Meredith Harrison, Sean DuBois, Nicholas Roma, Joshua Holden Elmer, Bruce Ferraro, Matthew Krinock, Darren Traub, Maria Tatiana Martinez-Baladejo, Dustin Wong, Christina Spoleti, Diyor Suyumov, Alec James Divito, Shani Varghese Daniel, Shilpa Salpekar, Christine Marchionni, Maaz Siddiqui, Christian Nathaniel Schill, Rebecca E. Bates, Troy D. Lovett, Isha Kaza, Anna Ng-Pellegrino, Stanislaw P. Stawicki

© The Editor(s) and the Author(s) 2023

The rights of the editor(s) and the author(s) have been asserted in accordance with the Copyright, Designs and Patents Act 1988. All rights to the book as a whole are reserved by INTECHOPEN LIMITED. The book as a whole (compilation) cannot be reproduced, distributed or used for commercial or non-commercial purposes without INTECHOPEN LIMITED's written permission. Enquiries concerning the use of the book should be directed to INTECHOPEN LIMITED rights and permissions department (permissions@intechopen.com).

Violations are liable to prosecution under the governing Copyright Law.

Individual chapters of this publication are distributed under the terms of the Creative Commons Attribution 3.0 Unported License which permits commercial use, distribution and reproduction of the individual chapters, provided the original author(s) and source publication are appropriately acknowledged. If so indicated, certain images may not be included under the Creative Commons license. In such cases users will need to obtain permission from the license holder to reproduce the material. More details and guidelines concerning content reuse and adaptation can be found at http://www.intechopen.com/copyright-policy.html.

Notice

Statements and opinions expressed in the chapters are these of the individual contributors and not necessarily those of the editors or publisher. No responsibility is accepted for the accuracy of information contained in the published chapters. The publisher assumes no responsibility for any damage or injury to persons or property arising out of the use of any materials, instructions, methods or ideas contained in the book.

First published in London, United Kingdom, 2023 by IntechOpen
IntechOpen is the global imprint of INTECHOPEN LIMITED, registered in England and Wales, registration number: 11086078, 5 Princes Gate Court, London, SW7 2QJ, United Kingdom

British Library Cataloguing-in-Publication Data
A catalogue record for this book is available from the British Library

Additional hard and PDF copies can be obtained from orders@intechopen.com

Updates in Anesthesia - The Operating Room and Beyond
Edited by Anna Ng-Pellegrino and Stanislaw P. Stawicki
p. cm.
Print ISBN 978-1-80355-576-8
Online ISBN 978-1-80355-577-5
eBook (PDF) ISBN 978-1-80355-578-2

We are IntechOpen, the world's leading publisher of Open Access books

Built by scientists, for scientists

6,400+
Open access books available

174,000+
International authors and editors

190M+
Downloads

156
Countries delivered to

Our authors are among the
Top 1%
most cited scientists

12.2%
Contributors from top 500 universities

WEB OF SCIENCE™

Selection of our books indexed in the Book Citation Index
in Web of Science™ Core Collection (BKCI)

Interested in publishing with us?
Contact book.department@intechopen.com

Numbers displayed above are based on latest data collected.
For more information visit www.intechopen.com

For EU product safety concerns:
IN TECH d.o.o., Prolaz Marije Krucifikse Kozulić 3, 51000 Rijeka, Croatia,
info@intechopen.com or visit our website at intechopen.com.

Meet the editors

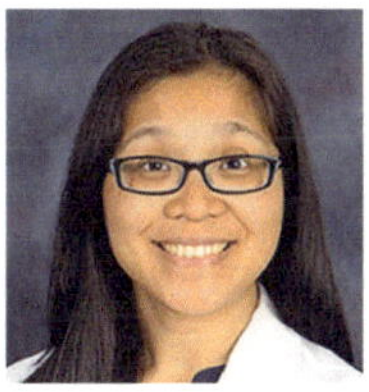

Anna Ng-Pellegrino is a board-certified cardiac anesthesiologist and the Director of Perioperative Research at the Department of Research and Innovation, St. Luke's University Health Network, Pennsylvania, USA. She is a mentor to medical students, student nurse anesthetists, residents, and postdoctoral research fellows. Her research interests and quality projects focus on perioperative medicine, including outcomes from enhanced recovery after surgery (ERAS) protocols, regional and pain medicine, ambulatory surgery, and safety monitoring for the patient floor in the hospital setting. Her authorship contributions can be seen in research articles, books, and abstracts.

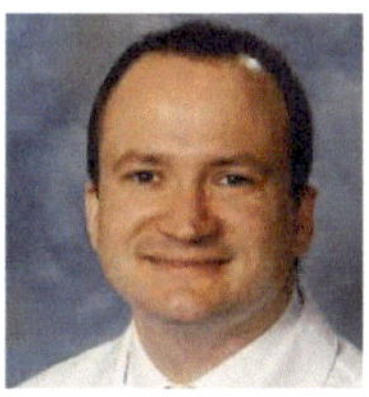

Dr. Stanislaw P. Stawicki, MD, MBA, is a professor of surgery and Chair of the Department of Research and Innovation, St. Luke's University Health Network, Pennsylvania, USA. A specialist in trauma, general surgery, and surgical critical care, he has co-authored nearly 700 scholarly works, including more than 25 books. In addition to national and international medical leadership roles, Dr. Stawicki is a member of numerous editorial boards and grant evaluation/review bodies. His areas of expertise include patient safety, medical innovation, blockchain technology, medical education, academic leadership, mentorship, trauma/critical care, and sonography.

Contents

Preface

Modern anesthesiology is a product of a century-long evolutionary process. A transition from "the art" to "the science" of anesthesiology has been taking place since the early 1900s, with novel applications of medical, surgical, and basic science knowledge, and successful implementation of technological advances. Further rapid growth took place following World War II when advances from the military experience of the most devastating war in human history became integrated into everyday clinical practice. In parallel, a unique synergy emerged between surgery and anesthesiology – a trend that continues to this day, now including various other procedural-oriented specialties.

With improvements in technology came improvements in anesthesia safety, with a plethora of scientific and technological advances. Today, anesthesiology is at the forefront of clinical innovation, providing leadership and direction to all the other specialty areas that intersect its domain within the collective Venn diagram of modern medicine. Among key developments of the recent past, concepts such as "prehabilitation" (work on conditioning/preparing the patient's mind and body weeks before surgery), "perioperative surgical home" (a construct wherein perioperative care is delivered on a continuum of preoperative to intraoperative to postoperative stages) and finally the "hospital at home" concept, have important implications for both the role and scope of practice of anesthesiologists of the future. Finally, it would be remiss not to mention the importance of enhanced recovery after surgery (ERAS) protocols, their more recent proliferation, and their beneficial effect on patient outcomes.

Modern-day anesthesiology encompasses many highly differentiated subspecialties, including critical care, neuroscience, pediatrics, geriatrics, cardiothoracic, obstetrics, regional and acute pain management. In this book, we would like to take the reader on a stimulating adventure through current and state-of-the-art anesthesia practice and its subspecialties. Within this broader context, we must emphasize the importance of collaboration and teamwork between anesthesia and various surgical and medical specialties when taking care of a patient, whether it is in the setting of trauma and critical care, in patients with psychiatric disorders, or when managing patients undergoing life-threatening complications requiring emergent airway and/or complex resuscitation efforts.

This book pays homage to, and recognizes, the importance of anesthesiology and anesthesiologists to our modern healthcare systems. It also highlights the various present and future roles undertaken by anesthesiologists, both in the operating rooms and beyond. We also emphasize the embrace of multidisciplinary and multi-specialty approaches, both of which are inherently natural and seamless to the modern practice of anesthesiology. As the editors of this unique collection of chapters, it is our hope that we are accurately and effectively portraying modern anesthesiology as a truly unifying force within the fabric of the contemporary healthcare environment.

Anna Ng-Pellegrino
Department of Anesthesiology,
Research and Innovations Department,
St. Luke's University Health Network,
Bethlehem, PA, USA

Stanislaw P. Stawicki
Department of Research and Innovation,
St. Luke's University Health Network,
Bethlehem, PA, USA

Section 1

Introduction

Chapter 1

Introductory Chapter: Modern Anesthesiology as a Unifying Force

Anna Ng-Pellegrino and Stanislaw P. Stawicki

1. Introduction

Modern anesthesiology has gained recognition as a leader in promoting patient safety and quality of care in the medical profession, with novel technological developments continually pushing for better clinical outcomes [1, 2]. There is also a tremendous amount of intellectual diversity within modern anesthesiology, including various schools of thought, subspecialties, interdisciplinary approaches, and a strong tradition of innovation (**Figure 1**). However, this has not always been the case [3]. As recently as a century ago, patients feared undergoing surgery because of the low likelihood of waking up from the anesthetic [4–6]. Not only did the options of inhaled anesthetic agents at that time impose many adverse reactions (changes in mentation, arrhythmias, liver toxicity), but anesthesia was administered via mask inhalation, hence, with an unprotected airway. The risk of aspiration of stomach contents was prevalent, leading to aspiration pneumonias and death [4].

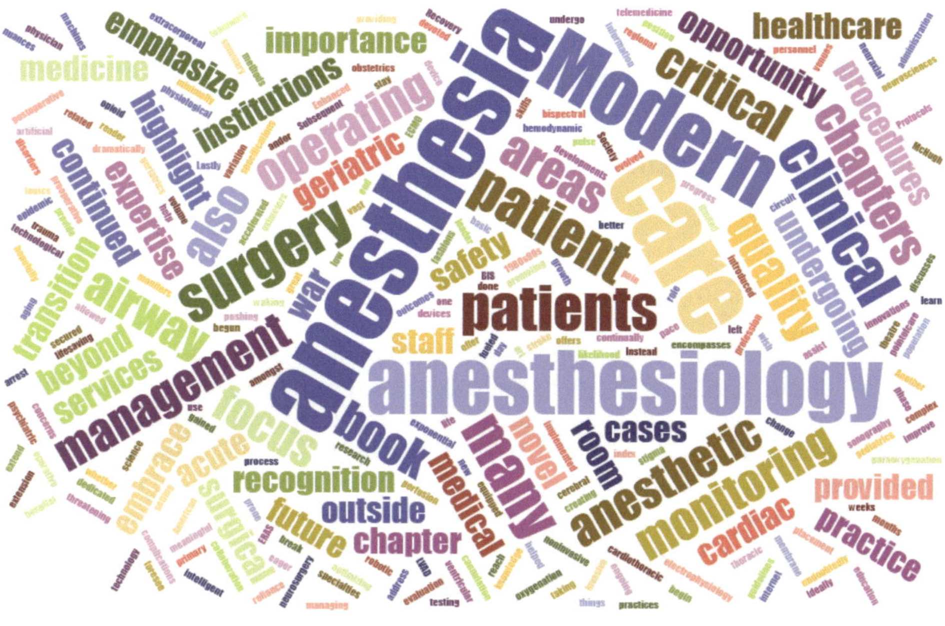

Figure 1.
Word cloud reflecting the breadth of topics within the current book.

IntechOpen

Anesthesia evolved dramatically from the 1900s, as there came to be successful implementations and novel applications of medical, surgical, and basic science knowledge with technological advances [3, 7, 8]. An extraordinary breakthrough occurred in 1926 when Arthur Guedel introduced the concept of a cuffed endotracheal tube through his experiments with submerging dogs underwater and under anesthesia [9]. The 1930s also provided the initial foundations for the modern concept of morbidity and mortality conferences, as anesthesia docs set up meetings with the coroner to learn about patient deaths from anesthesia [4].

2. Rapid growth and development

Modern anesthesiology dates back to the post-World War II era, with advances from the military experience of the most devastating war in human history becoming integrated into everyday clinical practice [8, 10]. A unique synergy emerged between surgery and anesthesiology – a trend that continues to this day [11]. This trend was further augmented by the influx of the newly available medical workforce, rich with experiences from the war theater [10]. From 1940s to 2000, the pace of progress, fueled by exponential growth in basic and clinical research, further accelerated the transition from "the art" into "the science" of anesthesiology [8, 12].

During the same time, patient safety organizations grew in number nationally and internationally. Increasingly more sophisticated anesthetic devices and adjunctive tools were created in this era [13, 14]. With improvement in technology came improvements in safely administering anesthesia through creative advances in airway equipment (video laryngoscopy), ventilators (safety valves and flowmeters set to prevent delivery of a hypoxic mixture to the patient), infusion pumps, and regional/neuraxial anesthetic kits [13, 14]. Monitors standardized to specifications by the American Society of Anesthesia were introduced and implemented in the 1980s–90s in the US. Subsequent innovations in monitoring devices allowed one to process hemodynamic and physiological information in noninvasive fashions (pulse oximeters, cerebral perfusion monitors, stroke volume variation monitoring, bispectral index (BIS) monitoring, modern point-of-care sonography) [2, 15–17]. Computer technology helped to improve the quality of care in the preoperative assessment stage and provided new opportunities for anesthesia training and simulation for crisis management [3, 18, 19].

3. Innovation: the core of anesthesiology's DNA

More than 13 million surgeries were performed in the United States from 2019 to 2021 [6]. In the 2000s–2010s, more than 50% of surgical, diagnostic, and interventional procedures are being performed outside of the operating room (OR), including settings such as cardiac catheterization labs, MRI suites, interventional radiology departments, and dental suits. The last three decades showed tremendous growth in the role anesthesia plays in perioperative management. The preadmission testing clinic evolved into a concept known as a perioperative surgical home, where anesthesia staff conducts the management of the preoperative, intraoperative, and postoperative care of a patient [20]. By having patients undergo "prehabilitation", where they concentrate on conditioning/preparing their mind and body weeks before surgery, would help to maximize wellness and reduce both complications and postoperative rehabilitation needs [21–23]. In addition, multidisciplinary care pathways and Enhanced Recovery after Surgery (ERAS) protocols are being created that incorporate precision medicine and improve patient outcomes [24, 25]. This new role in anesthesia helped to break down the stigma that anesthesia services are limited to the operating room. Instead, being equipped with a vast knowledge of acute care and lifesaving skills, anesthesia personnel are provided with the opportunity to help transition their quality of care and expertise into meaningful change outside of the operating room.

Modern day anesthesiology also encompasses many dedicated subspecialties, with a focus on critical care, neurosciences, pediatrics, geriatrics, cardiothoracic, obstetrics, and regional and acute pain management [26–31]. As editors of this book, we would like to take the reader on an adventure that will stimulate one's mindset on what is "current and state-of-the-art" in anesthesia practice and its subspecialties. With regards to airway management, a plastic surgery group in Europe provided a unique take on the use of supraglottic airways devices (i-gel LMA™, Intersurgical, UK) in the prone position. Another chapter discusses novel methods to provide paraoxygenation while an airway is being secured. The reader will hopefully embrace our chapters that focus on the anesthetic management of patients undergoing complex cardiac procedures, such as electrophysiology cases, left ventricular assist device (LVAD) placement, and extracorporeal circuit membrane oxygenation (ECMO) cannulation. As more surgical subspecialties have begun to offer minimally invasive and/or robotic procedures, chapters are devoted in this book to highlight Enhanced Recovery after Surgery (ERAS) Protocols in thoracic and neurosurgery cases. To address care for the aging population in the US, many institutions are creating guidelines for optimizing their care before surgery. The book chapter by McHugh offers a great summary of what is being done in the evaluation of the geriatric patient in the preoperative testing phase. To highlight concerns with the ongoing opioid epidemic in the US, there is a dedicated discussion of methods to curtail narcotic use in acute pain management, chronic pain management (interventional procedures), and regional pain management (local anesthetic nerve blocks) chapters. Lastly, we wish to emphasize the importance of collaboration and teamwork with surgical and medical specialties when taking care of a patient, whether it is in the setting of trauma and critical care, in patients with psychiatric disorders, or when managing patients who undergo life-threatening complications, such as cardiac arrest after neuraxial anesthesia.

4. Anesthesia beyond anesthesiology

The reach of modern anesthesiology does not begin, nor does it end in the operative theater. The future of anesthesia care will undoubtedly focus on topics such as the continued extension of anesthesia-related services to venues outside of the OR and the continued reliance on technology to further improve patient safety and quality of care, such as with telemedicine, the use of artificial intelligent machines, or the "internet of things" (IOT) construct [32–37]. Furthermore, as the world reflects on climate change and methods to prevent ongoing environmental harm, more anesthesia practices may turn to ways to achieve a "greener" operating room, such as minimizing the use of volatile agents and utilizing more total intravenous anesthesia (TIVA) [38, 39]. There is even an opportunity for anesthesia practices to extend beyond a patients' hospital stay. Many institutions foresee their anesthesia staff providing care weeks to months after surgery, as the "primary postoperative physician" [40, 41]. In addition, the concept of remote monitoring has extended into the home, to provide a "hospital at home" model of care [42, 43]. This highlights the use of anesthesia standard monitors to use at home and have the vital signs tracked over to a virtual remote center.

The clinical realm of anesthesia also does not end with anesthesiology-trained clinicians. For one the concept of "conscious sedation" has been extended to surgeons, gastroenterologists, dentists, intensivists, and emergency medicine physicians, among other specialties [44–46]. Ideally, further education can be provided by anesthesia staff to those eager to learn more about the nuances of airway management and anesthesia administration. Eventually, areas of clinical overlap may develop, with multi-specialty participation in "unified super-specialty areas" – such specialty and content expertise unification can currently be seen in areas such as critical care medicine, traumatology, geriatric medicine, and pain/palliative care [47–50].

5. Synthesis and conclusion

This book recognizes the important role that anesthesiologists play within our increasingly complex and moderm healthcare system. It also highlights the various present and future roles that anesthesiologists will partake, both in the operating rooms and beyond. We also emphasize the embrace of multidisciplinary and multi-specialty approaches, both of which are inherently natural and seamless to the modern practice of anesthesiology. It is our hope, as the Editors of this unique collection of chapters, that we accurately and effectively portray modern anesthesiology as a true unifying force within the fabric of the contemporary healthcare environment.

Author details

Anna Ng-Pellegrino[1,2*] and Stanislaw P. Stawicki[2]

1 Department of Anesthesiology, St. Luke's University Health Network, Bethlehem, Pennsylvania, United States

2 Department of Research and Innovation, St. Luke's University Health Network, Bethlehem, Pennsylvania, United States

*Address all correspondence to: anna.ngpellegrino@sluhn.org

IntechOpen

© 2023 The Author(s). Licensee IntechOpen. This chapter is distributed under the terms of the Creative Commons Attribution License (http://creativecommons.org/licenses/by/3.0), which permits unrestricted use, distribution, and reproduction in any medium, provided the original work is properly cited.

References

[1] Vanhonacker D, Verdonck M, Nogueira Carvalho H. Impact of closed-loop technology, machine learning, and artificial intelligence on patient safety and the future of Anesthesia. Current Anesthesiology Reports. 2022;**12**(4):451-460

[2] Cipriano A et al. Reducing telemetry use while improving patient outcomes: University health network experience with the implementation of oximetry-based monitoring system. International Journal of Academic Medicine. 2018;**4**(2):112

[3] Moon JS, Cannesson M. A century of technology in Anesthesia & analgesia. Anesthesia & Analgesia. 2022;**135**(2S):S48-S61

[4] Liu LL, Larson MD. Patient safety during anesthesia: 100 years of progress documented in Anesthesia & Analgesia. Anesthesia & Analgesia. 2022;**135**(2S):S37-S47

[5] Klafta JM, Roizen MF. Current understanding of patients' attitudes toward and preparation for anesthesia: A review. Anesthesia & Analgesia. 1996;**83**(6):1314-1321

[6] Hansson N et al. No silver medal for Nobel prize contenders: Why anesthesia pioneers were nominated for but denied the award. Anesthesiology. 2016;**125**(1):34-38

[7] Matioc AA. An Anesthesiologist's perspective on the history of basic airway management: The "modern" era, 1960 to present. Anesthesiology. 2019;**130**(5):686-711

[8] Kurup V and Barash P. History of Anesthesiology. A Guide to Anesthesiology for Medical Students. 2018;**2018**:4-5

[9] Thomson J, Arthur E. Guedel (1883-1956): Self-trained Pioneer. Anesthesiology-Philadelphia Then Hagerstown. 2000;**93**(3, SUPP/2):A1163-A1163

[10] Muravchick S, Rosenberg H. Austin Lamont and the evolution of modern academic American anesthesiology. The Journal of the American Society of Anesthesiologists. 1996;**84**(2):436-441

[11] Roberts CG. Some signposts of surgical Progress. Journal of the National Medical Association. 1949;**41**(1):3

[12] Frader JE, Caniano DA. Research and innovation in surgery. In: Surgical Ethics. New York: Oxford University Press; 1998. pp. 216-241

[13] Meyer J-U et al. Advanced technologies and devices for inhalational anesthetic drug dosing. Modern Anesthetics. 2008;**182**:451-470

[14] Saracoglu KT et al. Anesthesia machines and Anesthetic breathing system. In: Improving Anesthesia Technical Staff's Skills. Cham: Springer International Publishing; 2022. pp. 117-123

[15] Kelly N et al. Clinician-performed ultrasound in hemodynamic and cardiac assessment: A synopsis of current indications and limitations. European Journal of Trauma and Emergency Surgery. 2015;**41**:469-480

[16] Stawicki S et al. Use of the esophageal echo-Doppler to guide intensive care unit resuscitations: A retrospective study. IJCCM. 2007;**11**:54-60

[17] Kissin I. Depth of anesthesia and bispectral index monitoring. Anesthesia & Analgesia. 2000;**90**(5):1114-1117

[18] Marcks V, Hayes K, Stawicki SP. Operating room trauma simulation: The St. Luke's university health network experience. International Journal of Critical Illness and Injury Science. 2020;**10**(1):4

[19] Southwick K et al. Screen-based simulation as a novel recertification tool for certified registered nurse Anesthetists. Clinical Simulation in Nursing. 2023;**75**:11-19

[20] Kain ZN et al. The perioperative surgical home as a future perioperative practice model. Anesthesia & Analgesia. 2014;**118**(5):1126-1130

[21] Carli F, Scheede-Bergdahl C. Prehabilitation to enhance perioperative care. Anesthesiology Clinics. 2015;**33**(1):17-33

[22] Wynter-Blyth V, Moorthy K. Prehabilitation: Preparing patients for surgery. BMJ: British Medical Journal (Online). 2017:358. DOI: 10.1136/bmj.j3702

[23] Durrand J, et al. Prehabilitation. Perioperative Medicine–Current Controversies. 2016. p. 15-47

[24] Malige A, Sokunbi G. Efficacy of an enhanced recovery after surgery (ERAS) protocol for Orthopedic spinal fusion procedures. International Journal of Academic Medicine. 2020;**6**(3):252-253

[25] Frenzel Z, Fontem R, Gifford A. Implementation of an enhanced recovery after surgery protocol for video-assisted Thoracoscopic surgery lobectomy decreases perioperative opioid use. International Journal of Academic Medicine. 2020;**6**(3):260-261

[26] Capdeville M et al. The educational evolution of fellowship training in cardiothoracic anesthesiology–perspectives from program directors around the United States. Journal of Cardiothoracic and Vascular Anesthesia. 2018;**32**(2):607-620

[27] Cladis F, Yanofsky S. Education in pediatric anesthesiology: The evolution of a specialty. International Anesthesiology Clinics. 2019;**57**(4):3-14

[28] Shapiro DM et al. History and evolution of regional anesthesiology and acute pain medicine fellowship training. Regional Anesthesia & Pain Medicine. 2020;**45**(4):311-314

[29] Newman MF, Mathew JP, Aronson S. The evolution of anesthesiology and perioperative medicine. Anesthesiology. 2013;**118**(5):1005-1007

[30] Prielipp RC, Cohen NH. The future of anesthesiology: Implications of the changing healthcare environment. Current Opinion in Anesthesiology. 2016;**29**(2):198-205

[31] Teplick R, Rosenthal M. The evolution of the anesthesiologist: Novel perioperative roles and beyond. Anesthesiology Clinics. 2009;**27**(1):157-165

[32] Varughese S, Ahmed R. Environmental and occupational considerations of anesthesia: A narrative review and update. Anesthesia and Analgesia. 2021;**133**(4):826

[33] Bellini V et al. Artificial intelligence: A new tool in operating room management. Role of machine learning models in operating room optimization. Journal of Medical Systems. 2020;**44**(1):20

[34] Stawicki S. Blockchain in Healthcare: From Disruption to Integration. Vol. 10. Switzerland AG: Springer Nature; 2023

[35] Stawicki SP et al. Roadmap for the development of academic and medical applications of blockchain technology: Joint statement from OPUS 12 global and litecoin cash foundation. Journal of Emergencies, Trauma, and Shock. 2019;**12**(1):64

[36] Kelley KC et al. Answering the challenge of COVID-19 pandemic through innovation and ingenuity. In: Coronavirus Disease-COVID-19. Cham: Springer International Publishing; 2021. pp. 859-873

[37] Chauhan V et al. Novel coronavirus (COVID-19): Leveraging telemedicine to optimize care while minimizing exposures and viral transmission. Journal of Emergencies, Trauma, and Shock. 2020;**13**(1):20

[38] Wong SSC et al. Total intravenous anesthesia (TIVA) with propofol for acute postoperative pain: A scoping review of randomized controlled trials. Asian Journal of Anesthesiology. 2020;**58**(3):79-93

[39] Miller TE, Gan TJ. Total intravenous anesthesia and anesthetic outcomes. Journal of Cardiothoracic and Vascular Anesthesia. 2015;**29**:S11-S15

[40] Bridges KH, McSwain JR, Wilson PR. To infinity and beyond: The past, present, and future of tele-anesthesia. Anesthesia & Analgesia. 2020;**130**(2):276-284

[41] Coppens M, Van Caelenberg E, De Regge M. Postoperative innovative technology for ambulatory anesthesia and surgery. Current Opinion in Anaesthesiology. 2021;**34**(6):709-713

[42] Leff B et al. Satisfaction with hospital at home care. Journal of the American Geriatrics Society. 2006;**54**(9):1355-1363

[43] Shepperd S et al. Randomised controlled trial comparing hospital at home care with inpatient hospital care. II: Cost minimisation analysis. BMJ. 1998;**316**(7147):1791-1796

[44] Leroy P, Gorzeman M, Sury M. Procedural sedation and analgesia in children by non-anesthesiologists in an emergency department. Minerva Pediatrica. 2009;**61**(2):193-215

[45] Soifer BE. Procedural anesthesia at the bedside. Critical Care Clinics. 2000;**16**(1):7-28

[46] Amornyotin S. Sedation and monitoring for gastrointestinal endoscopy. World Journal of Gastrointestinal Endoscopy. 2013;**5**(2):47

[47] Krell K. Critical care workforce. Critical Care Medicine. 2008;**36**(4):1350-1353

[48] Bassette E et al. Hospice and palliative medicine fellowship after surgical training: A roadmap to the future of surgical palliative care. Journal of Surgical Education. 2022;**79**(5):1177-1187

[49] Bach JA et al. The right team at the right time–multidisciplinary approach to multi-trauma patient with orthopedic injuries. International Journal of Critical Illness and Injury Science. 2017;**7**(1):32

[50] Kelley KC et al. Emergency trauma providers as equal partners: From "proof of concept" to "outcome parity". The American Surgeon. 2019;**85**(9):961-964

Section 2

Airway Management

Chapter 2

Hypoxia and Paraoxygenation

Suresh Kumar Singhal and Manisha Manohar

Abstract

Hypoxemia whether critical or not is a complication associated with airway management. The abruptness with which the hypoxic events can occur during airway management in anticipated as well as unanticipated difficult airways provide very little time to the airway managers to avoid the whirlpool of complications that can ensue if hypoxia persists. An understanding of the etiology and mechanisms of hypoxemia and the techniques that can ensure oxygenation for a prolonged time provide a safe window to think and execute the airway management plans. Paraoxygenation is one such technique that ensures an uninterrupted oxygen supply to the patient after the onset of apnoea and prolongs the safe apnoea time significantly.

Keywords: hypoxia, hypoxemia, paraoxygenation, apneic oxygenation, safe apnea time, NODESAT, THRIVE, barotrauma

1. Introduction

Perioperative hypoxia occurs due to variety of causes. An anesthesiologist has to diagnose as well as treat the hypoxic events in a very short frame of time before the development of critical hypoxemia. An understanding of the causes and the pathophysiology of types of hypoxia is a prerequisite for successful management of hypoxic episodes. The technique of Paraoxygenation, also known as apneic oxygenation has found use in anaesthesia as well as critical care. This technique can be easily applied in patient population at risk of hypoxia with easily available equipments like nasal prongs, end bronchial catheters, RAE tube inside the operating theatres. Although associated with various complications, Paraoxygenation prolongs the duration of apnea without desaturation and buys time for the airway management before the development of critical hypoxemia.

1.1 Literature search

PubMed, Googlescholar, manual searches were used to find the relevant articles. The following key words were used for the search: apnoeicoxygenation, paraoxygenation, difficult intubation, hypoxia, hypoxemia, aventilatory mass flow.

1.2 Aim

This chapter focuses on understanding the pathophysiology of hypoxia and the role of paraoxygenation in various aspects of anaesthesiology and critical care.

Hypoxia

I. Definition

II. Classification

III. Clinical effects of hypoxia

Paraoxygenation

I. Physiologic basis

II. Prerequisite

III. Techniques

IV. Clinical application

V. Complications

2. Hypoxia

2.1 Definition

Although used synonymously quite often, the term hypoxia and hypoxemia are different and should be used in appropriate clinical scenarios. Hypoxemia is the arterial PO2 below what is expected normal for a patient's age while hypoxia is decreased level of tissue oxygenation. Hypoxia and Hypoxemia do not always coexist e.g., Hypoxia in cyanide poisoning is due to the defective utilisation of oxygen despite having normal oxygen levels in the blood.

2.2 Classification of hypoxia

1. Hypoxic hypoxia (Hypoxemia): is defined as arterial Pao2 less than 60 mmHg or SaO2 < 90%. Hypoxemia is one of the most feared and common complication related to tracheal intubation that can occur suddenly in the perioperative period. Hypoxemic episodes can occur during induction, maintenance, extubation and post extubation period (**Figures 1** and **2**).

2.2.1 Causes of hypoxemia

i. Hypoxemia due to the patient factors: Airway obstruction in unconscious patient is mostly due to tongue falling back against posterior pharynx and is commonly seen in patients with history of obstructive sleep apnea. Secretions/blood in the airway, laryngospasm, bronchospasm, glottic edema due to airway instrumentation, aspiration of vomitus, retained throat pack, external pressure on the trachea due to a neck hematoma can lead to critical hypoxemia.

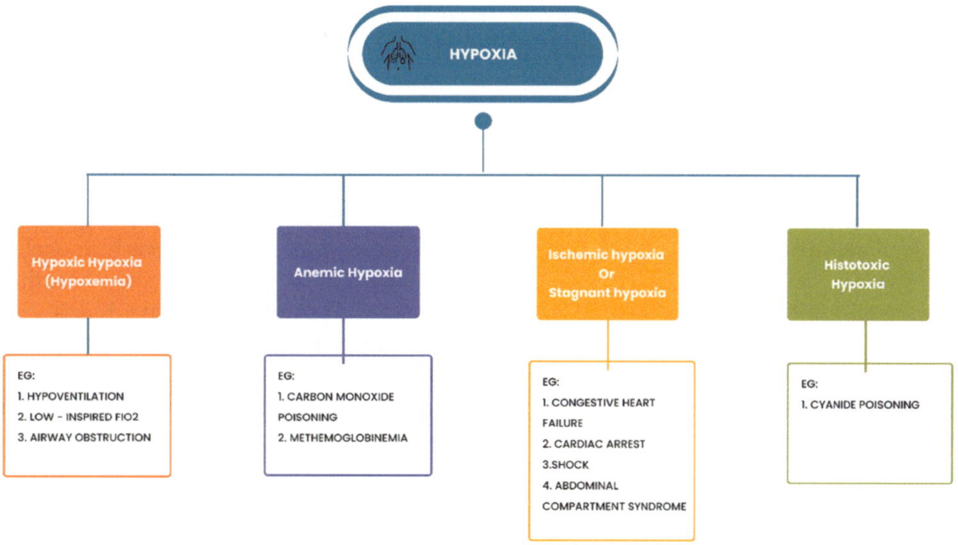

Figure 1.
Classification of hypoxia.

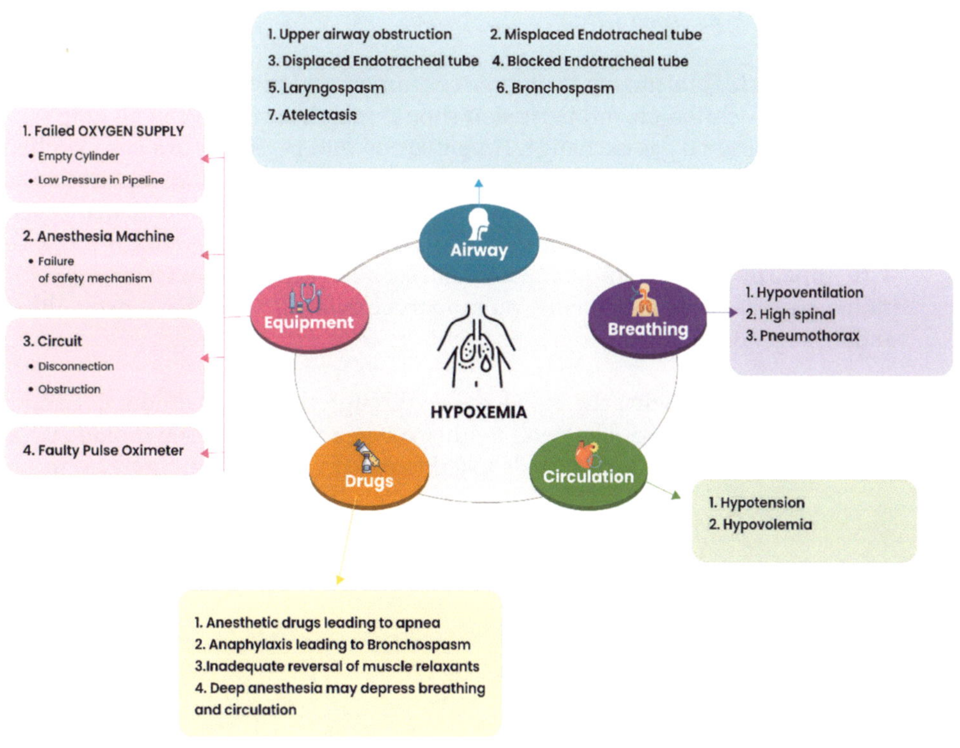

Figure 2.
Common causes of perioperative hypoxemia.

ii. Hypoxemia due to the equipment factors: Delivery and monitoring of the anaesthetic gases to the patient is done through a series of equipment. Any fault with the functioning of the equipment e.g.: pipeline, oxygen cylinder, anaesthesia machine, anaesthesia circuit, pulse oximetry can lead to the development of hypoxemia

2.3 Clinical effects of hypoxemia

The cardiovascular response to hypoxemia is a product of neural, humoral and direct effects. The neural reflex which is excitatory is mediated by aortic, carotid chemoreceptors, baroreceptors and central cerebral stimulation while the humoral reflex which is vasoconstrictive is mediated by release of catecholamines and renin angiotensin release. The direct local vascular effect of hypoxia is seen late and is manifested as inhibitory and vasodilatory effect. Mild arterial hypoxemia causes generalised activation of the sympathetic nervous system and release of catecholamines leading to an increase in heart rate, stroke volume and myocardial contractility. With the onset of moderate hypoxemia local vasodilation begins to predominate and systemic vascular resistance and blood pressure begin to decrease, however heart rate increases due to the hypotension induced stimulation of baroreceptors. With severe hypoxemia the local depressant effect dominates and blood pressure falls rapidly, pulse slows down, shock develops and heart either fibrillates or becomes asystolic [1] (**Figure 3**).

2.3.1 Mechanisms of hypoxemia [2]

a. V/Q mismatch/Q mismatch is the most common underlying mechanism for hypoxemia. Ventilation and perfusion should match each other in all lung regions for optimal gas exchange. If ventilation and perfusion are not matched gas exchange is affected. Low V/Q will impair oxygenation since ventilation is insufficient to fully oxygenate the blood. The degree of impairment will depend on the degree of V/Q mismatch. Alveolar arterial oxygen difference is increased with impairment of v/q ratio. Hypoxemia seen in chronic obstructive pulmonary disease, emphysema, pulmonaryembolism, asthma is mostly due to underlying V/Q mismatch

b. Right to left shunt: when the blood passes through the lungs without coming in contact with the ventilated alveoli neither oxygen nor the carbon dioxide is released from the blood. This leads to a decrease in Pao2 and an increase in

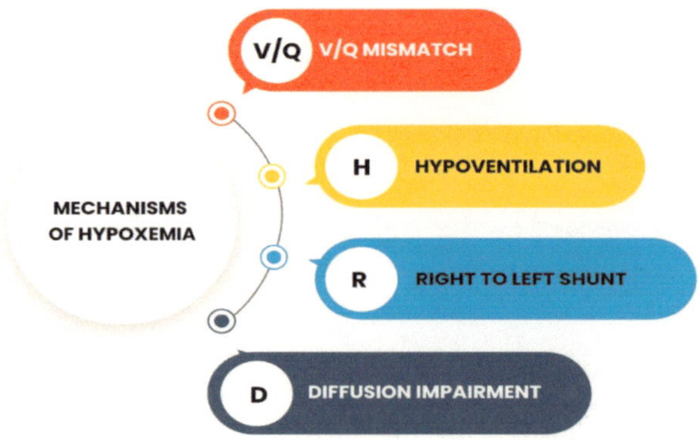

Figure 3.
Mechanisms of hypoxemia.

Paco2 and the condition is called SHUNT. Hypoxemia seen in pulmonary carbon dioxide is largely due to the right to left shunting of the blood

c. Diffusion impairment: impaired diffusion across the alveolar capillary membrane either due to fibrosis or vascular abnormality leads to slow diffusion of gases across the membrane. Hypoxemia seen in pulmonary fibrosis or in pulmonary edema is due to undergoing diffusion impairment

d. Hypoventilation: Paco2 more than 45 mmHg is the hallmark of hypoventilation. Adequate ventilation is required both for oxygenation as well as removal of carbon dioxide. Hypoventilation leads to a low PAO2 which subsequently leads to low Pao2.One of the characteristic features of hypoxemia cause due to hypoventilation is that it is corrected by administration of oxygen even if hypoventilation and hypercapnia persists.

2. *Anaemic hypoxia*: Anaemic hypoxia is characterised by decreased oxygen carrying capacity of the blood either due to low haemoglobin or due to presence of abnormal haemoglobin (carboxyhaemoglobin, methaemoglobin). A reduction in the haemoglobin concentration of the blood is accompanied by a corresponding decline in the oxygen carrying capacity of the blood. Although Pao2 is normal in anaemic hypoxia, the absolute quantity of the oxygen transported per unit volume of the blood is diminished. As the anaemic blood passes through the capillaries the usual quantity of oxygen is removed from it and Pao2 and saturation in the venous blood decline to a greater extent than normal. Presence of carbon monoxide in the blood leads to the formation of carboxyhaemoglobin there by reducing the amount of oxyhaemoglobin. The arterial oxygen decreases in proportion to the increase in carboxyhaemoglobin reflecting the ability of Carbon monoxide to block oxygen binding to haemoglobin.

3. *Ischemic or stagnant hypoxia or Hypokinetic hypoxia*: Decreased cardiac output or sluggish blood flow either due to heart failure, shock, or haemorrhage leads to stagnant hypoxia. The blood remains in the tissues for a greater period of time leading to increased extraction of oxygen. The Pao2 is usually normal but the venous and the tissue po2 values are reduced as a consequence of reduced tissue perfusion and greater tissue extraction.

4. *Histotoxic hypoxia*: is due to the inability of the tissue to utilise oxygen despite adequate availability of oxygen in the blood. Cyanide induced inhibition of cytochrome oxidase halts the process of oxidative metabolism in mitochondria leading to an increased uptake of pyruvate by mitochondria resulting in excess production of lacticacid.

The process of intubation inherently makes the patient prone to hypoxemia due to the reduced functional residual capacity (FRC) insupine position, hypoventilationdue to anaesthetic agents and deliberately induced apnoeawith musclerelaxants. Hypoxemia can develop with startling abruptness during the perioperative period without giving much time for the patient rescue. Oxygenating a patient prior to the induction of anaesthesia is called Preoxygenation. Adequate preoxygenation prolongs the duration of apnoea without desaturation (DAWD) by building up the oxygen reserve in the functional residual capacity which acts like a reservoir from where the oxygen can be extracted and delivered to blood thereby avoiding the desaturation to critical levels. Preoxygenation is currently the standard of care in all patients undergoing general anaesthesia. However, conventional preoxygenation techniques may be inadequate in providing a safe apnoeic period (time from apnoea onset to spo2 90%) in all patient's population especially the one with high oxygen requirements (paediatric, obstetric, obese) or those with difficult airways. In order to supplement preoxygenation and to prolong the safe apnoea time further Para oxygenation or apnoeic oxygenation can be used as a useful adjunct to preoxygenation.

3. Paraoxygenation

Para oxygenation is the technique of providing uninterrupted oxygen supply to the patient after the onset of apnoea in order to prolong the safe apnoea time especially in patients with difficult airways to provide adequate time to the anaesthesiologist for uninterrupted execution of the attempts to secure the airway. Paraoxygenation is also known as apnoeic oxygenation.

3.1 Physiologic basis of para oxygenation:

Aventilatory mass flow [3]/diffusion respiratio [4]/apnoeic diffusion of oxygen [5]: The oxygen consumption of a health adult is 250 ml/min while the carbon dioxide production is 200 ml/min. Inapnoeic patients the extraction of oxygen from the alveoli continues at the rate of 250 ml/min while carbon dioxide delivery to the alveoli is 21 ml/min thereby causing the alveolar pressure to become sub atmospheric leading to a generation of pressure gradient which enables the movement of additional administered oxygen provided the airway is patent· Preoxygenation facilitates the process of apnoeic oxygenation by denitrogenating the alveoli. In the absence of adequate preoxygenation, the persistence of nitrogen in the lungs along with the accumulating carbon dioxide will diminish the pressure gradient available for the mass flow of oxygen into the alveoli thereby hastening the onset of hypoxemia. The persistent delivery of 100 percent oxygen prevents the renitrogenation of the alveoli during the apnoea. The sub atmospheric pressure also promotes carbon dioxide transfer from blood to the alveoli. The degree of oxygen extraction from the alveoli exceeds the degree of carbon dioxide return to the alveoli since carbon dioxide is buffered in the body but with time the alveolar accumulation of carbon dioxide reaches a critical level beyond which the pressure gradient is reduced thereby reducing the aventilatory mass flow of oxygen.

3.2 Prerequisite for para oxygenation

1. *Patent upper airway*: A patent airway is an absolute prerequisite for successful paraoxygenation. This allows the oxygen to be delivered to the hypopharynx and be entrained into the trachea Patient should be positioned to maximise upper airway patency using ear to sternal notch positioning. During the apnoeic period, upper airway obstruction should be prevented by using the airway manoeuvres like head tilt, chin lift, jaw thrust or by using the oropharyngeal airway/nasopharyngeal airway.

2. *Adequate preoxygenation*: The benefit of apnoeic diffusion oxygenation is dependent on achieving maximal preoxygenation before apnoea.

3. *Placement of a device to deliver oxygen*: Para oxygenation can be achieved by using any device that administers oxygen into the respiratory tract including, nasal

cannula, nasopharyngeal catheter, rigid bronchoscope, catheter placed in trachea, endobronchial catheters, front of neck catheter, channels located in direct and video laryngoscopes.

4. *Oxygen source*: Auxiliary port in the anaesthesia machine or an oxygen cylinder in case of intubations done in out of operating room settings can be used for the oxygen denitrogenating supply.

3.3 Techniques

Various techniques for administration of paraoxygenation have been described. Oxygen can be delivered at different locations in the upper and lower airway during apnoea: Devices can be placed at following sites: Nares, nasopharynx, oropharynx, oral cavity, trachea, Primarybronchi (**Figure 4**).

1. NODESAT: Nasal oxygenation during efforts securing a tube

2. Direct pharyngeal insufflation

3. THRIVE: Trans nasal humidified rapid insufflation ventilatory exchange

4. Other techniques: Apnoeic oxygenation with nasopharyngeal catheters, intratracheal catheters, Bilateral or unilateral endobronchial catheters, buccal oxygen delivery with modified RAE tube, channels located in direct and videolaryngoscopes,

3.3.1 NODESAT: Nasal oxygenation during efforts securing a tube.

NODESAT was first described by Levitan [6], as a method to extend the safe apnea time during rapid sequence anaesthesia in the emergency department. Inappropriately sized nasal cannula is used to administer the standard unwarmed and dry oxygen at the rate of 15 litres/min while attempts for intubating the trachea by conventional

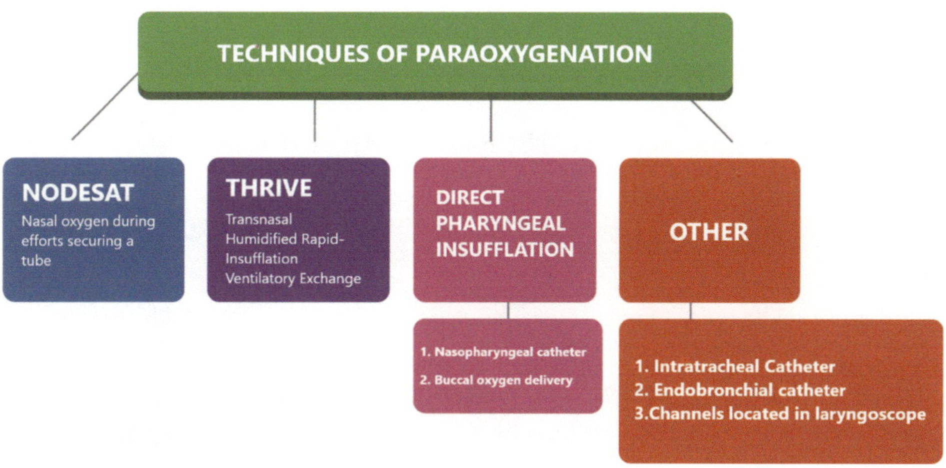

Figure 4.
Techniques of paraoxygenation.

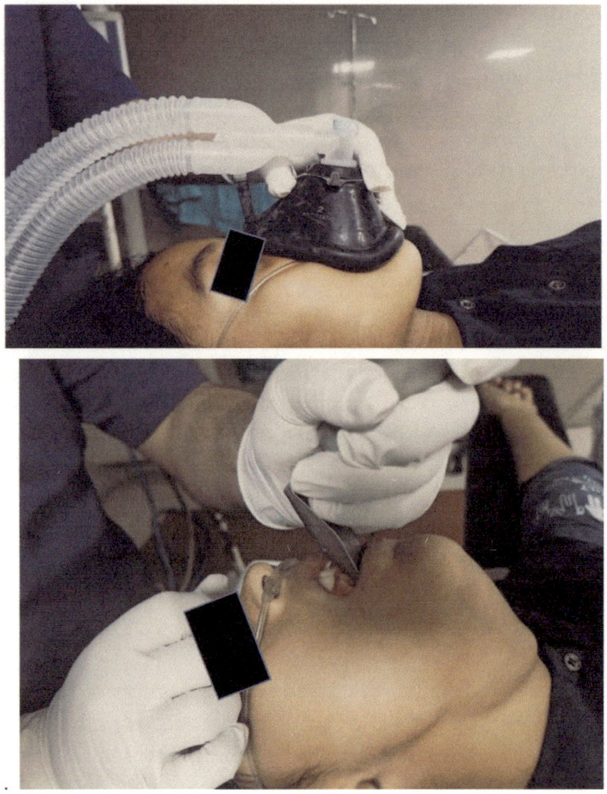

Figure 5.
(a) NODESAT during preoxygenation; (b) NODESAT during intubation.

laryngoscopy or video laryngoscopy or flexible fibreoptic bronchoscope are being made. Unlike other techniques, this technique does not require any special equipment and can be easily done in the operating theatre with nasal prongs and auxiliary oxygen port. However, they can impair the face mask seal during bag mask ventilation. The administration of dry, cold oxygen at high flows can lead to mucosal injury and mucociliary dysfunction (**Figure 5**).

3.3.2 Direct pharyngeal oxygen insufflation:

Para oxygenation can be achieved by using any device that administers oxygen to the pharynx (**Figure 6**).

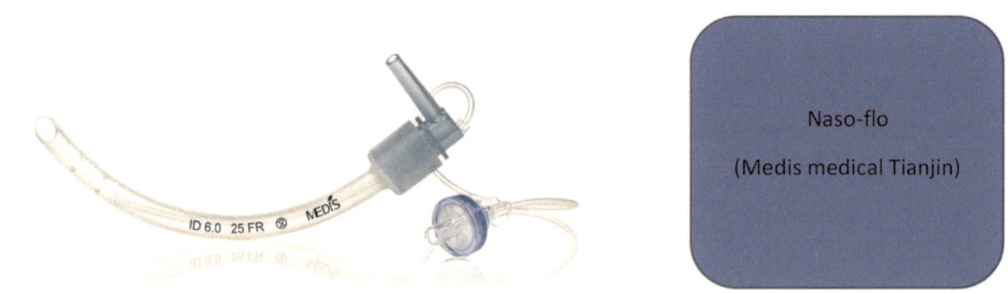

Figure 6.
Naso-Flo *(Medis medical CO Ltd).*

Nasopharyngeal catheter: A nasopharyngeal catheter advanced into the nasopharynx can be used to deliver oxygen during apnoea. The distance from the nares to the tragus of the ear is measured as taken as depth of the catheter insertion. Achar et al [7] found nasopharyngeal catheters to be more effective than nasal prongs in delivering oxygen during apnoea. The Naso-Flo®(Medis medical CO Ltd) is soft silicone nasopharyngeal airway device that allows for direct oxygen delivery into the pharynx, while humidification vents positioned towards the distal tip facilitate heat and moisture transfer.

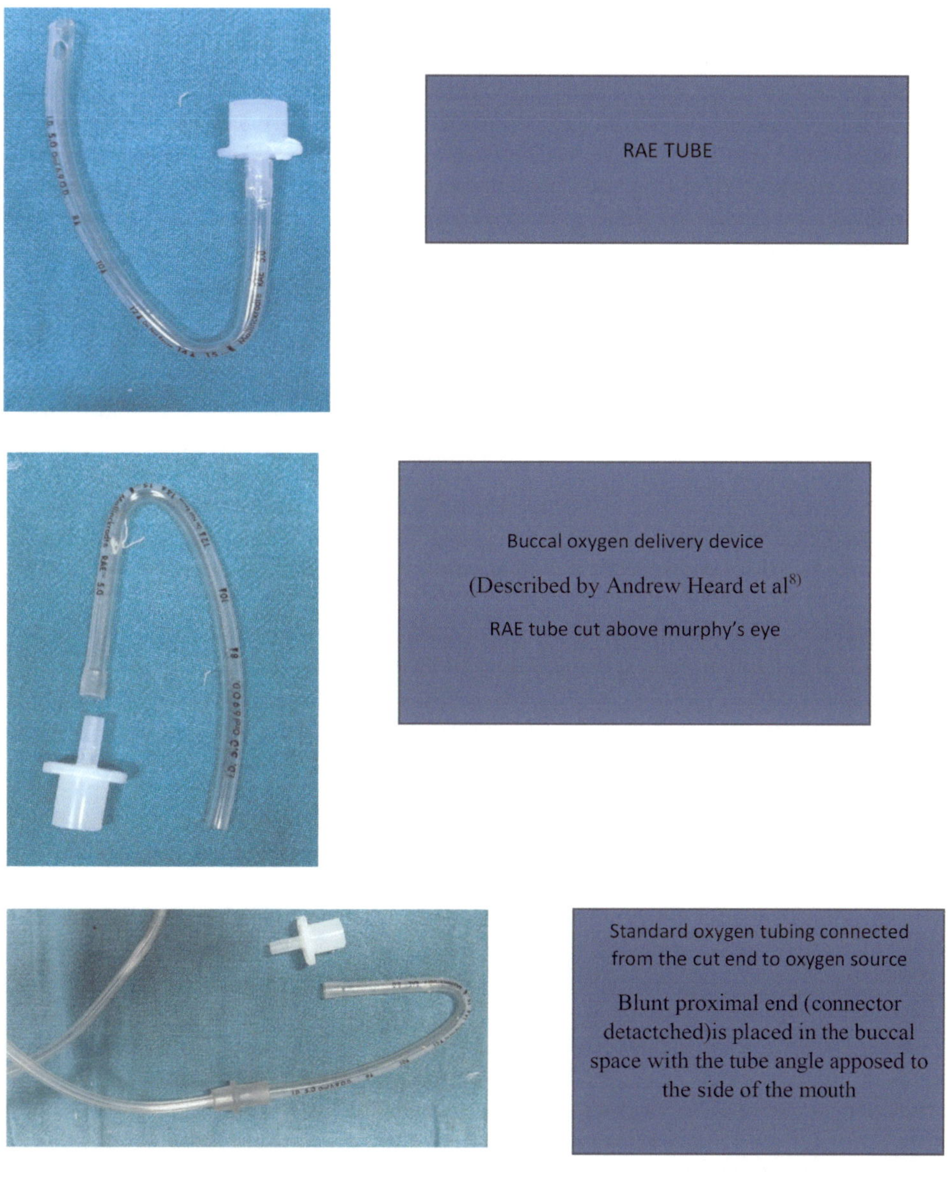

Figure 7.
Buccal oxygen delivery device. As described by Andrew Heard et al. [8] (a) RAE tube (b) RAE tube cut above murphy's eye (c) Standard oxygen tubing connected from the cut end to the oxygen source. The Blunt proximal end (connector detached) is placed in the buccal space with the tube angle apposed to the side of the mouth.

Buccal oxygen delivery: An inexpensive, readily available method of apneic oxygenation was described by Andrew Heard et al. [8]. A 3.5 mm south facing Ring Adair and Elwin (RAE) tube was cut above the murphy's eye. Standard oxygen tubing was connected from the cut end to the auxiliary oxygen outlet on the anaesthesia machine. The blunt proximal end was placed in the buccal space with the tube angle opposed to the left side of the mouth. The tube was fixed to the external cheek to maintained the position. This method of buccal oxygen delivery provided a viable alternative to the nasal route (**Figure** 7).

3.3.3 THRIVE: Trans nasal humidified rapid insufflation ventilatory exchange:

Patel and Nourae, in 2013, introduced the delivery of warm and humidified high flow nasal oxygen using OPTIFLOW™ system (Fischer and Paykellhealth care LTD Auckland, newzealand). Not only the apnea time were prolonged but the rate of rise of carbondixoide was found to be one third of what was expected [9]. This suggested a physiology supplementing classic apneic oxygenation. The clearance of carbondioxide can be explained by the interaction of cardiogenic oscillations and turbulent primary supraglottic vortex [10].

Primary supraglottic vortex: High-flow nasal oxygen enters the nose at 70-90 L/min, loops around the soft palate, and exits through the mouth. This creates a highly turbulent 'primary supraglottic vortex" which has the following effects:

It replenishes the pharynx with oxygen and prevents entrainment of room air.

It effectively bypasses the upper airways which ordinarily account for approximately 50% of the resistance of the entire respiratory system to airflow [11]. By effectively breathing 'directly from the glottis', work of breathing is reduced by approximately 50% [12].

It also generates a positive airway pressure which in turn reduces upper airway collapsibility and distal airway atelectasis [13].

The primary vortex does not, however, extend deep into the trachea and cannot by itself account for the observed level of gaseous exchange.

Cardiogenic oscillations: The compression and expansion of the small airways is brought about by the blood leaving and entering the thoracic cavity with each heartbeat [14]. The typical amplitude of a 'cardiogenic breath' is around 7-15 ml per heartbeat [10]. Ordinarily, cardiogenic oscillations result in small-volume mass movement of gases within the trachea.

During THRIVE, this small volume is flushed into the supraglottic vortex during cardiogenic 'expiration', is removed, and replaced by 100% oxygen. Cardiogenic 'inspiration' moves this oxygen towards the distal airways and also entrains turbulence, which enhances intratracheal mixing. e.g.

Volume of a 'cardiogenic breath' to be 12 ml per heartbeat,

Heart rate:70 beats per minute.

840 ml of gas which contains CO2 is removed, and is replaced with 100% oxygen. This is not enough to achieve full CO2 clearance. That is why carbondioxide still accumulates during THRIVE, but at a slower rate than with classical apnoeic oxygenation.

THRIVE is administered through a standard commercially available high flow oxygen delivery system e.g. Optiflow (Fischer and Paykel health care), Airvo, Airvo2 (Fischer and Paykel health care). It consists of a flowmeter, humidifier, heating system, heated non condensing circuit, and an oxygen connector for gas supply. Some

DOI: http://dx.doi.org/10.5772/intechopen.106827

of the ventilators. e.g Bellavista ventilators, IMT medical, Switzerland available in the market have an inbuilt system that provides the high flow oxygen therapy as well as invasive ventilation modes (**Figures 8–10**).

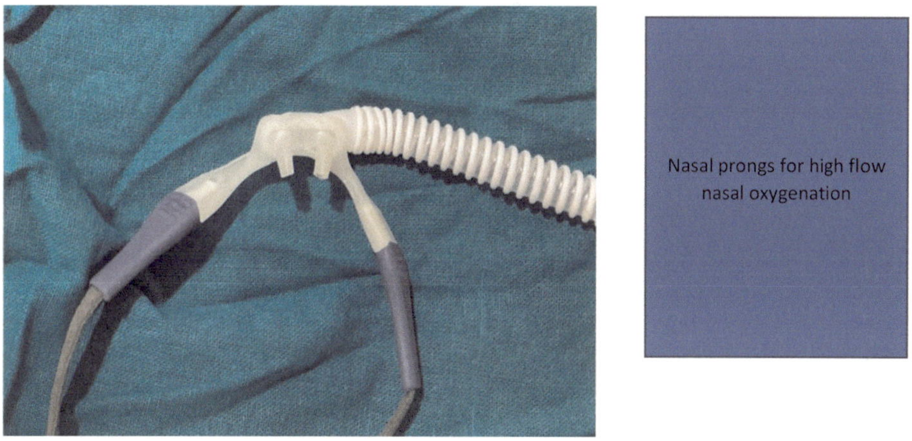

Figure 8.
Nasal prongs for high flow nasal oxygenation.

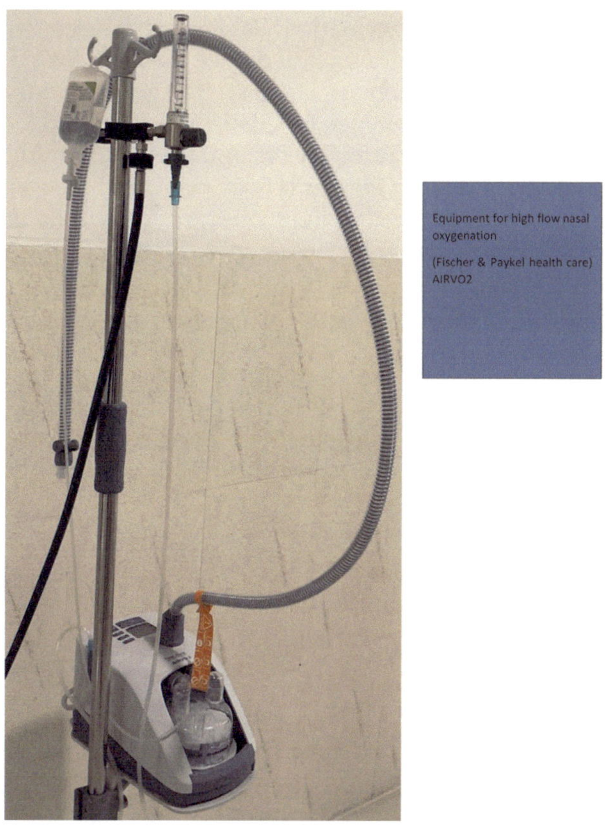

Figure 9.
Equipment for high flow nasal oxygenation (Fischer & Paykel health care) AIRVO2.

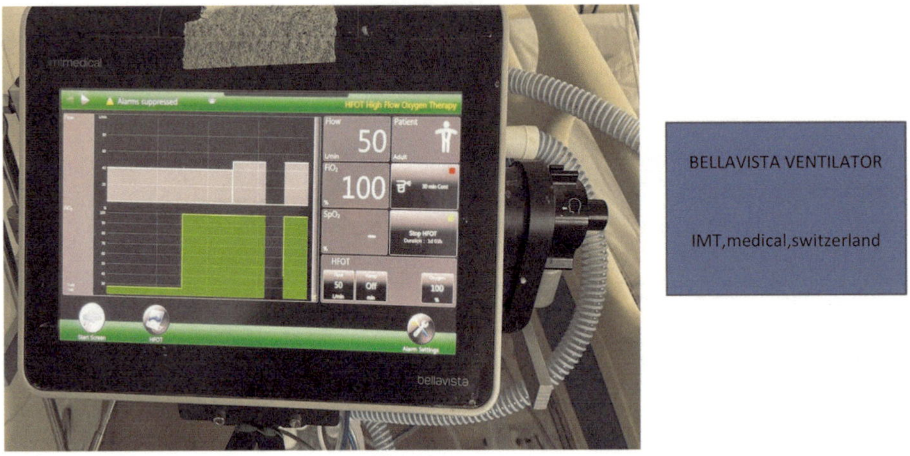

Figure 10.
Bellavista ventilator (IMT, medical, Switzerland).

3.3.4 Others

Endobronchial catheters: Endobronchial catheters are placed in the main stem bronchi. The catheter placedeither in right or left main stem bronchi or in both the bronchi can be used for apnoeic oxygenation. Babinski et al. used two polyethylene catheters (2.5 mm OD) with angulation of 20 degree for the right side and 30 degree for the left were placed in the bronchi under fibreoptic guidance for endobronchial apnoeic oxygenation. Humidified oxygen was delivered at 0.6 to0.7 L/min. The authors found the adequate oxygenation was maintained till 30 minutes with a mean co2 rise at rate 0.6mmhg/min [15] (**Figure 11**).

Dual use laryngoscopes: Dual use laryngoscopes are specifically designed to allow for the insufflation of oxygen during laryngoscopy. The miller port American profile

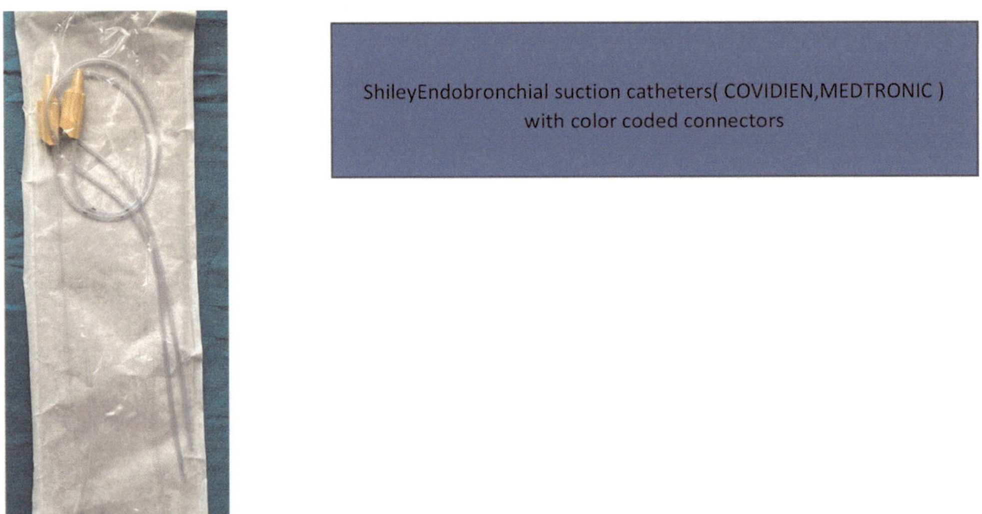

Figure 11.
ShileyEndobronchial suction catheters(COVIDIEN, MEDTRONIC) with color coded connectors.

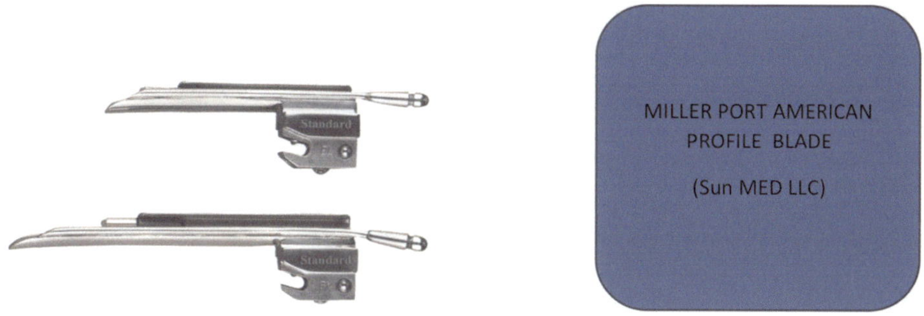

Figure 12.
Miller port American profile blade (Sun MED LLC).

conventional blade (Sun Med LLC) is commercially available laryngoscope that has an integrated tube that permits the delivery of oxygen and other gas mixtures during laryngoscopy (**Figure 12**).

Tracheal tube introducer: An Eschmann tracheal tube introducer was used by Millar et al. for administering apnoeic oxygenation. Two holes were drilled at both the end of the Eschmann gum elastic bougie (SIMSportex, Hythe Kent, UK) and apnoeic oxygenation was tested on an anaesthetic simulator model. The modified bougie was positioned 2–3 cm beyond the vocal cords with 8 l/min of oxygen flowing through it. The time taken for the oxygen saturation to fall was significantly prolonged when modified gum elastic bougie was used for apnoeic oxygenation [16]. COOKS airway exchange catheter (AEC) has a blunt tip which is a traumatic to internal structures. The lumen and distal side ports are designed to deliver oxygen. The removable Rapi-Fit Adapter permits oxygen delivery during an airway exchange procedure. Although cook's airway is intended for tracheal tube exchange, it can also be used to paraoxygenate the airways (**Figure 13a–c**).

Intratracheal catheters: A retrospective study was conducted by Rudlof and Hohenhorst [17] analysing 47 patients who underwent apnoeic oxygenation at 0.5 l/min using a catheter inserted into the trachea. The median Spo2 at the end of the apnoeic period was found to be 100 percent. The mean apnoea time was found to be 24.7 min with no adverse effects.

3.4 Clinical applications of paraoxygenation/apnoeic oxygenation

See **Figure 14.**

3.4.1 Routine elective endotracheal intubation

Para oxygenation through nasal or nasopharyngeal catheter prolongs the safeapnoea time and also decreases the degree of desaturation during induction of anaesthesia and endotracheal intubation in adult ASA 1–2 patients undergoing anaesthesia for elective surgery [18]. Apnoeic oxygenation has been shown to be associated with increased per intubation oxygen saturation, decreased rate of hypoxemia and first pass intubation success [19]. During one lung ventilation, apneic oxygenation of the deflated lung through a suction catheter can reduces the likelihood of hypoxemia and need for resumption of double lung ventilation [20, 21].

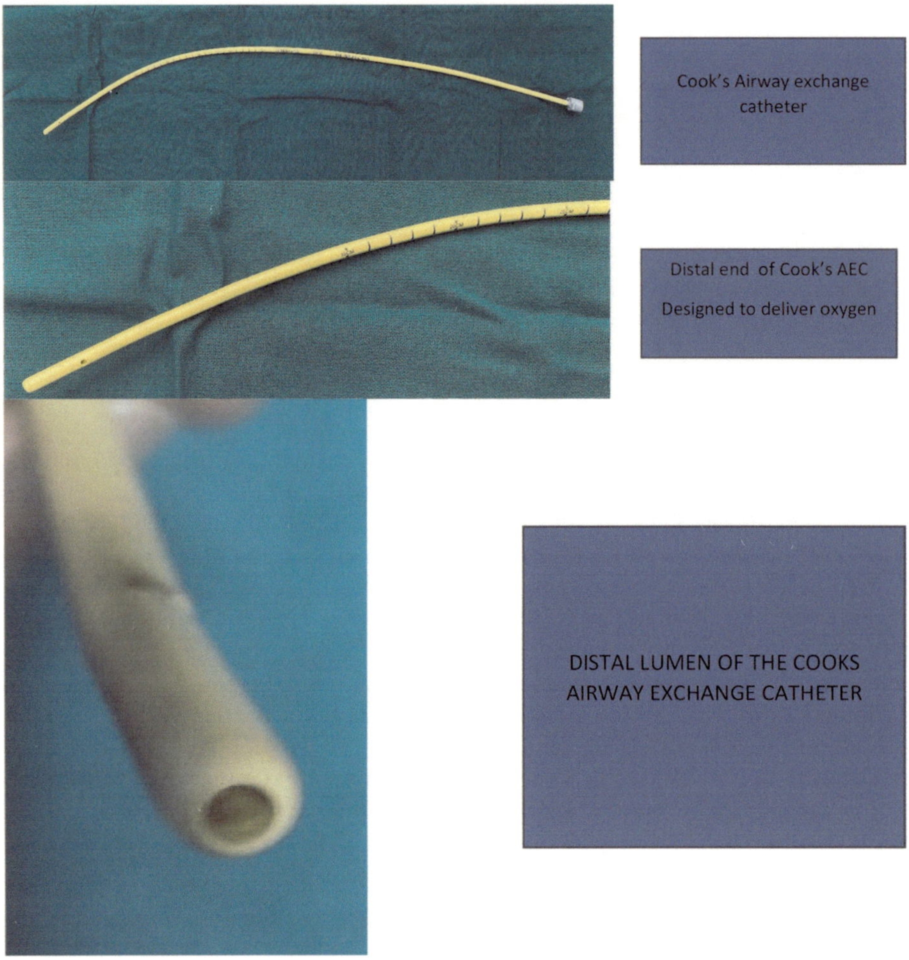

Figure 13.
Cooks airway exchange catheter (cook medical). (a) Cook's Airway exchange catheter; (b) Distal end of Cook's AEC Designed to deliver oxygen; and (c) distal lumen of the cooks airway exchange catheter.

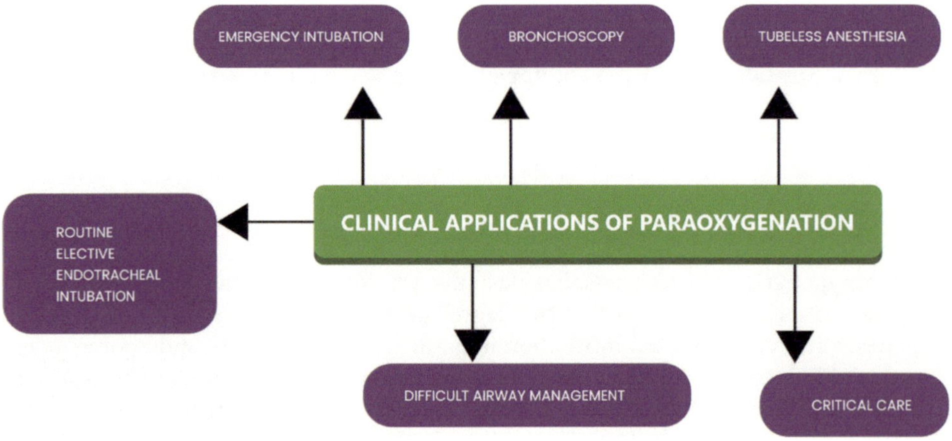

Figure 14.
Clinical applications of paraoxygenation.

3.4.2 Difficult airway management

Awake intubation: Awake fibreoptic intubation is indicated in cases with anticipated difficult airways. Even though the procedure can be done with local anaesthesia, sedation is often required to improve the patient tolerance and cooperation. Sedative induced apnea, can lead to hypoventilation, and upper airway obstruction during awake fibreoptic intubation in difficult airway resulting in critical oxygen desaturation. Paraoxyygention can be used as an effective tool to ensure adequate oxygenation while the airway is being navigated by the scope. Schroeder et alevaluated a special oropharyngeal oxygenation device (OOD), allowing a continuous laryngeal oxygen insufflation during and parallel with bronchoscopy [22]. Apnoeic laryngeal oxygenation in a preoxygenated manikin with both oxygen insufflation via the OOD and the bronchoscope kept oxygen saturation in the test lung at 95% over 20 min. Oxygen insufflation via OOD or bronchoscope was found to be more effective than nasal oxygen insufflation.

Physiologically difficult airway: Peri intubation hypoxia is more common in physiologically difficult airways e.g., paediatric, obstetric and obese patient population. Obesity leads to decreased in function residual capacity, increases atelectasis and shunting in the dependent region of the lung. Resting metabolic rate, work of breathing and minute oxygen demand however are increased. This combination of the factors makes the obese patient prone to hypoxemia during the induction of the induction of anaesthesia. Oxygen insufflation at 15 l/min through nasopharyngeal airway and standard nasal cannula can significantly increase the safe apnea time during induction of anaesthesia in obese patients [23].

Although apnoeic oxygenation is extensively studied in the adult population, very few studies have been conducted on the paediatric population, there is evidence that apnoeic oxygenation is a simple easy to apply intervention that can decrease hypoxemia during paediatric endotracheal intubation. Not only it increases the time until desaturation but also reduced the overall incidence of hypoxia during laryngoscopy in paediatric population [24].

Difficult airway society and obstetric anaesthetist association guidelines issued in 2015 for the management of difficult tracheal in obstetric patients emphasised on the role of apnoeic oxygenation via nasal cannula, nasopharyngeal catheter or mask [25]. AIDA Arecommends the universal use of 15 L/min oxygen insufflation via nasal cannula for obstetric general anaesthesia they recommend the use of nasal prongs to insufflate oxygen during the apnoeic period in patients with difficult airway [26].

Tubeless anaesthesia: Managing the shared airway in the glottic and subglottic pathologies presents a challenge to the anaesthesiologist as well as the surgeon. Tubeless anaesthesia with apnoeic oxygenation allows a good access and visualisation of the glottis without oxygen desaturation. Apneic oxygenation enables tubeless anaesthesia for extended period of time. Vocalcordbiopsy, balloon dilation of subglottic stenosis has been done using this technique. Apnoeic oxygenation with nasal cannula and THRIVE has been found to be safe and feasible for the endoscopic management of subglottic stenosis in short glottic surgical procedures [27].

Bronchoscopy: Apnoeic oxygenation can be done in patient undergoing rigid bronchoscopy with passive oxygen insufflation through the side port of the bronchoscope or a tracheal catheter [28, 29]. High flow administration of oxygen via side sport of bronchoscope risk barotrauma if the path for gas egress becomes obstructed even for brief period.

Critical care: Recent guidelines for the management of airway in critical care patients have recommended that nasal oxygen should be applied throughout the airway management. If the standard nasal cannula is used it should be applied during preoxygenation with a flow of 5 L/min while awake and increased to 15 L/min when the patient loses conscious. A high flow nasal cannula can also be used if already in place [30].

Diagnosis of brain death: Apnoea test done in diagnosis of brain death involves the temporary suspension of mechanical ventilation. During this time oxygen is insufflate through the tracheal tube via a catheter to prevent hypoxemia.

3.4.3 Emergency intubation

Patients requiring emergency airway management are at a greater risk of hypoxemia due to underlying lung pathology, high metabolic requirements, high respiratory drive or inability to protect the airway. Rapid sequence intubation in critically ill patients is associated with episodes of hypoxia. Apneic oxygenation has been shown to reduce the incidence of desaturation in patient undergoing rapid sequence intubation in emergency [31]. A systematic review to investigate the effect of apnoeic oxygenation on incidence of clinically significant hypoxemia during emergency endotracheal intubation concluded that paraoxygentaion reduces the incidence of hypoxemia in emergency endotracheal intubation and supported the inclusion of apnoeic oxygenation in everyday practice (**Figure 15**) [32].

3.5 Complications of paraoxygenation

Hypercarbia: During Para oxygenation carbon dioxide cannot be vented out. Co2 levels continue to rise leading to an increase in PH and development of respiratory acidosis [15, 33, 34]. Paco2 levels increase with a speed of 1.1–3.4 mmHg. Mean CO2 levels can reach as high as 160 mmHg [33]. However, with THRIVE the rate of carbon dioxide accumulation is less than that seen in classic apnoeicoxygenation [9]. The

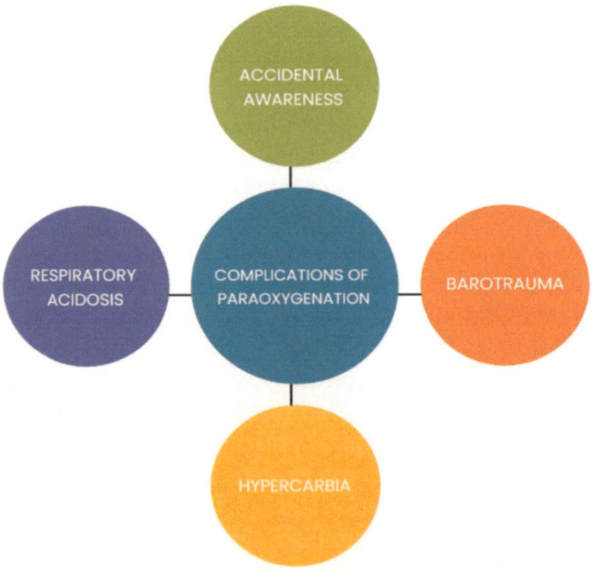

Figure 15.
Complications of paraoxygenation.

effects of hypercarbia are versatile ranging from tachycardia, increased cardiac output, increased cerebral blood flow. Prolonged apnoeic oxygenation should be avoided in patients with contraindication to hypercapnia e.g., cardiac arrythmia, hemodynamicinstability, raised intracranial pressure. Para oxygenation interrupts the early detection of rise of carbon dioxide. Since the end-tidal carbon dioxide monitoring cannot be done during apnea, transcutaneous carbon dioxide measurements may help in minimizing the risk and optimal utilization of Para oxygenation [35].

Acidosis: Gradual increase in the carbon dioxide levels leads to respiratory acidosis however, during testing for brain death in addition to respiratory acidosis, a mild metabolic acidosis of unknown cause also develops during apnoeic oxygenation [36].

Accidental awareness: Apnoeicoxygenation does not deliver volatile agents to the lung. Hence adequate anaesthesia during the airway management should be ensured to avoid accidental awareness [37]. Total intravenous anaesthesia {TIVA} can be used during paraoxygenation to avoid the accidental awareness during this procedure. Tubeless anaesthesia with apnoeic oxygenation for the short glottic procedures also requires the administration of intravenous anaesthesia to ensure adequate depth during the procedure.

NODESAT, direct pharyngeal insufflation delivers dry and cold oxygen to the respiratory tree. Administration of dry and cold gases can induce bronchoconstriction in patients with asthma [38]. Airway resistance is increased to reduce the airflow in the upper and trachea to protect the lungs from the challenge of dry and cold gases [39, 40]. Dry gases cause excessive water loss by the nasal mucosa [41]. This may reduce the nasal mucociliary clearance rate due to the changes in the rheological properties or adhesiveness of the nasal mucus and slowing of ciliary pulses [42]. High flow dry gases result in inspissated secretions that can cause life threatening airway obstruction [43].

Barotrauma: Apnoeic oxygenation is a widely accepted method for apnea testing in brain death. During the apnea testing, ventilator assistance is discontinued and oxygen is delivered into the trachea via an oxygen catheter placed at the level of carina while waiting for the spontaneous respiratory movements. Apnea testing related pneumothorax was first reported by Bar joseph et al. [44]. In order to avoid pneumothorax authors proposed that the oxygen flow rates should not exceed 6 l/min, oxygen catheter diameter should be narrower than the diameter of the endotracheal tube and the tip of the oxygen catheter should not exceed the tip of the endotracheal tube to avoid wedge position in the trachea. A case of pneumothorax and pneumomediatinum was reported by saposnik et al. [45] during apnea testing. Vivien et al. [46] proposed that a 12 french catheter should be advanced only 5 cm into the endotracheal tube and oxygen flow rates should not exceed 8 l/min to avoid pneumothorax during apnea testing. Barotraumacan occur if there is no clear route for egress of gases during apnoeicoxygenation.AT- piece or a self-inflating bag valve system can be used as an alternative technique to conductapnoeatest. Serious air leak syndromes have been reported with the use of high flow especially in paediatric age group. HFNC is being used as a respiratory support for preterm infants. HFNC is being used as an alternative to nasal continuous positive airway pressure (CPAP) and in particular to prevent postextubation failures. A case of tension pneumocephalus in a preterm infant was reported by Iglesias et al. [47] as a complication during HFNC ventilation. Significant neurological impairment was detected and support was eventually withdrawn. Clinicians need to be aware of this rare but possible complication during HFNC therapy, as timely diagnosis and treatment can prevent neurological sequelae. Paying close attention to flow rate, nasal cannula size and insertion, regularly checking insertion depth

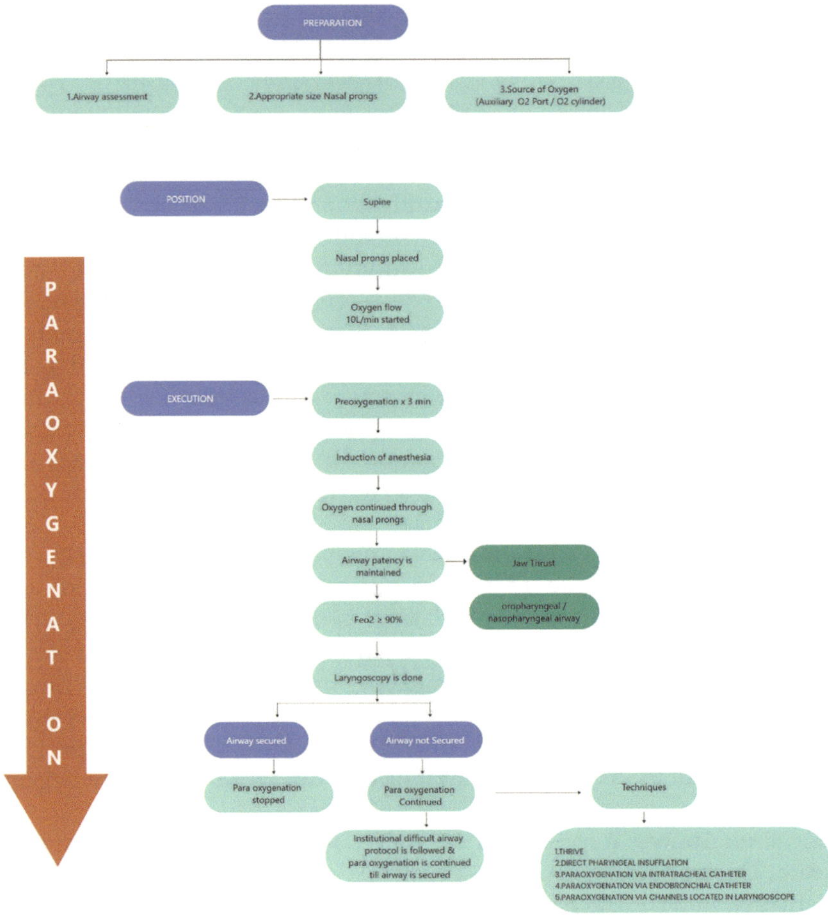

Figure 16.
Paraoxygenation: Preparation to execution.

can help to avoid these complications. Cases of pneumo-orbitus [48], epistaxis, subcutaneous emphysema, oesophageal rupture, gastric rupture [49, 50] have all been reported with use of apneic oxygenation.

4. Conclusion

Perioperative critical hypoxia is one of the most feared complication an anesthesiolgist may come across. These episodes often occur abruptly and demand prompt intervention to avoid irreversible damage. Management of these life-threatening situations requires simultaneous diagnosis and treatment of hypoxia. Differentiating between the patient factors and the machine factors leading to hypoxic event is imperative. Paraoxygenationor apneic oxygenation techniques can help to buy time, avoid panic and execute airway securing strategies by delaying the development of critical hypoxemia. Routine application of paraoxygenation techniques in everyday clinical practice and a knowledge of various equipments that can be used to administer paraoxygenation to the patient can help prevent the nightmare of critical hypoxic perioperative events (**Figure 16** and **Table 1**).

Technique	Device used	Advantages	Disadvantages
NODESAT	Nasal prongs	1.No special equipment required 2.Easily done in emergency and elective settings	Dry and cold oxygen delivery leading to mucosal injury
THRIVE	Commercially available devices (OPTIFLOW)	1.Humidified oxygen delivery 2.Higher flow than NODESAT upto 60 L/min 3. Carbon dioxide clearance	Costly equipment Not readily available
DIRECT PHARYNGEAL INSUFFLATION	1.Nasopharyngeal catheter 2.Buccal oxygen delivery	1.More effective than nasal prongs 2.Buccal delivery is an alternative to nasal route	Dry and cold oxygen delivery leading to mucosal injury
OTHER TECHNIQUES	1.Endobronchial catheters 2.Dual use laryngoscope	1.Endobronchial oxygenation During the laryngoscopy	Dry and cold oxygen delivery leading to mucosal injury

Table 1.
Summary of techniques of paraoxygenation.

Abbreviations

ASA	American society of anesthesiologist.
AEC	Airway exchange catheter.
AIDAA	All India difficult airway society.
DAWD	duration of apnea without desaturation.
FRC	Functional residual capacity.
HFNO	High flow nasal oxygenation.
NODESAT	Nasal oxygenation during efforts securing a tube.
OOD	Oropharyngeal oxygenation device.
PAO2	partial pressure of alveolar oxygen.
PaO2	partial pressure of oxygen in blood.
THRIVE	Trans nasal humidified rapid insufflation ventilatory exchange.
V/Q ratio	ventilation/perfusion ratio.

Author details

Suresh Kumar Singhal* and Manisha Manohar
Department of Anaesthesiology and Critical Care, Pt. B.D. Sharma Post Graduate Institute of Medical Sciences, Rohtak, India

*Address all correspondence to: ssinghal12@gmail.com

IntechOpen

© 2022 The Author(s). Licensee IntechOpen. This chapter is distributed under the terms of the Creative Commons Attribution License (http://creativecommons.org/licenses/by/3.0), which permits unrestricted use, distribution, and reproduction in any medium, provided the original work is properly cited.

References

[1] Wilson WC, Bneumof JL. Physiology of Airway Management. 4th ed. Philadelphia: Elsevier; 2018. pp. 144-145

[2] Brian P. Respiratory Physiology and Pathophysiology. 9th ed. Philadelphia: Elsevier; 2020. pp. 376-379

[3] Bartlett RG, Brubach HF, Specht H. Demonstration of aventilatory mass flow during ventilation and apnea in man. Journal of Applied Physiology. 1959;**14**: 97-101

[4] Draper WB, Whitehead RW, Spencer JN. Studies on diffusion respiration: Alveolar gases and venous blood pH of dogs during diffusion respiration. Anesthesiology. 1947;**8**: 524-533

[5] Holmdahl MH. Pulmonary uptake of oxygen, acid–base metabolism, and circulation during prolonged apnoea. Acta Chirurgica Scandinavica. Supplementum. 1956;**212**:1-128

[6] Levitan RM. NO DESAT! Nasal oxygen during efforts securing a tube. Emergency Physicians Monthly. 2010. https://www.epmonthly.com/article/no-desat/

[7] Achar SK, Pai AJ, Shenoy UK. Apneic oxygenation during simulated prolonged difficult laryngoscopy: Comparison of nasal prongs versus nasopharyngeal catheter: A prospective randomised controlled study. Anesthesia, Essays and Researches. 2014;**8**:63-67

[8] Heard A, Toner AJ, Evans JR, Aranda Palacios AM, Lauer S. Apneic oxygenation during prolonged laryngoscopy in obese patients: A Randomised, Controlled Trial of Buccal RAE Tube Oxygen Administration. Anesthesia and Analgesia. 2017;**124**(4): 1162-1167

[9] Patel A, Nouraei SA. Transnasal humidified rapid-insufflation ventilatory exchange (THRIVE): A physiological method of increasing apnoea time in patients with difficult airways. Anaesthesia. 2015;**70**:323-329

[10] Nouraei R et al. Tubeless Ventilation – THRIVE What is Transnasal Humidified Rapid-Insufflation Ventilatory Exchange (THRIVE). ENT Audiology News. 2018;**27**:2

[11] Sandhu GS, Nouraei SAR. Laryngeal & Tracheobronchial Stenosis. San Diego, USA: Plural Publishing; 2015

[12] Delorme M, Bouchard PA, Simon M, et al. Effects of high flow nasal cannula on the work of breathing in patients recovering from acute respiratory failure. Critical Care Medicine. 2017;**45**: 1981-1988

[13] Parke R, McGuinness S, Eccleston M. Nasal high-flow therapy delivers low level positive airway pressure. British Journal of Anaesthesia. 2009;**103**: 886-890

[14] Slutsky AS, Brown R. Cardiogenic oscillations: A potential mechanism enhancing oxygenation during apneic respiration. Medical Hypotheses. 1982;**8**: 393-400

[15] Babinski MF, Sierra OG, Smith RB, Leano E, Chavez A, Castellanos A. Clinical application of continuous flow apneic ventilation. Acta AnaesthesiolScand. 1985;**29**:750-752

[16] Millar FA, Hutchison GL, Glavin R. Gum elastic bougie, capnography and

apnoeic oxygenation. European Journal of Anaesthesiology. 2001;**18**:51-53

[17] Rudlof B, Hohenhorst W. Use of apneic oxygenation for the performance of pan-endoscopy. Otolaryngology and Head and Neck Surgery. 2013;**149**: 235-239

[18] Grude O, Solli HJ, Andersen C, Oveland NP. Effect of nasal or nasopharyngeal apneic oxygenation on desaturation during induction of anaesthesia and endotracheal intubation in the operating room: A narrative review of randomised controlled trials. Journal of Clinical Anesthesia. 2018;**51**: 1-7

[19] Oliveira JE, Silva L, Cabrera D, Barrionuevo P, Johnson RL, Erwin PJ, et al. Effectiveness of apneic oxygenation during intubation: A systematic review and meta-analysis. Annals of Emerging Medicine. 2017;**70**: 483-494

[20] Jung DM, Ahn HJ, Jung SH, et al. Apneic oxygen insufflation decreases the incidence of hypoxemia during one-lung ventilation in open and thoracoscopic pulmonary lobectomy: A randomised controlled trial. Journal of Thoracic and Cardiovascular Surgery. 2017;**154**: 360-366

[21] Sanchez-Lorente D, Gomez-Caro A, Jimenez MJ, Molins L. Apnoeic oxygenation on one-lung ventilation in functionally impaired patients during sleeve lobectomy. European Journal of Cardiothoracic Surgery. 2011;**39**:e77-e79

[22] Schroeder DC, Wetsch WA, Finke SR, Dusse F, Böttiger BW, Herff H. Apneic laryngeal oxygenation during elective fiberoptic intubation - a technical simulation. BMC Anesthesiology. 2020;**20**(1):300

[23] Moon TS, Tai K, Kim A, et al. Apneic oxygenation during prolonged laryngoscopy in obese patients: A Randomised, Double-Blinded,Controlled Trial of Nasal Cannula Oxygen Administration. Obesity Surgery. 2019; **29**:3992-3999

[24] Dancy MA. Efficacy of apneic oxygenation during paediatric endotracheal intubation. Pediatric Emergency Care. 2021;**37**(10):528-532

[25] Frerk C, Mitchel VS, McNarry AF, et al. Guidelines for management of unanticipated difficult intubation in adults. British Journal of Anaesthesia. 2015;**115**(6):827-848

[26] Myatra SN, Shah A, Kundra P, Patwa A, Ramkumar V, Divatia JV, et al. All India Difficult Airway Association 2016 guidelines for the management of unanticipated difficult tracheal intubation in adults. Indian Journal of Anaesthesia. 2016;**60**(12):885-898

[27] Youssef DL, Paddle P. Tubeless anesthesia in subglottic stenosis: Comparative review of apneic low-flow oxygenation with thrive. The Laryngoscope. 2022;**132**(6):1231-1236

[28] Pathak V, Welsby I, Mahmood K, Wahidi M, MacIntyre N, Shofer S. Ventilation and anaesthetic approaches for rigid bronchoscopy. Annals of the American Thoracic Society. 2014;**11**: 628-634

[29] Cheatle CA, Chambers KB. Anaesthesia for bronchoscopy. Anaesthesia. 1955;**10**:171-172

[30] Higgs A, McGrath BA, Goddard C, Rangasami J, Suntharalingam G, Gale R, et al. Guidelines for the management of tracheal intubation in critically ill adults. British Journal of Anaesthesia. 2018; **120**(2):323-352

[31] Wimalasena Y, Burns B, Reid C, Ware S, Habig K. Apneic oxygenation was associated with decreased desaturation rates during rapid sequence intubation by an Australian helicopter emergency medicine service. Annals of Emergency Medicine. 2015;**65**(4): 371-376

[32] Pavlov I, Medrano S, Weingart S. Apneic oxygenation reduces the incidence of hypoxemia during emergency intubation: A systematic review and meta-analysis. The American Journal of Emergency Medicine. 2017; **35**(8):1184-1189

[33] Eger EI, Severinghaus JW. The rate of rise of PaCO2 in the apneic anesthetized patient. Anesthesiology. 1961;**22**:419-425

[34] Dragoumanis CP, Papaiannou V, Foutzitzi S, Prassopoulous P, Pneumatikos I. Apnoeic oxygenation for elimination of respiratory motion artefact in an intubated patient undergoing helical computed tomography pulmonary angiography. Journal of Radiology and Case Report. 2008;**2**:5-7

[35] Ng I, Krieser R, Mezzavia P, Lee K, Tseng C, Douglas N, et al. The use of Trans nasal Humidified Rapid-Insufflation Ventilatory Exchange (THRIVE) for pre-oxygenation in neurosurgical patients: A randomised controlled trial. Anaesthesia and Intensive Care. 2018;**46**:360-367

[36] Frumin MJ, Epstein RM, Cohen G. Apneic oxygenation in man. Anesthesiology. 1959;**20**:789-798

[37] Pandit JJ, Andrade J, Bogod DG, et al. The 5th National Audit Project (NAP5) on accidental awareness during general anaesthesia: Summary of main findings and risk factors. Anaesthesia. 2014;**69**:1089-1101

[38] Berk JL, Lenner KA, McFadden ER Jr. Cold-induced bronchoconstriction: Role of cutaneous reflexes vs. direct airway effects. Journal of Applied Physiology. 1987;**63**(2):659-664

[39] Fontanari P, Burnet H, Zattara-Hartmann MC, Jammes Y. Changes in airway resistance induced by nasal inhalation of cold dry, dry, or moist air in normal individuals. Journal of Applied Physiology. 1996;**81**(4):1739-1743

[40] Fontanari P, Zattara-Hartmann MC, Burnet H, Jammes Y. Nasal eupnoeic inhalation of cold, dry air increases airway resistance in asthmatic patients. The European Respiratory Journal. 1997; **10**(10):2250-2254

[41] Van Oostdam JC, Walker DC, Knudson K, Dirks P, Dahlby RW, Hogg JC. Effect of breathing dry air on structure and function of airways. Journal of Applied Physiology. 1986;**61**(1):312-317

[42] Salah B, Dinh Xuan AT, Fouilladieu JL, Lockhart A, Regnard J. Nasal mucociliary transport in healthy subjects is slower when breathing dry air. The European Respiratory Journal. 1988;**1**(9):852-855

[43] Wood KE, Flaten AL, Backes WJ. Inspissated secretions: A lifethreatening complication of prolonged noninvasive ventilation. Respiratory Care. 2000; **45**(5):491-493

[44] Bar-Joseph G, Bar-Lavie Y, Zonis Z. Tension pneumothorax during apnea testing for the determination of brain death. Anesthesiology. 1998;**89**(5): 1250-1251

[45] Saposnik G, Rizzo G, Deluca JL. Pneumothorax and pneumoperitoneum

during apnea test: How safe is this procedure. Arq. Neuropsiquitar. 1998;**58**: 905-908

[46] Vivien B, Haralambo MS, Riou B. Barotrama during apnea testing for the determination of brain death. Annales Francaises d'Anesthesie et Reanimation. 2001;**20**(4):370-373

[47] Iglesias-Deus A, Perez-Munuzuri A, Lopez-Suarez O, Crespo P, Couce ML. Tension pneumocephalus induced by high-flow nasal cannula ventilation in a neonate. Archives of Disease in Childhood Fetal and Neonatal Edition. 2017;**102**:F173-F175

[48] O'Brien BJ, Rosenfeld JV, Elder JE. Tension pneumo-orbitus and pneumocephalus induced by a nasal oxygen cannula: Report on two paediatric cases. Journal of Paediatrics and Child Health. 2000;**36**:511-514

[49] Alifano M, Veyrie N, Rabbat A. Pneumothorax, pneumomediastinum and hemorrhagic shock complicating oxygen administration through a nasopharyngeal catheter. Annals of Thoracic Surgery. 2010;**90**:2061

[50] Yao HH, Tuck MV, McNally C, Smith M, Usatoff V. Gastric rupture following nasopharyngeal catheter oxygen delivery-a report of two cases. Anaesthesia and Intensive Care. 2015;**43**: 244-248

Chapter 3

Anesthesia in Plastic Surgery: Intersurgical I-gel Placement in a Prone Position

Judith Adrianne Deutsch, Kata Šakić, Dinko Bagatin, Johann Nemrava and Tomica Bagatin

Abstract

Anesthesia is a specialization which in past history has branched off of surgery. It needs to be very creative in its delivery, in order to accommodate the many operating positions, needed by the surgeon. The patient positions must also be safe and adequate for proper ventilation, throughout the operative procedure. There are times when multiple positions must be used, turning the patient over, even several times. Careful planning and team discussions prior to an operation are absolutely necessary, to form anesthetic and operative plans. The aim of the supraglottic airway device (Intersurgical i-gel) prone position induction method is to describe, detail and present its safe efficacy for certain planned operative procedures. Patient fasting preparation is a must, nil by mouth for 8 h. This method and sequence alleviates the use of muscle relaxants for patient rotation. This increases patient safety by keeping muscle tone normal, reduced drug use, minimizing rotation of the patient, and reduces possible injury of patient and among staff involved in rotating. Some may say induction in the prone position may be unsafe due to aspiration risks, but knowing anatomy and gravitational physics, in the event of any secretions projected, they will project forwards onto the operating table (through the gastric port of the i-gel), not into the tracheal area. This similar technique and principle are seen and used for the recovery position, to aid in free drainage of fluid from within the oral cavity. The method is used for a variety of operations worldwide and introduced in 2018 at Poliklinika Bagatin (PB). Approximately, 80 prone position inductions or 10% of all general anesthesias are performed every year at PB. More than 240 anesthesized patients in the prone position with an i-gel have used this method, since it was introduced. All have been with excellent results, minimal risk and appropriate ventilation of patients. I-gel placement in prone position was successful everytime. This method is advantageous to avoid multiple rotations of patients and avoid the use of muscle relaxants, otherwise used, with classic endotracheal intubation methods. The exact process will be discussed in more detail and described within the chapter.

Keywords: i-gel, prone position, patient safety, reduced rotation, faster preparation, esthetic plastic procedures, liposuction

IntechOpen

1. Introduction

Creative anesthesia and patient safety are the goals of accommodating surgeons and providing superior anesthesia. The entire team have the same focus, to complete an operation in the best possible manner and with exceptional results. Plastic surgery has high expectations for perfect results. There are numerous operative procedures being offered in esthetic plastic surgery, requiring various forms of anesthesia, in various positions. The anesthesia provided may be local, local with sedation (local potentiated), regional blocks and general. The choice of delivery can involve the patient's desires, but must be a safe method, in order to maximize comfort during the procedure. Some procedures may last several hours, and in these cases a balance between the patient's desires, comfort and safety must be weighed out, for the most optimal choice. Preoperative consultations and plans are discussed between the patient, surgeon, anesthesiologist and the entire team, to define the type of optimal anesthesia to be delivered, as well as surgical technicalities and specifics (instruments, devices, sutures) needed.

Preoperative preparations with the anesthesiologist can be challenging with patients who have specific disorders, chronic disease, previous operations, increased age, mobility issues, various drug therapies being taken, allergies and more. Preoperative testing, thromboprophylaxis, intraoperative active body warming, hydration are among other vitally important features of preoperative and intraoperative preparations that need to be considered.

Today many patients undergoing anesthesia, wish to complete as much as possible, while under one anesthesia. This needs to be assessed by both the surgeon and anesthesiologist for safety, logistics and feasibility. At times, a combination of operations, two body regions, can be performed. This significantly increases the duration of the anesthesia and operation. In some cases, this may not be possible, and a recommendation is made for the procedures to be performed separately.

The vast offerings of procedures in esthetic plastic surgery most commonly include: total body liposuction, abdominoplasty, breast enhancement, breast reduction, breast lift, areolar corrections, septorhinoplasty, face lifting, lip lift, eyebrow lift, blepharoplasty, auricular corrections, chin implants, and lipofilling.

Many individual clinics may be specialized in other specific types of esthetic plastic operations, offering even more procedures, not mentioned here. However, the list is comprised of the more common available procedures worldwide and what is offered at Poliklinika Bagatin (PB). Furthermore, these various procedures can involve different positions, which are challenging for the anesthesiologist and their team. Therefore, good preparation is key. The prone position can be a safe and great alternative induction position, reducing patient rotations, avoiding the use of muscle relaxants and increasing patient and staff safety.

2. Methods and procedures

A deeper understanding of the methods and procedures, used worldwide and at PB, using prone position induction will be described. A detailed refresher of anatomy is recommended, for the anatomical placement differences between the endotracheal (ET) tube and i-gel intubation devices.

Anatomy of the airway is vitally important and needs to be protected, during any procedure. The pharynx is comprised of the nasopharynx, oropharynx and

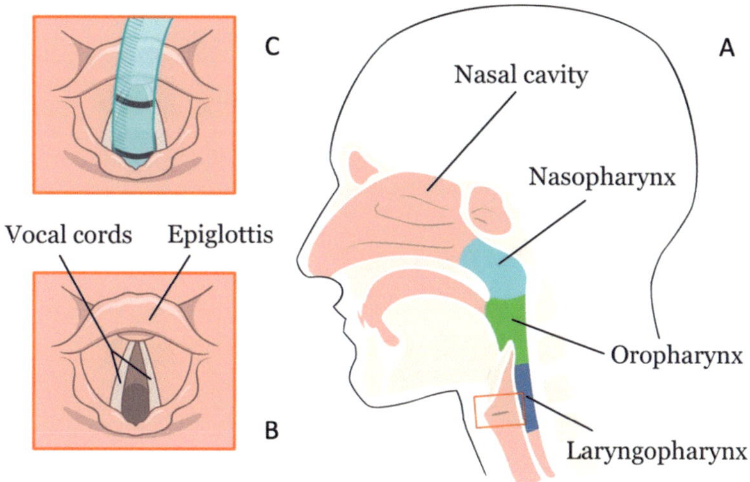

Figure 1.
(A) Sagittal plane anatomy head; (B) vocal chords, epiglottis image without ET tube; (C) image of ET tube in place following intubation.

laryngopharynx (**Figure 1A**) [1, 2]. The upper section, nasopharynx connects the nasal passages to the airway. The middle section, the oropharynx forms the mouth. While the lower portion, the laryngopharynx is the area with the entrance into the trachea passing the vocal chords (**Figure 1B**) [1, 2].

The process of intubation can comprise of an endotracheal tube, which is the most secure method of separating the airway from the gastrointestinal passages, or the use of laryngeal devices, which adequately ventilate but do not separate these passages (**Figure 2A** and **B**) [1, 2]. Both methods require complete sedation of the patient and placement onto an anesthetic machine for controlled or assisted ventilation. Standard monitoring (blood pressure, ECG, and pulse oximetry) should always be used, regardless of the anesthesia type and method chosen. Placement onto an anesthetic machine gives more diverse information, such as end tidal CO_2, tidal volume, respiratory rate, various airway pressures and concentrations of anesthetic gases. Even more advanced monitoring (arterial pressures) can be used, depending on the complexity and duration of the procedure being performed, more often used within the hospital setting rather than outpatient clinics.

Other methods used at PB, such as local, local with added sedation (local potentiation) and regional blocks are used with mask or nasal oxygen tubing in spontaneously breathing patients. The various anesthetic methods can be used on their own or in combination, for optimum pain control coverage during and after procedures. Both surgeons and anesthesiologists can perform the local and regional anesthetic methods. However, intubation requires specific training and skills, and is usually reserved for anesthesiologists.

Placement of the ET tube involves the use of a laryngoscope, to move away soft tissues and the base of the tongue, gently lifting the epiglottis, in order to visualize the entrance into the trachea (**Figure 1B**) [1, 2]. The ET tube is then advanced, with care, into the trachea, passing the vocal cords (**Figure 1C**) [1, 2]. Fixation and final placement of the ET tube is confirmed by chest auscultation hearing equal breath sounds on either side of the chest and then securing it with medical tape or a tie.

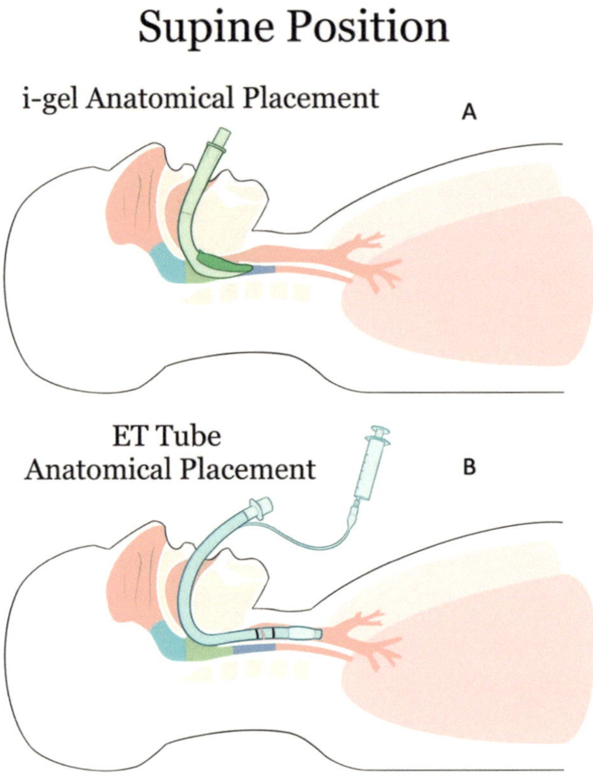

Figure 2.
(A) i-gel following intubation; (B) ET tube following intubation.

Proper auscultation and fixation prevent accidental one lung ventilation and possible barotrauma (**Figure 2B**) [1, 2].

There are various generations of laryngeal devices available, however all have similar principles in their placement, with a variation in fixation of position (with or without a cuff). They all cover the entrance into the trachea and the esophagus. They do not separate or prevent spillage over into the tracheal area, which can cause concerns, potentially causing aspiration of fluids into the respiratory system (**Figure 2A**) [1, 2]. However, proper patient preparation can reduce spillage into this area.

The i-gel is a unique device, which is elegantly simple and requires no balloon inflation (**Figure 3**) [3].

Assistance to perform a mandibular thrust aids in the opening of the mouth. The placement of the i-gel follows the curvature of the tongue and the device is advanced into position after passing the tongue base. There usually is a final jolt, felt in the hand when the i-gel reaches its final snug position, felt similarly in supine and prone position placement. Thereafter it can be taped or tied to remain in position. The final choice, of which intubation method and device will be used, is decided by the anesthesiologist.

Created in 2007, the i-gel is a versatile device capable of providing safe effective anesthesia in fasted patients, as mentioned earlier. The various operations it can be used for are for those lasting up to 4 h, ideally for procedures of the neck down and used with caution involving abdominal distention and pressures [3]. Prone position I-gel use adds a new dimension of possibilities for additional procedures on the backside of patients. The list of possible procedures can span from esthetic plastic

DOI: http://dx.doi.org/10.5772/intechopen.106538

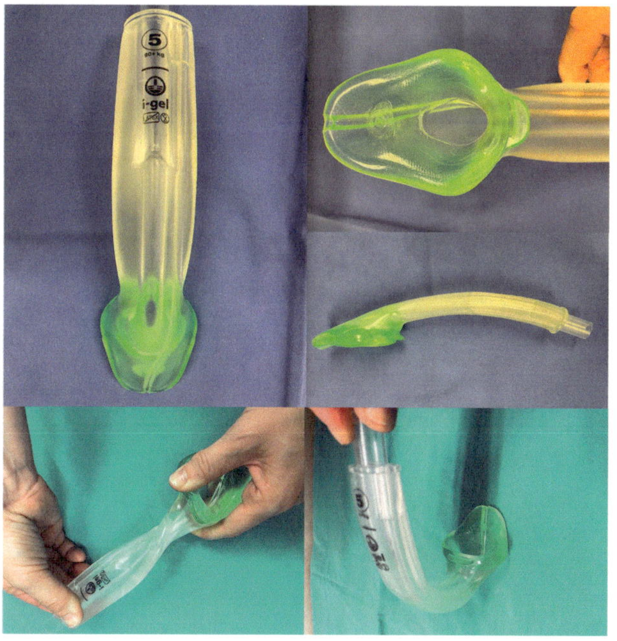

Figure 3.
Intersurgical i-gel laryngeal device (flexibility).

to abdominal, vascular, orthopedic, urology, gynecology, fiberoptic guidance, and numerous beneficial pediatric uses [3]. As with any anesthetic method complications can always arise. They can be of various intensities, from mild to severe, and these are mentioned further into the chapter. The anesthesiologist must weigh out the risks and benefits prior to every anesthesia they perform.

3. Comparison of supine and prone intubations

The supine position, laying flat on the back with the head placed in a neutral position, is the most common intubating position. The patient, following intubation with either an ET tube or laryngeal device, can be moved into desired postions, to facilitate the operative areas. Caution with laryngeal device use, as some movements may cause displacement.

When performing a supine induction with an ET tube, a hypnotic, an opiate, and a muscle relaxant (paralytic) are given to aid in its placement. This completely relaxes (paralyzes) all the muscles in the body. In contrast, a supine induction with an i-gel requires just a hypnotic and opiates. Following intubation, the patient can then be placed into desired positions, extreme caution must be used not to cause injury, when the patient is fully relaxed and paralyzed.

The anesthesiologist is the voice of the team and sets the start of patient positioning and movements. All movements must be thoroughly planned and synchronized. This ensures that everyone involved moves at the same time, to avoid injuries.

Prone position induction begins with the patient placing themselves onto the operating table, in the most comfortable head and body position. A good visual image is, as if they are sunbathing (**Figure 4**).

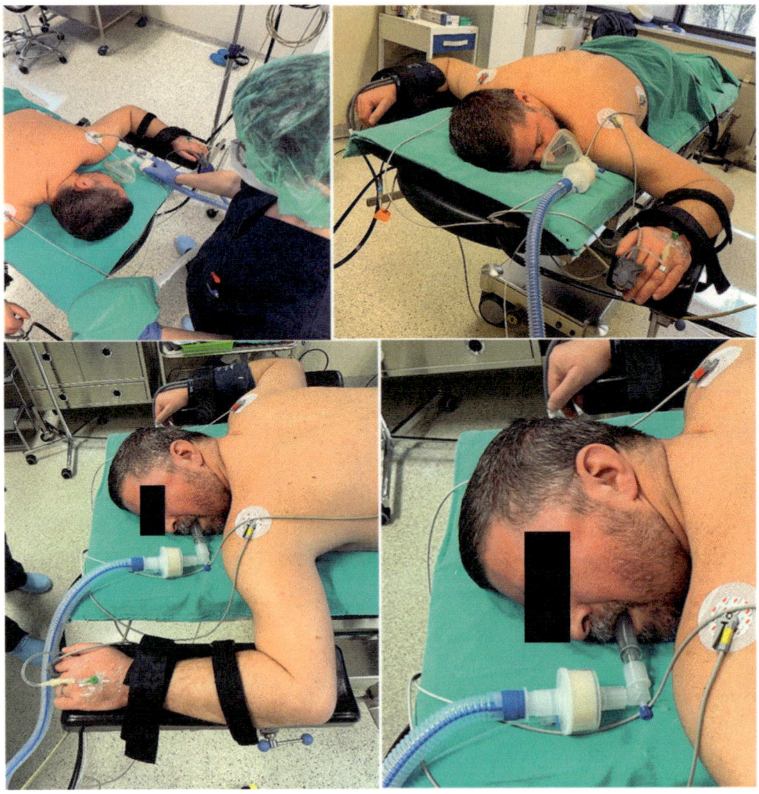

Figure 4.
Patient oxygenation in prone position. Patient in prone position with i-gel.

Their hands and arms are placed in extensions, in a somewhat relaxed forwards position. An added benefit of this method, is that the patient positions themselves, avoiding pressure points that can cause injury. This is especially important, when lying in position for a greater length of time. The induction can begin, when the patient has found their most comfortable body and head position. Another advantage is determining can they tollerate such a position. High BMI patients may have difficulty in ventilation but this can be visualized prior to anesthesia. Finding their most comfortable position is key. The operating table can be adjusted to help further. At PB, patients with an increased BMI are routine. Extreme BMI (over 40 kg/m^2) patients are advised beforehand, to reduce weight and are guided by a nutritionist to prepare them, for future procedures.

Prone positioning induction, following patient position, intravenous access (can be placed earlier) and monitoring attachment, begins with preoxygenation. A mask with flowing oxygen is placed near the mouth of the patient, not too close to the mouth as to cause discomfort or stress. A hypnotic and an opiate drug are used. When the patient has lost eyelash reflexes and is asleep, the laryngeal device (i-gel) can be placed. The anesthetic technician assists in a gentle mandibular thrust, in order to open the mouth, while the anesthesiologist places the device into the pharynx. The use of your index finger to gently move the tongue away, if needed, to aid in i-gel placement is helpful. The sensation of the device „sitting into position "is similar as when applying the device in the supine position. Attachment to the anesthetic machine, parameters and quality check of ventilation are the same. Often fixation of the i-gel is not necessary in the prone position, as the position itself prevents the i-gel displacement. The eyes, ears, and neck flexion/extension need to be checked. The operating table is then tilted up to 10–20° angle, in an anti-Trendelenburg position (head slightly higher than feet). This reduces potential secretions draining from the gastrointestinal tract. In the event of visible drooling, gentle suctioning around, through the gastric port and the main i-gel channel can be done. Remember that all patients using this technique need to be well fasted. It is also advisable to have a stretcher bed near by, in the event you need to turn the patient quickly over onto their back, for any reason.

The avoidance of muscle relaxants (paralytics), reduced rotations, better patient and staff protection are some of the reasons why many centers worldwide, and PB, are using this prone method, for planned and well fasted patients, in selected operations. At PB, only the Intersurgical i-gel is used for the prone position method.

Magnetic resonance imaging (MRI) can show anatomical coverage in a prone position, with the head turned to the right side (**Figure 5**, Courtesy of Special Hospital AGRAM, Zagreb, Croatia) [4].

The imaging done in this position, may have been the first of its kind. When compared to supine MRI imaging, the anatomy is similar. Unfortunately, due to the limitations of the radio frequency (RF) head coil, an image with a i-gel in place,

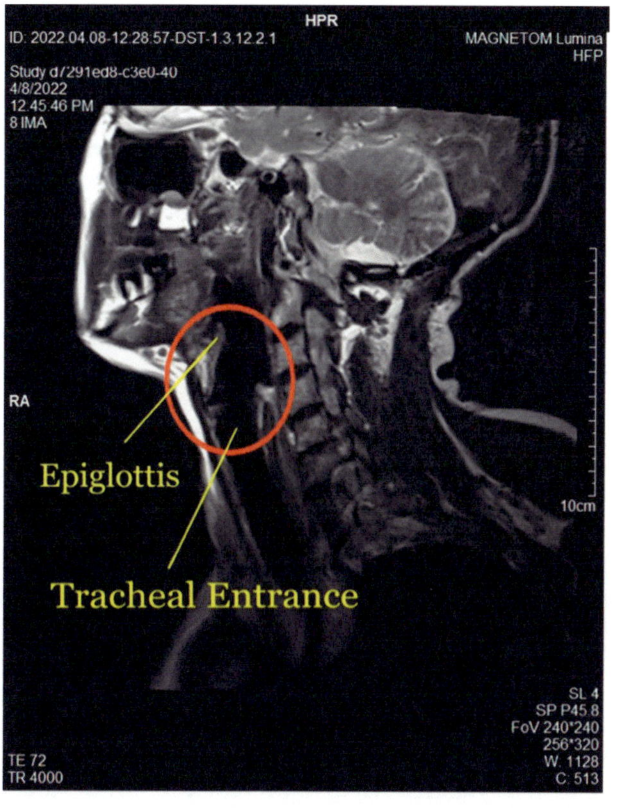

Figure 5.
MRI image of prone position with head turned to the right side (courtesy of Special Hospital AGRAM, Zagreb, Croatia).

in a prone position, was unattainable for safety reasons. Limited head and i-gel device space, in a prone position, were the main factors.

4. Possible complications of prone position

The prone position, as with any intubating position, can have various complications [5–9]. The most common complications can be secretional aspiration, air leakage—improper fit of the i-gel device, increased abdominal and thoracic pressures, tongue swelling, tongue cyanosis, and hypoglossal nerve injury [10–15]. Mentioned earlier, is the importance of a patient being well fasted, to avoid obvious food aspirational risks. Secretions in a fasted patient can also cause aspiration, but to a reduced effect. This can be avoided to gently aspirate around and through the i-gel, if present.

Air leakage around the i-gel can occur, reducing tidal voume and compromising ventilation, if the i-gel is too small. A properly sized i-gel can alleviate this issue (sizing by weight on packaging).

Heavy BMI patients can have ventilation difficulty, due to increased abdominal and thoracic pressures. The anti-Trendelenburg position can be increased to reduce these pressures and aid in better ventilation. An added benefit, of the patient positioning themselves, is the ability to observe position tolerance, while they are still awake. For the increased BMI patients, in prone, the increased operation table adjustment was enough, to normalize the higher thoracic pressures, to have adequate ventilation throughout the procedures.

Patients with gastroesophageal reflux disease (GERD) have been done successfully, in prone with the i-gel during the first phase of a liposuction procedure at PB. However, upon rotation into a supine position they are intubated with an endotracheal tube, for the remainder of the operation. This is also true for planned extended liposuction with abdominoplasty. Following rotation into supine, a switch is made from i-gel to ET, with the addition of an urinary catheter to monitor output, as well as hydration.

Continuous suctioning through the i-gel port is not recommended. This could have an effect on ventilation values and the patient's attempts to breath spontaneously. Patients can and should be encouraged to breath spontaneously while in the prone position. This is also an effective method, for heavy BMI patients, to reduce abdominal and thoracic pressures.

Intersurgical the manufacturer of the i-gel device recommends a maximum 4 h of use [3]. This is mainly due to pressure sores developing in the parynx where the i-gel comes into direct contact with the mucosa and base of the tongue. With prone position the i-gel pressure points are in different areas as compared to the supine position. Therefore, an extended length of usage time is possible, up to an additional 2–3 h, after rotating from prone to supine. At PB, this is done often and with minimal or no issues. There have been a few incidences of regional numbness of the tonuge, minor swelling, throat soreness, which resolved in a few days or weeks, without permanent damage, and with no special interventions necessary. In some instances, a low dose of dexamethasone (8 mg) was sufficient to reduce swelling, if present. The patients were explained the causative factor and followed up, with all of them making a full recovery of these minor injuries. There have been documented complications, at other institutions, with laryngeal devices of premolar toothloss, tongue cyanosis and hypoglossal nerve injury [11, 14, 15]. However, at PB these more serious complications have not been observed. The majority of these serious complications involved classic laryngeal mask devices, not the i-gel, since the i-gel was created in 2007 [3].

All in all, PB has had great success using the prone position induction method, for over 3 years, with minimal complications. As with all induction methods, anethesiologists must have a back up plan and always be prepared for the unexpected.

5. Induction for esthetic plastic procedures

At PB a variety of esthetic plastic procedures are available. Some larger operations requiring general anethesia, may rotate patients several times, while for others only one patient position is necessary. For operations involving the head, neck, ears, face an ET intubating method is used, while for breast augmentation, reduction and lifting a laryngeal device (i-gel) is preferred. For some procedures, a combination of both can be used. The final choice lies in the decision of the anesthesiologist, however, for longer operative times, an ET tube is preferred [5, 6].

Since 2019, at Poliklinika Bagatin 756 various procedures have been performed during the pandemic era (**Table 1**).

Computer simulations using the VECTRA XT 3D, aid in displaying visual results of some postoperative procedures, before and after imaging. The VECTRA captures body images, 360° measurements and imaging, taking only a few seconds to produce a simulated image [16–18]. This is an added benefit where reconstructive plans can be worked out in detail with the surgeon and patient before the actual operation.

During the pandemic era, this was a challenging time. New protocols and safety precautions had to be created and followed. More online consultations were performed, followed by shorter in person visits, to reduce exposure risk. Masks, sanitizing gel, body temperature control, ozone devices, constant cleaning of offices, examination and operating rooms were the norm. Paradoxically, there was an increased interest in esthetic plastic procedures during this period. Perhaps, this was due to working from home. Patients were able to avoid taking off sick days for procedures, recovery was in the privacy of their home and not as noticeable, as it would be having to return to their workplace. The percentages of the most common procedures performed at Poliklinika Bagatin, during the pandemic era, are presented in **Figure 6**.

As seen from the table and graph, the prone position is used for total body liposuction (with or without abdominoplasty). The operations usually begin on the backside of the patient and following completion, the patients are turned around to complete

Total body liposuction	45
Liposuction + Abdominoplasty,	32
Abdominoplasty	7
Breast augmentation (all types)	304
Septorhinoplasty	218
Ritidectomy (face lifting)	30
Other procedures	120
Total operations	756

Table 1.
Esthetic plastic operative procedures poliklinika bagatin from November 2019 to January 2022 (the pandemic era).

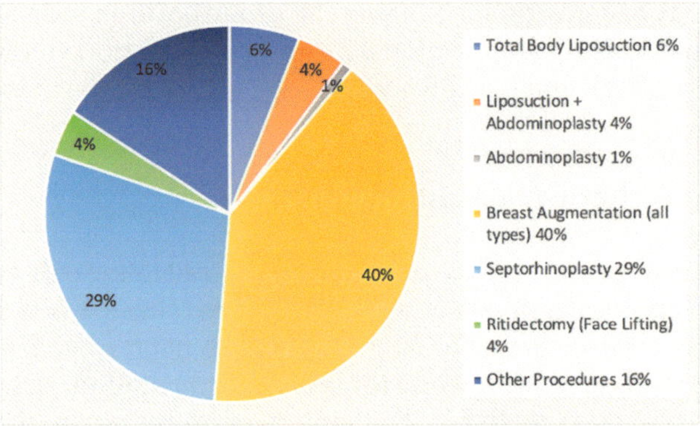

Figure 6.
Esthetic plastic operative procedures Poliklinika Bagatin during the pandemic era.

the frontside [19, 20]. At this point, following roation, a decision will be made to the length of the procedure, whether to keep the i-gel in place for the remainder of the operation, or if an ET tube will be placed. If abdominoplasty is planned, an ET tube is placed (the procedure can be lengthy and last more than 4 h). However, if only liposuction is planned, often the i-gel will remain, as the procedure will last up to 2 h more in the new supine position.

Other uses of the i-gel are with breast augmenation procedures, in estimated operative times up to 4 h. If more time is expected, such as with reduction, lifting and lipofilling, then an ET tube is preferred.

Ritidectomy (Face Lifting), septorhinoplasty, cleft lip corrections, palatal expansion, and various dental procedures require intubation with an ET tube.

As a private clinic, PB needs to provide safe anesthesia and surgery at a highest level. Providing a method without the use of muscle relaxants reduces recovery time, reduces muscle fatigue, and helps patients be prepared for discharge. However, in the event they are not ready, other arrangements are in place to care for them until they can safely go home [7].

6. Conclusion

This chapter reflects on a successful 3 year period, at PB, in which the prone position induction was introduced in 2018, for certain esthetic plastic procedures. The clinic has benefited from easier patient preparation, less patient rotation, reduced muscle relaxant (paralytic) drug use and increased safety for patients and staff.

Some clinicians may not believe in the i-gel as a reliable laryngeal device, and may reserve its use only for emergencies. However, the i-gel is an unique and extremely useful device, with a wider scope of delivery, that has changed anaethesia today [21]. This chapter explains that the i-gel can be used in uncommon induction positions safely. Future analysis of pulmonary pressure differences using the i-gel in prone and supine position, in the same patient after roation, are being gathered. Also, a study to compare tongue complications in prone and supine, with an i-gel in situ for 4 h is being developed. There are numerous fascinating aspects to observe and present with this method of intubation. Its use has been very reliable and valuable [9]. However, most importantly are the patient, staff and clinic benefits, using this safe and secure method, for a variety of procedures. PB finds the i-gel a remarkable and useful device, and will continue to use it and the prone position induction method, for years to come, after their successful introduction.

7. Discussion

After researching the use of i-gel in the prone position, we have found its usefulness in Japan, India, Germany, Netherlands, Denmark, Spain, Portugal, Poland, Croatia and even sporadic uses in the UK. A special thank you to all the colleagues who gave feedback about the use of i-gel in prone position. Initial experiences with this method, I personally observed in Porto, Portugal at the CICA Centar (a beautifully organized 1 day ambulatory surgery clinic) in 2014, and its use was routine. This method used Worldwide is intended for shorter duration procedures performed dorsally on the back, arms, legs ideally for any back side region. As asked by one editor, could it be used for spinal operations? Indeed, potentially it could be used for minor spinal procedures which are shorter in length, and not expected to develop serious complications intraoperatively, which would require converting to a deeper and more secure form of airway control and anesthesia. In the Netherlands this method of prone i-gel use is used for selected spinal operations since 2013 [22]. It is an excellent method to consider, for example, in lipoma excision, pilonidal sinus, achilles tendon heel repair, prone jackknife position for hemorroids, certain radiological exams or total body liposuction. Anesthesiologists are constantly faced with risks, never knowing when something may go awry. In general, being ultra prepared and choosing the least risky route, with patient safety as a leading determinate, are the mainstays of anesthetics. Throughout history most innovative new devices, techniques, methods, etc.... have been created to simplify and make our work easier. The technique, for PB, has been shown to be safe, reliable and a valuable alternative to the classic intubation and rotational methods being used. Regardless of the method used, patient's safety should come first. Remember, there can be many routes to get to our final destination, but get there safely. The ultimate choice lies with the anesthesiologist.

Author details

Judith Adrianne Deutsch[1*], Kata Šakić[2,3], Dinko Bagatin[4], Johann Nemrava[4] and Tomica Bagatin[5]

1 Anaesthesiology, Resuscitation and Intensive Care, Polyclinic Bagatin, Croatia

2 Faculty of Dental Medicine and Health Osijek, Anaesthesiology, Resuscitation and Intensive Care, University of Osijek, Croatia

3 School of Medicine University of Zagreb, Polyclinic Bagatin, Croatia

4 Faculty of Dental Medicine and Health Osijek, General and Plastic Reconstructive and Aesthetic Surgery, University of Osijek, Polyclinic Bagatin, Croatia

5 Faculty of Dental Medicine and Health Osijek, University of Osijek, Polyclinic Bagatin, Croatia

*Address all correspondence to: judita10000@gmail.com

IntechOpen

© 2022 The Author(s). Licensee IntechOpen. This chapter is distributed under the terms of the Creative Commons Attribution License (http://creativecommons.org/licenses/by/3.0), which permits unrestricted use, distribution, and reproduction in any medium, provided the original work is properly cited.

References

[1] Vrabac L. Chapter Text Illustrator, Fig. 1, 2, 3. Zagreb, Croatia: University of Zagreb, Faculty of Engineering and Computing (FER); 2022

[2] Netter FH. Atlas of Human Anatomy. 7th ed. Elsevier; 13 March 2018. ISBN-13: 978-0323393225. ISBN-10: 0323393225

[3] Intersurgical Ltd. I-gel. Crane House, Molly Millers Lane, Wokingham, Berkshire, UK; T:+44(0)118 9656 300, F: +44(0)118 9656 356, info@intersurgical.com, www.intersurgical.com

[4] Special Hospital AGRAM, Department of Radiology, Magnetic Resonance Imaging, Zagreb, Croatia.

[5] Edgcombe H, Carter K, Yarrow S. Anaesthesia in the prone position. British Journal of Anaesthesia. 2008;**100**(2): 165-183. DOI: 10.1093/bja/aem380

[6] Feix B, Sturgess J. Anaesthesia in the prone position. Continuing Education in Anaesthesia Critical Care and Pain. 2014;**14**(6):291-297. DOI: org/10.1093/bjaceaccp/mku001

[7] Meltzer B. A Guide to Patient Positioning. Outpatient Surgery. Association of Operating Room Nurses 2005Recommended practices for positioning the patient in the perioperative practice setting In: Standards, Recommended Practices, and Guidelines Denver, CO; 2008. Available from: http:// www.aorn.org

[8] Taxak S, Gopinath A. Insertion of i-gel airway in prone position. Minerva Anesthesiologica. 2010;**76**(5):381. PMID: 20395902. Available from:https://igelevidence.intersurgical.com/. (2010)

[9] Weksler N, Klein M, Rozentsveig V, Weksler D, Sidelnik C, Lottan M, et al. Laryngeal mask in prone position: Pure exhibitionism or a valid technique. Minerva Anesthesiologica. 2007;**73** (1-2):33-37 PMID: 17356505

[10] Agrawal S, Sharma JP, Jindal P, Sharma UC, Rajan M. Airway management in prone position with an intubating laryngeal mask airway. The Journal of Clinical Anesthesia. 2007;**19**(4):293-295. DOI: 10.1016/j.jclinane.2006.09.009. PIMD: 17572326

[11] Chau SW, Wang FY, Wu CW, Lu DV, Shen YC, Hung CW, et al. Premolar loss following insertion of a classic laryngeal mask airway in a patient in the prone position. Journal of Clinical Anesthesia. 2011;**23**(7):588-589. DOI: 10.1016/J.jclinane.2010.08.024. PMID: 22050808

[12] Mohammad S, Hashemain R, Nouraei N, Radpay B. Comparison of igel and laryngeal mask airway in anesthetized paralyzed patients. International Journal of Critical Illness and Injury Science. 2014;**4**(4):288-292. DOI: 10.4103/2229-5151.147520

[13] Kannanjia A, Srivastava U, Saraswat N, Mishra A, Saxena S. A preliminary study of i-gel: A new supraglottic airway device. Indian Journal of Anaesthesia. 2009;**53**(1):52-56. [PubMed] [Google Scholar].

[14] Twing S, Brown JH, Williams R. Swelling and cyanosis of the tongue associated with use of a laryngeal mask airway. Anaesthesia and Intensive Care. 2000;**28**:449-450. [PubMed][Google Scholar]

[15] Stewat A, Lindsay WA. Bilateral hypoglossal nerve injury following the use of laryngeal mask airway.

Anaesthesia. 2002;**57**:264-265. [PubMed] [Google Scholar]

[16] Moss C. Vectra Imaging Breast Augmentation and Virtual Rhinoplasty, 2022. Available from: http:// www.chrismoss.com.au.

[17] Canfield Scientific, Inc. Vectra XT 3D Imaging. 4 Wood Hollow Road, Parsippany, NJ, 07054, USA; T: 800 815 4330, 973 434 1200, F: 973 887 1249. Available from: http://info@canfieldsci.com, http://www.canfieldsci.com

[18] Hoyos A, Perez ME, Guarin DE, Montenegro A. A report of 736 high-definition lipoabdominoplasties performed in conjunction with circumferential VASER liposuction. Plastic and Reconstructive Surgery. 2018;**142**(3):662-675. DOI: 10.1097/PRS.0000000000004705

[19] Hoyos AE, Millard JA. VASER-assisted high definition lipoplasty. Aesthetic Surgery Journal. 2007;**27**(6):594/604. DOI: 10.1016-j.asj.2007.08.007

[20] Bagatin D, Bagatin T, Deutsch J, Šakić K, Nemrava J, Isomura E, et al. VASER Liposuction. How to Get Natural Results with Ultrasound Assisted Liposuction? Rijeka: IntechOpen; 2021. DOI: 10.5772/intechopen.100154

[21] Kubo Y, Kiyama S, Suzuki A, Kondo I, Uezono S. Use of supraglottic airway devices in the prone position. Journal of Anesthesia and Clinical Research Open Access. 2017;**8**(12). DOI: 1000797. Available from: https://www.longdom.org/open-access/use-of-supraglottic-airway-devices-in-the-prone-position-2155-6148-1000797.pdf

[22] Welsch P, Volk T. Retrospective audit: Use of the laryngeal mask airway in prone patients undergoing elective surgery on the spine—An acceptable alternative? Clinical Anaesthesia. Anasth Intensivmed. 2013;**54**:172-180

Section 3

Cardiac Anesthesia

Chapter 4

The Field of Cardiac Electrophysiology

Nicholas Roma, Joshua Elmer, Bruce Ferraro, Matthew Krinock and Darren Traub

Abstract

Cardiac electrophysiology is a unique and growing field that has made numerous advances in the past 15 years. Specifically, the field is advancing in terms of types of procedures as well as scope of practice. Pacemakers, implantable cardioverter-defibrillators (ICDs), and ablations have been the cornerstone of the field and continue to treat more and more conditions. This chapter will convey a birds-eye view of the types of the procedures in electrophysiology, the indications/contraindications, and the advances in the past 15 years. Additionally, local vs. general anesthesia in these procedures as well as the indication for the type of anesthesia will be discussed. The overall aim of this chapter is to present a unique viewpoint of cardiac electrophysiology as well as elaborate on the various types of anesthesia in this field.

Keywords: pacemaker, implanted cardioverter defibrillator, ablation, atrial fibrillation, electrophysiology

1. Introduction

Over 50 years ago, the cardiac action potential was first applied to clinical medicine [1]. This action potential includes four separate phases: resting, rapid depolarization, rapid repolarization, and a plateau phase with each of these phases correlating to a different ion channel as well as a different physiologic event in the heart [2]. The field of cardiac electrophysiology addresses and treats inherent faults within the heart's action potential as well as structural causes of cardiac arrhythmias. Historically, arrhythmias were classified into three distinct categories: abnormal impulse generation, abnormal impulse conduction, simultaneous impulse generation/conduction [3]. Although the types of arrythmias could be distinguished, all abnormal rhythm pathophysiology were found to consistently be related to an abnormal action potential. For example, in 1991 a study was performed proving that the action potential is prolonged in hypertrophied hearts signifying the relationship between the action potential and damaged tissue [4]. Furthermore in cardiomyopathy, K+ channels have been shown to be altered also prolonging the cardiac action potential [5]. Finally in long QT syndrome a link to a specific gene affecting a specific ion channel was identified affecting the action potential and thus demonstrating that arrhythmias

IntechOpen

can occur in structurally normal hearts if there is an abnormality in the cell's ion channels [6].

The relationship between ion channel/action potential abnormality and related cardiac structure is the foundation of cardiac electrophysiology. Pharmacology, procedures, and patient care have come from this relationship. As intensive research has been performed since the original thesis of ion channels and arrythmias, advances in the field have grown at an extremely rapid rate. Pacemakers (transcutaneous and permanent), catheter-based ablations for all type of arrythmias, cardioversions, and non-invasive cardiac monitoring have become the new norm in electrophysiology. Additionally, advances in anesthesiology have allowed shorter procedure times, more efficient procedures, and less risk. This chapter will highlight some of the most important procedures, indications for these procedures, current advances, and the role anesthesiology plays in cardiac electrophysiology.

2. The most common procedures of cardiac electrophysiology

2.1 Catheter ablations

In 1886, Walter Gaskell discovered specialized muscle fibers between the atria and the ventricle caused an irregular rhythm when cut—which was the first indication of an electrical system within the heart [7]. This has since become the basis of procedures such as cardiac or catheter ablations in electrophysiology. Presently, catheter ablations are used for almost every type of cardiac arrhythmia including: paroxysmal supraventricular tachycardia (SVT), atrial fibrillation, atrial flutter, and ventricular arrhythmias including frequent premature ventricular contractions and ventricular tachycardia.

2.1.1 Atrial fibrillation

Atrial fibrillation is the most common cardiac arrythmia in clinical practice with 6–12 million people predicted to suffer from this condition in the United States by 2050 [8]. The condition stems from ectopic beats typically from the pulmonary veins causing the atria to rapidly contract [9]. This arrythmia can lead to a multitude of complications including adverse remodeling as well as increased stroke risk from clot formation in stagnant blood. Atrial fibrillation is divided into three types: paroxysmal (lasting less than 7 days and self-terminating), persistent (longer than 7 days), and permanent (where there is decision to make no attempt at restoration of sinus rhythm). Typically, rapidly acting anti-arrhythmic agents especially amiodarone are first-line treatment for paroxysmal atrial fibrillation to attempt conversion. Cardioversion, an electric shock sent through the heart to reset the electrical circuit, is second line if pharmaceuticals do not work. Finally, since 85–95% of patients have their atrial fibrillation stemming from pulmonary veins, ablating these specific spots can be quite successful [10]. Treatment success rate of ablations for paroxysmal atrial fibrillation is between 65 and 75% [11]. Unfortunately, persistent atrial fibrillation is much less successful with a procedure success rate of roughly 45% [12]. Regardless, ablation therapy can be an effective treatment for atrial fibrillation particularly when combined with an anti-arrhythmic agent. A short procedure over continuous medical management can be beneficial to young and healthy individuals with a new diagnosis as well as the older population to avoid an overuse of medication.

The goal of atrial fibrillation ablation is to ablate or burn the connection between the pulmonary veins and the left atrium, often referred to as pulmonary vein isolation (PVI). The type of anesthesia during the procedure has also shown specific benefits. General anesthesia is preferred to IV sedation for PVI as this allows for less patient movement and improved ability to electrically map cardiac tissue with improved catheter contact [13]. Utilizing general anesthesia can improve efficacy rates and provide better patient outcomes in atrial fibrillation ablations.

At the start of atrial fibrillation ablations, a Transesophageal Echocardiogram (TEE) is performed after intubation. Of note, a paralytic is not used after intubation due to observation of the diaphragm. The TEE is utilized to look for thrombus in the Left Atrium as this is a direct contraindication to the procedure. If no thrombus is present, the procedure can continue. An additional preventive measure is esophageal temperature. Esophageal temperature is utilized because of the high frequency/temperature of the catheter used to physically ablate the pathway. This catheter reaches such high temperatures that a major potential complication of an ablation is esophageal injury. Any acute change to the temperature could indicate injury has occurred. Complications in atrial fibrillation ablations include: atrial-esophageal fistula, stroke, tamponade, and pulmonary vein stenosis. These complications were found in roughly 2.9% of the cases [14].

2.1.2 Atrial flutter

Atrial flutter is best known for the saw-tooth pattern seen on EKG. This saw tooth pattern represents the abnormal electrical circuit occurring in the heart and causing rapid beating of the atrium. Atrial flutter is ideal for ablation due to the typical anatomical landmarks found in the right atrium where the ectopic beats are from. Due to this, the success rate of an atrial flutter ablation is 95% [15]. Given the high success rate of catheter ablation of atrial flutter and the difficulty of medically treating this arrythmia, ablation of atrial flutter has now moved into first-line treatment. Atrial flutter ablations are very similar to atrial fibrillation ablations in terms of anesthetic considerations. TEE still occurs after intubation and no paralytic is used after initial intubation to determine diaphragm status. Additionally, an esophageal temperature catheter is placed as atrial flutter ablations have a similar risk of esophageal injury due to high temperature/frequency being used. Other complications of atrial flutter ablations are in line with atrial fibrillation ablations including stroke, tamponade, and vascular complications.

2.1.3 SVT

Paroxysmal SVT is broken down into pathway mediated tachycardia, AV nodal reentrant tachycardia and focal atrial tachycardia [10]. Pathway mediated tachycardias and AV nodal re-entrant tachycardia are disorders of impulse conduction, while focal atrial tachycardia is caused by a trigger, re-entry, or abnormal automaticity [16]. Typically, patients can present with a multitude of symptoms including palpitations, shortness of breath, and decreased exercise tolerance. The pathway of treatment for these patients starts with calcium/beta blockers or class Ic/III anti-arrhythmic agents. Depending on patient preference and success of medical therapy, catheter ablation can also be performed [17]. The focus of this type of ablation is the pre-mapping which finds the specific ectopic location or abnormal pathway in the atria and/or ventricles. This site is then ablated using radiofrequency energy or cryo-therapy with an 85–90% success rate for cessation/cure of the arrythmia [10]. SVT ablations differ in anesthetic management. These ablations do not require intubations as the goal for this procedure is to have the patient follow commands during the procedure. During the catheter placement and ablation, the patient may be sedated more, but after these instances the patient should be able to follow commands. The overall goal is to have the patient alternate between an asleep-awake-asleep cycle with the overall goal being a dissociated patient.

Arterial lines (A-lines) in EP ablations are on a case-by-case basis. If the patient has medications that require an A-line then one will be placed. One consideration that holds true is if the patient has an ejection fraction (EF) <35%, an A-line should be placed. This A-line will allow the possibility of acute intervention if needed. Additionally, for all ablations post-operative management is similar. Patients should lay supine for 4–6 hours to prevent bleeding from the catheter sites with a pressure dressing applied. After this period of time, the patient is typically discharged to the cardiac floor for further monitoring (**Table 1**).

2.2 Implantable devices

2.2.1 Pacemakers

The traditional pacemaker provides an external electrical stimulus by which myocytes may be depolarized, eliciting contraction of the heart muscle (**Figure 1**) [18]. Pacemakers function when the intrinsic pacing system of the heart fails to pace effectively and quickly enough to provide an adequate cardiac output for the patient. Muscle contraction takes place almost instantaneously following electrical impulse through the process of excitation-contraction coupling. The components of the traditional pacemaker include a pulse generator, housing a battery and electrical components, and leads, which project from the device housing into the myocardium to provide the site of impulse delivery [19]. These leads in the modern pacemaker also have the capacity to sense the heart's native electric activity in specific chambers to determine when the pacemaker should provide the external stimulus, and whether that external stimulus is necessary [19].

There are many indications for the use of conventional pacemakers and these indications continue to expand with new technology. Pacemaker implantation can be considered for patients with sinus node dysfunction, acquired AV nodal conduction and HIS Purkinje pathology, neurocardiogenic syncope, neuromuscular diseases impacting cardiac tissue conduction, and congestive heart failure [19]. Equipment and techniques for pacemaker implant continue to evolve and improve the safety of this procedure but like any invasive procedure there are inherent risks associated with the procedure. Implantation of the actual pacemaker is started with a small (~5 cm)

Procedure	TEE after intubation	Esophageal Temp Probe	Level of Sedation	Arterial Line indicated
Atrial Fibrillation Ablation	Yes	Yes	Constant	Case by Case
Atrial Flutter Ablation	Yes	Yes	Constant	Case by Case
SVT Ablation	No	No	Cyclic	Case by Case

Table 1.
Summary of anesthesiology in ablation procedures.

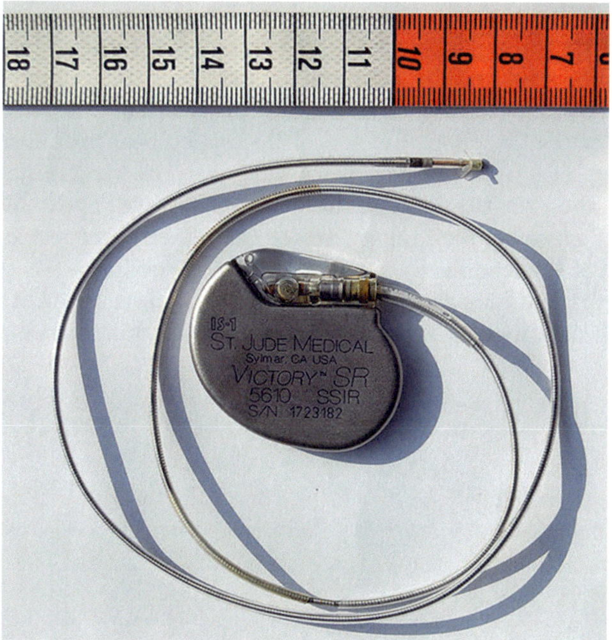

Figure 1.
A pacemaker [Fruitsmaak].

incision in the upper chest. Then a wire is thread through the vein and into the heart. This wire connects directly to the pacemaker to generate the electric signal that is required to physically pace the heart. The type of pacemaker as well as indication of the pacemaker will determine the specific chamber(s) where the wire(s) is placed. A common placement for the wire is in the right atrium and can be confirmed via chest x-ray. Prior studies have demonstrated varying complication rates for pacemaker implantation ranging from 3 to 10% [20]. The studies have shown that both patient characteristics and center volumes impact procedural complication rates. The most frequently reported major complication related to pacemaker implants are lead related re-interventions, while hematoma is the most reported minor complication. Other possible complications can include infection, cardiac perforation, pneumothorax, and lead dislodgement [20].

Within the last 10 years, leadless cardiac pacemakers have come onto the scene as a potential alternative option to traditional cardiac pacemakers [21]. These devices were designed to offer a leadless system to avoid many of the short and long-term complications that occur with transvenous pacemaker leads. A leadless device is much smaller than a traditional pacemaker in size and these devices will continue to miniaturize. The leadless device features electronics, a lithium battery, and electrodes. Uniquely from a conventional pacemaker, however, is the fact that the device housing includes both the pulse generator and the electrode which delivers that impulse to the cardiac tissue. An attachment end is used to screw in or attach via prongs into the endocardium. Different from the traditional pacemaker, the leadless model is installed via a sheath beginning in the femoral vein and extending up to the right ventricle which can be seen on chest x-ray [21].

While leadless pacemakers share some features of transvenous pacemakers, they are much more recent in their development, and are not able to be utilized for the full range of indications of transvenous pacemakers. Leadless pacemakers are rate adaptive and may modify pacing upon detecting a patient exercising. These devices have a battery life of approximately 10 years and are externally programable, a featured shared with traditional pacemaker devices. The first leadless cardiac pacemaker was a ventricular only system: it senses and acts on a ventricle, has inhibitory activity, and features a rate response function. A newer pacemaker, the Medtronic Micra AV is able to sense the atria and pace the ventricle for patients in sinus rhythm with heart block (**Figure 2**) [22]. This newer technology, which can be seen on chest x-ray, indicates the advancement of the leadless pacemaker and the capability it has (**Figure 3**) [23].

Leadless pacemakers have a growing list of indications for use as the technology further evolves. Indications include permanent atrial fibrillation with AV block,

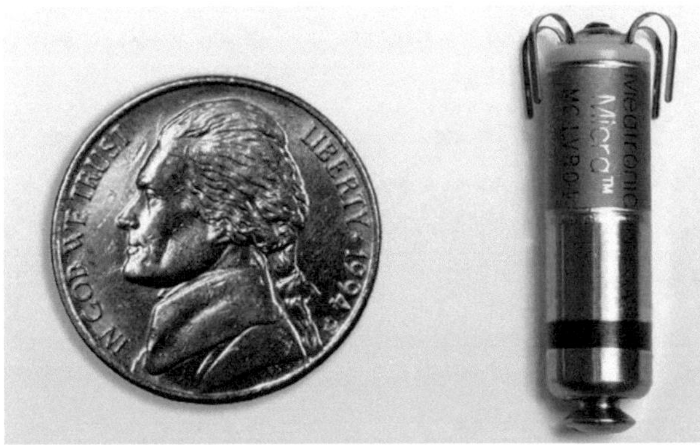

Figure 2.
Micra leadless pacemaker [Metropolitan Heart and Vascular Institute].

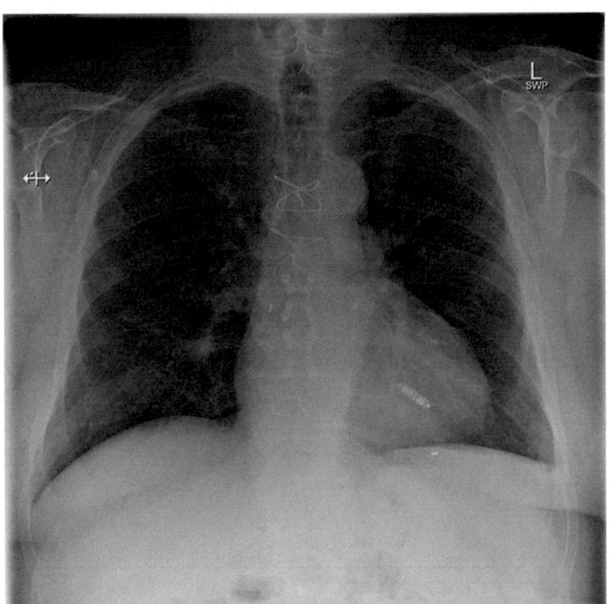

Figure 3.
Leadless pacemaker on chest X-ray (Khader et al. [23]).

second- or third-degree block in patients with normal sinus rhythm, and sinus bradycardia [24]. As uses for the leadless pacemaker expand, so does understanding of the possible complications of this device. Major complications include cardiac injury, complications at the site of entry in the groin, thromboembolism, presyncope, syncope, cardiac failure, and acute myocardial infarction, among others. Classically, the most reported of these major complications are problems at the site of catheter entry as well as perforation of the myocardium, which differs from the higher rates of electrode dislodgement, site infections, and lead fractures seen in transvenous pacemakers [21, 25]. In a study on a specific model of leadless device, the micra transcatheter pacing study, complications were reported from the 12-months post-implantation of the leadless device [26]. This study involved 745 patients at 56 centers in 19 different countries and compared prospective data on the Micra leadless system with historical data on transvenous pacemakers. Overall, the leadless system had a lower risk of major complications by a difference of 48% mostly related to the reduction in system revision. Last, no major infections have been attributed to the Micra leadless device at 12 months, which is encouraging given the infection risk seen with transvenous pacemakers [26].

As with any new technology, many opportunities exist for improvement of the leadless pacemaker. For one, improving safety of the device, and in particular, the installation process, would further set the leadless pacemaker apart from its transvenous counterpart. Specifically, modifying how the device attaches into the myocardium is one such way that has been suggested to reduce perforation risk. In addition, development of improved battery lifespan or a charging system for the battery within the pacemaker will allow for a longer device usage with fewer repeat procedures [27]. Aside from improvements in safety, the uses for the leadless pacemaker may also continue to expand with time. In fact, efforts are already underway to develop an atrial leadless pacemaker in addition to dual chamber pacing, two areas which can increase the number of patients who may benefit from such a device [28].

2.2.2 *Implantable cardioverter-defibrillator*

Conventional transvenous implantable cardioverter defibrillators (ICDs) consist of similar components to a transvenous pacemaker: a battery, a pulse generator, and leads, which ultimately provide a pathway for shock delivery to cardiac tissue [29]. To deliver a shock, charge first accumulates within the capacitor of the device before being expelled through the leads to reach the myocardium. In addition to delivering a shock in instances of ventricular arrythmia, modern ICDs feature pacing activity similarly to pacemakers. Therapies for arrhythmia delivered by ICDs come in multiple forms, with synchronized versus asynchronized shocks as well as overdrive pacing. Synchronized and asynchronous shocks work to terminate abnormal rhythms, such as ventricular fibrillation and ventricular tachycardia, through electrical cardioversion. In contrast, overdrive pacing can be utilized in ventricular tachycardia, where the ICD transiently delivers pacing at a rate above the rate of tachycardia to cease the arrythmia. These ICD devices come in single chamber and dual chamber systems, with dual chamber systems able to discriminate between atrial and ventricular arrythmias and provide pacing output to both chambers [29]. Finally, cardiac resynchronization therapy defibrillators can be used to simultaneously pace the right and left ventricle in patients with heart failure believed to be exacerbated by conduction system disease.

Indications for an ICD include use as primary and secondary prevention. Primary prevention involves placing a defibrillator to prevent cardiac arrest in patients with known cardiac conditions that place them at increased risk for lethal ventricular arrhythmias. These conditions include but are not limited to: ischemic and non-ischemic cardiomyopathy with left ventricular ejection fraction <35%, long QT syndrome, Brugada syndrome, hypertrophic cardiomyopathy and arrhythmogenic right ventricular cardiomyopathy [30]. Secondary prevention indications include those patients who have already suffered a cardiac arrest from ventricular tachycardia or ventricle fibrillation and those patients with sustained ventricular tachycardia in the setting of structural heart disease [30]. Regarding the risks of transvenous ICDs, there are many overlaps with complications seen in transvenous pacemakers. Common risks of conventional ICD devices include lead-related issues which require revision, localized and systemic infections, cardiac perforation, and hematoma at the site of implantation [20].

Similarly, to the recent rise in leadless pacemakers as a potential alternative to transvenous pacemakers, subcutaneous ICD (S-ICD) devices have been recently developed to rival or improve upon transvenous ICD (TV-ICD) systems. These S-ICD devices are implanted within the subcutaneous tissue typically on the left side allowing for shock delivery of 80 Joules through tissue adjacent to the heart as opposed to leads directly projecting into the heart chambers (**Figures 4** and **5**) [31, 32]. This difference in function results in a different profile of complications; S-ICD complications include pocket infections and device erosion [33]. Conversely, complications of transvenous ICDs are predominantly due to its lead system and include perforation of cardiac tissue, tamponade, pneumothorax, and lead repositioning [34]. Of note, S-ICD devices may be used for many of the same indications of TV-ICDs, such as primary or secondary life-threatening arrythmia prevention or certain patients with congenital or inherited cardiac conditions (including hypertrophic cardiomyopathy, Brugada syndrome, and ischemic and non-ischemic cardiomyopathies, among others) [33]. Therefore, the advent of S-ICDs expands options for patients considering ICD implantation and allows patients and clinicians to work together in determining which risks may be best tolerated in the long term.

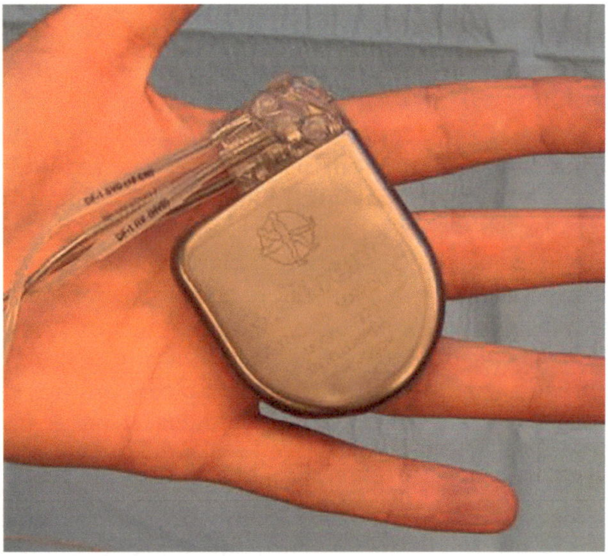

Figure 4.
Subcutaneous ICD [CardioNetworks].

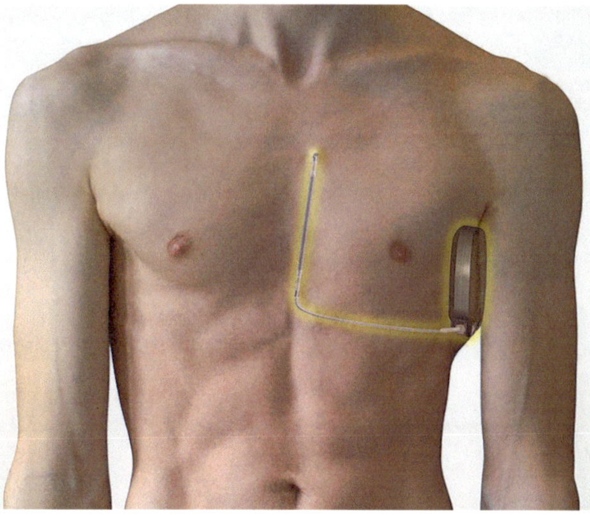

Figure 5.
Subcutaneous ICD location [Wikipedia].

2.2.3 Further anesthetic considerations for PM and ICD

Anesthesia for pacemaker and ICD placement traditionally required general anesthesia under the direction of an anesthesiology team. Modern approaches to sedation for device placement have involved use of a lower level of sedation and in some cases occur under a proceduralist directed, nurse administered (PDNA) model. In particular, the placement of traditional transvenous pacemakers and leadless pacemakers now favors this PDNA model to achieve conscious sedation in these patients [35]. However, the role of the anesthesiology team in such a procedure is largely determined by patient characteristics impacting the risk of such a procedure. ICD placement may also favor this PDNA model, due to an increasing push toward conscious sedation in ICD placement procedures. In fact, a conscious sedation model using opiates with benzodiazepines may be more favorable when compared to general anesthesia due to shorter procedure and recovery times as well as cost to patients [36]. In cases where sedation using Propofol is to be used, the risk of hypotension and respiratory depression must be considered. In these cases as well as cases involving deep sedation during device placement, it is recommended that proceduralists consider involvement of anesthesiology [35]. Additionally, differentiating between ICD and pacemakers on chest x-ray is imperative to ensure adequate anesthesiology pre-operative prep. To distinguish a pacemaker vs. ICD on chest x-ray, Pacemakers have small leads (**Figure 6a**), where ICD's have thick coiled segments at the end of their leads (**Figure 6b**) [37].

For patients with an active ICD, special considerations are needed for any additional procedures that these patients go through. For example, a magnet is placed over a patient with an ICD before incision and then removed after the procedure is performed. This magnet turns off the ICD shock function to ensure patient safety throughout the operation. In some cases, the ICD beeps to ensure the shock function has been disabled and will beep again when the magnet is removed. In other cases, a device representative will be present in the room to ensure the device's shock has been disabled and to interrogate the device as needed. Active pacemaker patients also have

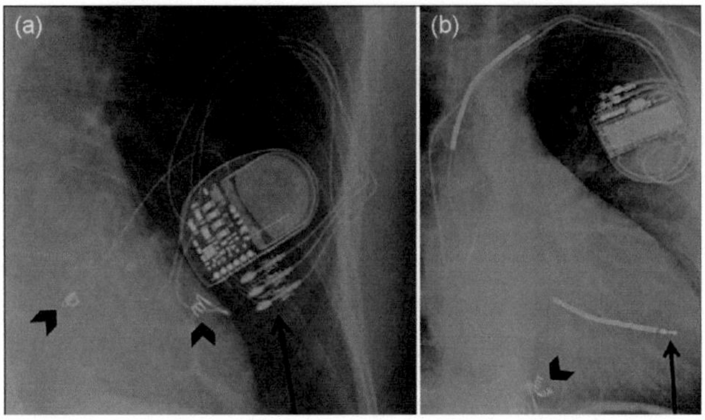

Figure 6.
(a) Chest X-ray ensuring lead placement in pacemaker is correct, and (b) ICD segmented coils being shown (Torres-Ayala et al. [37]).

special considerations before surgery that need to be considered. Device interrogation should be done before and after surgery if the surgery is directly affecting the device or if any complication occurs during the procedure involving the pacemaker. Additionally, similar to ICD's magnets can be used before surgery to place the pacemaker in asynchronous mode. However, before considering using a magnet for a pacemaker there are several considerations that need to be addressed including the dependency of the pacemaker for the patient, the type of surgery, and is the pacemaker obstructing the surgical field. ICD and pacemaker patients need these special considerations before procedures to ensure the success of the operation.

2.3 Noninvasive and invasive cardiac monitoring for arrythmias

Before noninvasive cardiac monitoring, many arrythmias would be missed due to the arrythmia not occurring at the specific moment the EKG was being taken. Today, various monitors allow clinicians to detect many arrythmias such as atrial fibrillation, atrial flutter, tachycardia-bradycardia syndrome, junctional rhythms, and many more outside of the office or hospital. Typically, if a patient presents with palpitations, subjective irregular heart rhythm, unexplained syncope, or other cardiac manifestations with a normal EKG; a Holter monitor or ambulatory extended monitor can be utilized. A Holter monitor or ambulatory extended monitory is a wearable device that has electrodes that record EKG's. The device can be worn between 1 day to 4 weeks but in general does not provide real time data. These devices have the downside of being cumbersome to the patient as they are bulky and limit daily activity (**Figure 7**) [38].

Mobile telemetry is similar to Holter and event recorders but involves real time monitoring by a data center that can notify a patient or physician immediately of an arrhythmia. An implantable cardiac loop recorder is a small device implanted under the skin that can track rhythm, rate, and even correlation with symptoms of the patient (**Figure 8**) [39, 40]. Implantation of loop recorders do not require IV sedation. Lidocaine is typically used to numb the area before the10–15 minute procedure. Loop recorders have a battery life up to 5 years and can store data and transmit the data almost immediately to a monitoring physician [39]. A study in 2007 showed that loop recorders were superior for the diagnosis of an arrythmia over the conventional treatment method of Holter monitor (24 hours), 4-week random EKG monitoring,

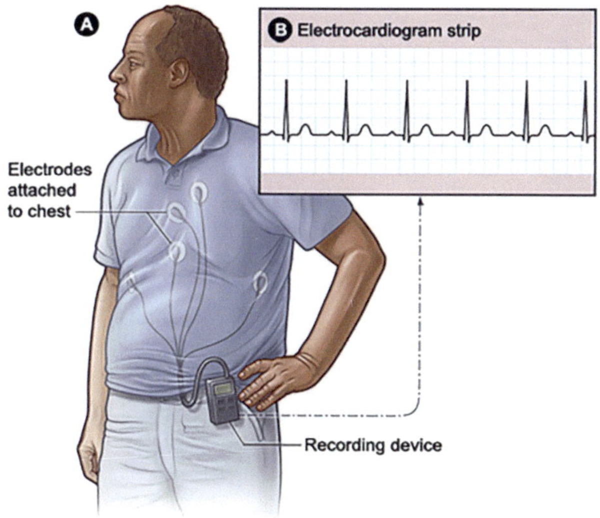

Figure 7.
Overview of Holter monitor being worn [National Heart Lung and Blood Institute].

and an EP study [41]. One of the primary uses for loop recorders in the modern era is detection of occult atrial fibrillation in patients with a cryptogenic stroke. Prospective studies have demonstrated that in patients with cryptogenic stroke, when a loop recorder is placed, atrial fibrillation will be discovered in up to 30% over 3 years of monitoring [42]. Loop recorders have shown a significantly higher diagnostic yield than periodic EKG monitoring or 24 and 48 hour Holter monitoring for these patient populations [43]. From a clinical standpoint, if a patient presents to the office with any cardiac manifestations pointing to a serious cardiac arrythmia that occurs rarely throughout a 12 month period, a loop recorder may be the most cost effective and efficient diagnostic tool.

3. Discussion

Cardiac electrophysiology is an ever-growing field. One of the possible advancements with EP is performing the procedures without fluoroscopy. Fluoroscopy allows the proceduralist to visualize the surgical field for ablations, pacemaker/ICD implantations, etc. The main concern with fluoroscopy is the amount of radiation exposure to the EP lab team. As Low As Reasonably Achievable (ALARA) is an implemented system to reduce radiation exposure in the lab. Certain recommendations utilizing this concept are a certain distance from the table, additional lead shielding, table height, and appropriateness of fluoroscopy [44]. As these measures are actively being done in EP labs, exposure of radiation is still imminent.

Advancements to utilize other imaging in substitution of fluoroscopy could potentially be the future of the EP lab. Imaging such as intracardiac echocardiography, cardiac MRI guidance, and 3D electromapping systems have all been proposed [45]. Using these styles of imaging could produce the same result with a much less radiation exposure risk for not only the patient, but also the physician and their team. Robotic

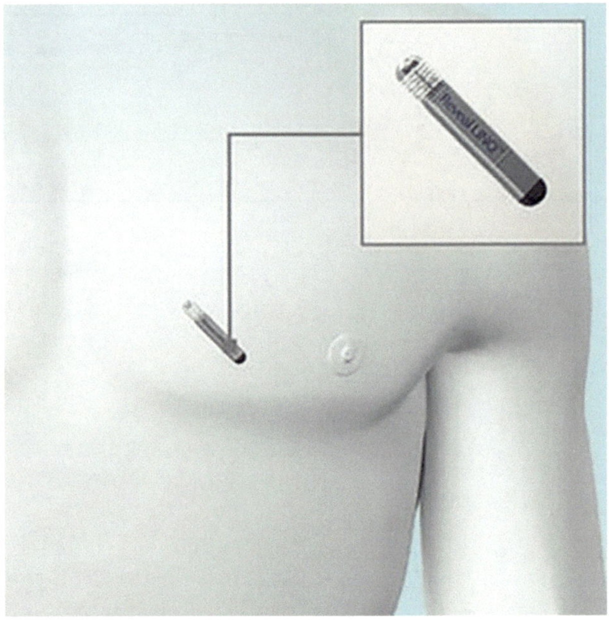

Figure 8.
Loop recorder and location of the monitor [Mobitz Heart and Rhythm Center].

surgery is also an option as this would eliminate the number of people required to be present in the room. Overall, these advancements are still far away as there needs to be a clear indication that success rate of the procedure nor the patient outcome would not falter, but a fluoroscopy-free EP lab could be the future of electrophysiology.

4. Conclusion

In conclusion, cardiac electrophysiology is an ever-growing field with many advances in recent years. The field itself has an extraordinary amount of depth and conditions that can be treated. Pacemakers, ablations, and ICDs are the forefront of electrophysiology, but the field is actively expanding into cardiac monitoring. The anesthesia management of EP procedures is quite extensive. Atrial fibrillation and Atrial flutter ablations require TEE pre-procedure as well as active esophageal temperature monitoring. SVT ablations do not require intubation, but require an extensive awake-sleep-awake cycle with the overall goal being a dissociated patient to actively monitor the patient during the procedure. ICD/pacemaker anesthesiology practice favors a PDNA model, but each patient is considered on a case-by-case basis. Anesthesiology and electrophysiology work hand in hand to give the best possible care for the patient and to ensure optimal patient outcomes.

Author details

Nicholas Roma[1*], Joshua Elmer[2], Bruce Ferraro[3], Matthew Krinock[3] and Darren Traub[3]

1 Department of Internal Medicine, St. Luke's University Health Network, Bethlehem, Pennsylvania, USA

2 Lewis Katz School of Medicine, Temple University, Philadelphia, Pennsylvania, USA

3 Department of Cardiology, St. Luke's University Health Network, Bethlehem, Pennsylvania, USA

*Address all correspondence to: nicholas.roma@sluhn.org

IntechOpen

© 2022 The Author(s). Licensee IntechOpen. This chapter is distributed under the terms of the Creative Commons Attribution License (http://creativecommons.org/licenses/by/3.0), which permits unrestricted use, distribution, and reproduction in any medium, provided the original work is properly cited. (cc) BY

References

[1] Grant AO. Cardiac ion channels. Circulation. Arrhythmia and Electrophysiology. 2009;**2**(2):185-194. DOI: 10.1161/CIRCEP.108.789081

[2] Roden ME, Dan M, Balser JR, George AL, Anderson ME. Caridac ion channels. Annual Review of Physiology. 2002;**64**:431

[3] Hoffman BF, Rosen MR. Brief reviews cellular mechanisms for cardiac arrhythmias. An Official Journal of the American Heart Association. 1981;**49**(1): 1-15. Available from: http://ahajournals.org

[4] Aronson R. Mechanisms of arrhythmias in ventricular hypertrophy. Journal of Cardiovascular Electrophysiology. 1991;**2**:249-261

[5] Beuckelmann DJ, Näbauer M, Erdmann E. Alterations of K+ currents in isolated human ventricular myocytes from patients with terminal heart failure. Circulation Research. 1993;**73**(2):379-385. DOI: 10.1161/01.RES.73.2.379

[6] Roden DM, George AL. The cardiac ion channels: Relevance to management of arrhythmias. Annual Review of Medicine. 1996;**47**:135-148. DOI: 10.1146/annurev.med.47.1.135

[7] Silverman ME, Grove D, Upshaw CB. Why does the heart beat? The discovery of the electrical system of the heart. Circulation. 2006;**113**(23):2775-2781. DOI: 10.1161/CIRCULATIONAHA.106.616771

[8] Lippi G, Sanchis-Gomar F, Cervellin G. Global epidemiology of atrial fibrillation: An increasing epidemic and public health challenge. International Journal of Stroke. 2021;**16**(2):217-221. DOI: 10.1177/1747493019897870

[9] Haissaguerre M, Jaïs P, Shah DC, Takahashi A, Hocini M, Quiniou G, et al. Spontaneous initiation of atrial fibrillation by ectopic impulses originating in the pulmonary veins. Cardiology in Review. 1999;**7**(2):65. DOI: 10.1097/00045415-199903000-00006

[10] Lee G, Sanders P, Kalman JM. Catheter ablation of atrial arrhythmias: State of the art. The Lancet. 2012;**380**(9852):1509-1519. DOI: 10.1016/S0140-6736(12)61463-9

[11] Kong MH, Piccini JP, Bahnson TD. Efficacy of adjunctive ablation of complex fractionated atrial electrograms and pulmonary vein isolation for the treatment of atrial fibrillation: A meta-analysis of randomized controlled trials. Europace. 2011;**13**(2):193-204. DOI: 10.1093/europace/euq384

[12] Brooks AG et al. Outcomes of long-standing persistent atrial fibrillation ablation: A systematic review. Heart Rhythm. 2010;**7**(6):835-846. DOI: 10.1016/j.hrthm.2010.01.017

[13] di Biase L et al. General anesthesia reduces the prevalence of pulmonary vein reconnection during repeat ablation when compared with conscious sedation: Results from a randomized study. Heart Rhythm. 2011;**8**(3):368-372. DOI: 10.1016/j.hrthm.2010.10.043

[14] Gupta A et al. Complications of catheter ablation of atrial fibrillation a systematic review. Circulation. Arrhythmia and Electrophysiology. 2013;**6**(6):1082-1088. DOI: 10.1161/CIRCEP.113.000768

[15] Willems S et al. Catheter ablation of atrial flutter guided by

Electroanatomic mapping (CARTO): A randomized comparison to the conventional approach. Journal of Cardiovascular Electrophysiology. 2008;**11**(11):1223-1230

[16] Characteristics E, Chen S, Chiang C, Yang C, Cheng C. Sustained atrial tachycardia in adult patients of radiofrequency ablation. Circulation. 1994:1262-1278

[17] Blomström-Lundqvist C et al. ACC/AHA/ESC Guidelines for the Management of Patients with Supraventricular Arrhythmias—Executive Summary: A Report of the American College of Cardiology/American Heart Association Task Force on Practice Guidelines and the European Society of Cardiology. Vol. 42. Elsevier Masson SAS; 2003. p. 8. DOI: 10.1016/j.jacc.2003.08.013

[18] Fruitsmaak S. St. Jude medical pacemaker with ruler. Wikipedia. 2007

[19] Mulpuru SK, Madhavan M, McLeod CJ, Cha YM, Friedman PA. Cardiac pacemakers: Function, troubleshooting, and management: Part 1 of a 2-part series. Journal of the American College of Cardiology. 2017;**69**(2):189-210. DOI: 10.1016/J.JACC.2016.10.061

[20] Kirkfeldt RE, Johansen JB, Nohr EA, Jorgensen OD, Nielsen JC. Complications after cardiac implantable electronic device implantations: An analysis of a complete, nationwide cohort in Denmark. European Heart Journal. 2014;**35**(18):1186-1194. DOI: 10.1093/EURHEARTJ/EHT511

[21] Reddy VY et al. Permanent leadless cardiac pacing. Circulation. 2014;**129**(14):1466-1471. DOI: 10.1161/CIRCULATIONAHA.113.006987

[22] Leadless Pacemaker. Metropolitan Heart and Vascular Institute; 2022

[23] Khader O, Thabet M, Knipe H. Leadless cardiac pacemaker. Radiopaedia.org. 2022. DOI: 10.53347/rID-57378

[24] Reynolds D et al. A leadless intracardiac transcatheter pacing system. The New England Journal of Medicine. 2016;**374**(6):533-541. DOI: 10.1056/NEJMOA1511643

[25] Sattar Y et al. Complications of leadless vs conventional (lead) artificial pacemakers—A retrospective review. Journal of Community Hospital Internal Medicine Perspectives. 2020;**10**(4):328. DOI: 10.1080/20009666.2020.1786901

[26] Duray GZ et al. Long-term performance of a transcatheter pacing system: 12-month results from the Micra Transcatheter pacing study. Heart Rhythm. 2017;**14**(5):702-709. DOI: 10.1016/J.HRTHM.2017.01.035

[27] Middour TG, Chen JH, El-Chami MF. Leadless pacemakers: A review of current data and future directions. Progress in Cardiovascular Disease. 2021. DOI: 10.1016/j.pcad.2021.06.003

[28] Vatterott PJ et al. Implant, performance, and retrieval of an atrial leadless pacemaker in sheep. Heart Rhythm. 2021;**18**(2):288-296. DOI: 10.1016/J.HRTHM.2020.09.022

[29] Glikson M, Friedman P. The implantable cardioverter defibrillator. Lancet. 2001;**357**:1107-1117

[30] Sorbera CA, Cusack EJ. Indications for implantable cardioverter defibrillator therapy. Heart Disease. 2002;**4**(3):166-170. DOI: 10.1097/00132580-200205000-00007

[31] ICD. CardioNetworks; 2007

[32] Robystarm07. S-ICD. Wikipedia; 2020

[33] Savarimuthu S, Roy S, Obeidat M, Harky A. Subcutaneous implantable cardioverter defibrillator: Can it overtake its transvenous counterpart. Pacing and Clinical Electrophysiology. 2021;**44**(8):1413-1420. DOI: 10.1111/PACE.14246

[34] Knops RE et al. Subcutaneous or Transvenous defibrillator therapy. New England Journal of Medicine. 2020;**383**(6):526-536. DOI: 10.1056/NEJMOA1915932/SUPPL_FILE/NEJMOA1915932_DATA-SHARING.PDF

[35] Gerstein NS, Young A, Schulman PM, Stecker EC, Jessel PM. Sedation in the electrophysiology laboratory: A multidisciplinary review. Journal of the American Heart Association. 2016;**5**(6). DOI: 10.1161/JAHA.116.003629

[36] Bollmann A, Kanuru NK, DeLurgio D, Walter PF, Burnette JC, Langberg JJ. Comparison of three different automatic defibrillator implantation approaches: Pectoral implantation using conscious sedation reduces procedure times and cost. Journal of Interventional Cardiac Electrophysiology. 1997;**1**(3):221-225. DOI: 10.1023/A:1009768806894

[37] Torres-Ayala SC, Santacana-Laffitte G, Maldonado J. Radiography of cardiac conduction devices: A pictorial review of pacemakers and implantable cardioverter defibrillators. Journal of Clinical Imaging Science. 2014;**4**(Dec):74. DOI: 10.4103/2156-7514.148269

[38] "Holter Monitor NIH," National Heart Lung and Blood Insitute. NIH; 2013

[39] Galli A, Ambrosini F, Lombardi F. Holter monitoring and loop recorders: From research to clinical practice. Arrhythmia & Electrophysiology Review. 2016;**5**(2):136-143. DOI: 10.15420/AER.2016.17.2

[40] Implantable Loop Recorder. Mobitz Heart and Rhythm Center. Mobitz; 2022

[41] Giada F et al. Recurrent unexplained palpitations (RUP) study. Comparison of implantable loop recorder versus conventional diagnostic strategy. Journal of the American College of Cardiology. 2007;**49**(19):1951-1956. DOI: 10.1016/j.jacc.2007.02.036

[42] Liao J, Khalid Z, Scallan C, Morillo C, O'Donnell M. Noninvasive cardiac monitoring for detecting paroxysmal atrial fibrillation or flutter after acute ischemic stroke: A systematic review. Stroke. 2007;**38**(11):2935-2940. DOI: 10.1161/STROKEAHA.106.478685

[43] Diederichsen SZ et al. Comprehensive evaluation of rhythm monitoring strategies in screening for atrial fibrillation: Insights from patients at risk monitored long term with an implantable loop recorder. Circulation. 2020;**141**(19):1510-1522. DOI: 10.1161/CIRCULATIONAHA.119.044407

[44] Rogers A, Brodt C. Minimizing radiation in the modern electrophysiology laboratory. Journal of Innovations in Cardiac Rhythm Management. 2018;**9**(8):3265-3270. DOI: 10.19102/icrm.2018.090805

[45] Purtell CS, Kipp RT, Eckhardt LL. Into a Fluoroless future: An appraisal of fluoroscopy-free techniques in clinical cardiac electrophysiology. Current Cardiology Reports. 2021;**23**(4). DOI: 10.1007/s11886-021-01461-y

Chapter 5

Extracorporeal Membrane Oxygenation: Beyond Conventional Indications

Akram M. Zaaqoq, Mariam Gabrial and Heidi J. Dalton

Abstract

Over the last several years, the use of extracorporeal membrane oxygenation (ECMO) has exponentially increased. As the technology advanced, the rate of devastating complications has decreased somewhat, and the utility of ECMO has expanded beyond its conventional uses in cardiogenic shock and acute respiratory distress syndrome (ARDS). Currently, ECMO can be deployed in the perioperative period with high-risk surgeries where cardiac or respiratory compromise is anticipated. Moreover, it can be utilized in difficult airway patients or patients undergoing airway surgeries, thoracic surgery patients, trauma victims and many other conditions previously excluded. The aim of this review is to highlight the ECMO-patient interaction, the indications for ECMO in the non-cardiac surgery population, ECMO management and potential complications.

Keywords: extracorporeal membrane oxygenation, ECMO, extracorporeal life support, ECLS, trauma, peripartum

1. Introduction

Fifty years ago, the first use of extracorporeal membrane oxygenation (ECMO) was for long-term respiratory support in an adult patient with post-traumatic acute lung injury [1]. Since that report, there has been an exponential increase in the use of ECMO for both circulatory and respiratory support. Due to the advances in technology, surgical techniques, and critical care medicine, ECMO has become part of standard care for many diseases in centers which can provide ECMO support. An analysis on ECMO data from 34 states enrolled in the Healthcare Cost and Utilization Project showed a significant increase in ECMO use from 2011 through 2014 [2], with an overall rate 1.34 per 100,000 patients per year. Similarly, the analysis of The Extracorporeal Life Support Organization (ELSO) international registry from 1989 to 2013 revealed an increase in ECMO use predominantly in adult patients [3].

This substantial increase and availability have expanded the utilization of ECMO beyond being a last-resort salvage intervention when other modalities are deemed insufficient. Currently, ECMO is deployed electively to mitigate the risk and ensure the safe and successful performance of high-risk procedures in at-risk patients. Elective initiation of ECMO has been associated with better outcomes than emergent rescue placement in the setting of cardiopulmonary arrest [4]. Further, by anticipating operative risks, a multidisciplinary team can decide on and prepare the most appropriate ECMO modality to provide support if needed. Venovenous (V-V) ECMO provides adequate gas exchange if the airway or the pulmonary function is compromised but cardiac function is adequate. However, venoarterial (V-A) ECMO will provide organ perfusion when both heart and lung function are inadequate. The perioperative use of ECMO requires an understanding of the basic physiology of ECMO, when to initiate the extracorporeal support, and how to manage and monitor for potential complications. This chapter will highlight common areas of ECMO management to provide the best care for those critically ill patients.

2. Methods

To address our research questions, we conducted a comprehensive review of the literature by using MEDLINE and EMBASE database on July 25th, 2022. The search strategy was focused on the indications for ECMO. Keywords and MeSH term relating to these categories were used to optimize the database search. We searched with keywords and MeSH term "Extracorporeal membrane oxygenation" OR "ECMO" OR "ECLS" AND "TREATMENT INDICATION". All relevant articles were screened. We included any related work that was published in English; explicitly described the approach and specific methods; and identified issues, challenges, strengths, and limitations. The search returned 265 titles from which 240 focused on different indications for ECMO and 25 centered around ECMO management and transport (Supplementary). We thoroughly reviewed and categorized the included articles according to their format and relevant clinical themes.

3. Basics and physiology of extracorporeal membrane oxygenation

3.1 Basics of extracorporeal membrane oxygenation

ECMO is an Extracorporeal Life Support (ECLS) modality, where deoxygenated blood flows into a membrane lung (oxygenator- where gas exchange occurs) and returns to the patient. The presence of the membrane lung (oxygenator) and a pump, which ensures circuit flow, are required features for ECMO. Other key components are cannulas, tubing, air-gas blender, and heat exchanger. Pressure and flow sensors are also commonly integrated into the ECMO circuit. The artificial lung is a microporous hollow fiber made from polymethylpentene (PMP) [5]. The blood surrounds the fibers and flows in the opposite direction of oxygen to obtain optimal gas exchange. The difference in partial pressure between the gas phase and the venous blood allows diffusion of oxygen (O_2) across the membrane into the blood and carbon dioxide (CO_2) from the blood into the fiber gas. The oxygenator is connected to, or integrated with, a heat exchanger that controls the blood temperature through conduction from warm water for warming or cooling with ice or other means. The most used pump is a centrifugal device that creates suction to drain blood and propels it forward to the return site. The positive pressure generated by the centrifugal head must be higher than the pressure in the returning site from the circuit to allow forward flow. There are multiple factors determining the blood flow through the ECMO circuit: preload (patient blood volume, vascular tone and patency, and the size and the location of the drainage cannula), afterload (size and location of the reinfusion cannula, patient blood pressure/systemic vascular resistance, the length of the tube between the pump and patient), and the resistance throughout the ECMO circuit (kinking of the tubes, connections, the degree of oxygenator clot burden). Viscosity and temperature may also affect blood flow and gas exchange.

ECMO cannulas are made from polyurethane and commonly have biocompatible hydrophilic coatings, although each manufacturer may use a different coating [6]. The drainage (inflow) cannulas are multi-stage with sizes that range from 8–32F. The return (outflow) cannulas are single stage with variable sizes and lengths based on the ECMO modality, the size of the accessed vessels, and the targeted ECMO flow. In V-V ECMO dual cannulation, femoro-femoral (V_f-V_f) configuration, the return cannula size used most in adults are 23–27F and should be placed so the distal port is at the level of the vena cava / right atrium junction. In femoral-jugular (V_f-V_j) configuration, the return cannula sizes are usually 17–25F short cannulas. In peripheral V-A ECMO, the return cannula sizes range from 15–21F. It is recommended that a distal perfusion cannula is additionally inserted (usually in the superficial femoral artery) to prevent lower limb ischemia. The size of the distal perfusion cannula often ranges from 6–8F. Finally, in dual-lumen (DL) V-V ECMO configuration, cannula sizes range from 13–32F.

3.2 Physiology of extracorporeal membrane oxygenation

There are two main modes for ECMO, V-V and V-A. However, hybrid modes such as V-AV can be adopted in certain clinical situations to provide extra support or to reduce risk such as differential hypoxia (North-South syndrome).

3.2.1 Venoarterial extracorporeal membrane oxygenation (V-A ECMO)

In V-A ECMO, deoxygenated venous blood is drained from the patient into the ECMO circuit, passes through the pump and oxygenator for gas exchange, and oxygenated blood is then returned to the patient's arterial circulation (**Figure 1a**). Thus, V-A ECMO provides both circulatory and respiratory support until either the heart recovers, more durable options become available, transplant occurs, or the decision is made that further care is futile and ECMO is withdrawn. The flow in V-A ECMO is adjusted to maintain adequate tissue perfusion but does not totally capture all of the native cardiac output. Providing oxygenated circulatory support reduces the requirements for vasopressors and inotropes that might increase myocardial oxygen demand, inhibit myocardial recovery or result in secondary organ damage. However, as flow back into the arterial circulation on V-A ECMO results in higher afterload than a normal physiologic state, V-A ECMO can exacerbate left ventricular (LV) failure and cause left atrial (LA) hypertension with resultant pulmonary edema or pulmonary hemorrhage. Failure of the aortic valve to open also increases risk of thrombosis from static blood in the LV [7]. As a result, offloading the LV in this circumstance is required via left ventricular venting techniques, such as low dose inotrope support or more invasive unloading efforts, through intra-aortic balloon pump, Impella device, atrial septostomy or direct placement of venting cannulas via the pulmonary vein, LA, or LV.

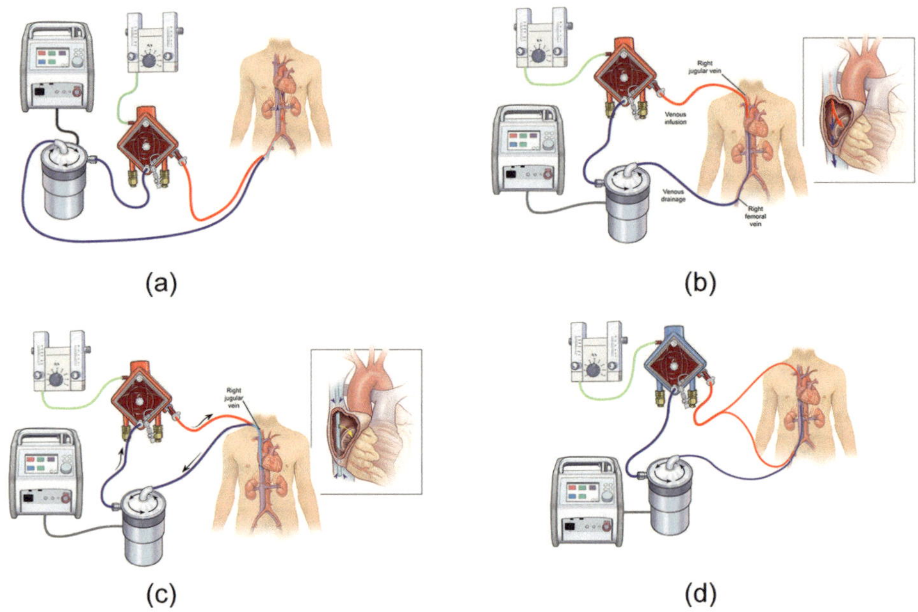

Figure 1.
Different modes and configurations of extracorporeal membrane oxygenation (ECMO). a: Venoarterial (V-A) ECMO; b: Two cannulas V-V ECMO; c: Double lumen venovenous (V-V) ECMO; and d: Veno-arteriovenous (V-AV) ECMO.

3.2.2 Venovenous extracorporeal membrane oxygenation (V-V ECMO)

In V-V ECMO, the flow is in series with the native lung and heart, hence V-V ECMO does not provide circulatory support (**Figure 1b** and **c**). It is usually utilized in patients with hypoxic and hypercapnic respiratory failure such as severe acute respiratory distress syndrome patients. By providing adequate oxygenation and ventilation, V-V ECMO reduces the injurious effect of mechanical ventilation and thus may provide the most optimal environment for lung recovery. The ECMO flow is adjusted to capture native cardiac output and maintain set gas exchange goals. Recirculation, defined as a portion of the oxygenated blood returning from the ECMO circuit being drawn back into the drainage cannula without reaching the systemic circulation, is common to some extent in all V-V support. Recirculation can be minimized by keeping return and drainage cannulas separated by 5–10 cm and is also usually less with double lumen cannulas. Recirculation is also exacerbated by anything that restricts forward flow from the right ventricle, such as pulmonary embolus or right ventricular failure. One unique configuration of V-V ECMO is the V-PA one, in which a double cannula is inserted into the pulmonary artery. This configuration has the advantage of right ventricular support, less recirculation of oxygenated blood, and single site access with subsequent easier mobility for the patient.

3.2.3 Hybrid configurations

Hybrid configurations for ECMO are considered when the patient on either V-V or V-A ECMO experience certain complications that further impact the heart or the lung functions during the ECMO support (**Figure 1d**). V-A ECMO provides circulatory and respiratory support. However, it increases the left ventricular afterload, impairs ventricular drainage, and predisposes the patient to pulmonary edema. As the heart recovers, differential oxygenation happens in the upper body because of partially impaired lung function [8]. This "North-South" phenomenon necessitate consideration of hybrid configuration such as V-AV ECMO to overcome [9]. In V-V ECMO, the development of myocardial dysfunction such as right ventricular failure, might require insertion of arterial return cannula to provide the required circulatory support, for example VV-A or VV-VA ECMO configuration [10].

3.2.4 Targets of extracorporeal life support

Targets for ECMO support depends on the indications for ECMO initiation, the patient clinical conditions, and the degree of underlying organ dysfunction. In V-A ECMO, the main goal is to maintain the organ-systems perfusion and to prevent organ-system failure until the heart recovers or more durable option is established. In V-A ECMO the ECMO flow determines the oxygen delivery to the tissues. Most centers aim for mixed venous oxygen saturation > 70% [11]. In addition to ECMO flow, increasing the oxygen carrying capacity can be increased by blood transfusion to higher hemoglobin goal or reducing the oxygen consumption by sedating the patient and establish invasive mechanical ventilation. On the other hand, in V-V ECMO the main goal is to establish adequate gas exchange to the tissues and allow resting settings on mechanical ventilation. Generally, tidal volume less than 4 cc/kg of IBW, plateau pressure around 25 cm H2O, and driving pressure < 14 [12].

3.2.5 Monitoring of extracorporeal membrane oxygenation

Monitoring of the ECMO circuit performance is of the utmost importance because it reflects the interaction between the patient and the machine, and changes noted earlier can prevent compromise of the patient's clinical status. Upon ECMO initiation, the flow that meets the patient's clinical needs and goals for hemodynamics and gas exchange is established. This becomes continuously monitored and adjusted to meet set goals. Serial correlations between the rotations per minute (RPM) and the resultant ECMO flow is important to be aware of, and when it changes (the same RPM achieving lower ECMO flows), this could indicate hypovolemia, vasodilation, blood loss, a kink in the circuit or anything that prevents drainage of blood to the circuit or return to the body. Ideally ECMO flows in adults should target above 2 LPM to avoid circuit clotting.

Additionally, multiple points of pressure measurements across the ECMO circuit are often continuously monitored and important to be aware of. Venous pressure (P vein, also called P1 or other names dependent on manufacturer) is the pressure in the drainage line, and it is usually a negative pressure measurement as the centrifugal pump suctions blood from the body. Normal values should be set based on maintaining negative pressure values <100 cm H20 across the pressure drop of the cannula. These values are provided by pressure flow charts for every cannula via the manufacturer. An increase in the venous pressure (more negative) is indicative of hypovolemia, kinking of the drainage line or clot in the drainage cannula. Arterial pressure (P artery) is the positive pressure in the reinfusion cannula and should not exceed 300 cm H_2O. An increase reflects an increase in the afterload (e.g., hypertension), kinking in the reinfusion line or a clot in the return cannula. Δ P is the pressure across the membrane lung and is measured at pre and post membrane lung sites. Values may change based on surface area and flow but should be tracked serially and often initially are less than 20 cm H2O. The increase in Δ P across the membrane lung may indicate significant clot in the oxygenator. The ability to be aware of and understand the significance of other changes is also important as an ECMO provider, with many courses available internationally and knowledge assessments available via industry (Innovative ECMO Concepts; ECMO advantage and others) as well as organizations such as ELSO, CHEST, ATS, SCCM, and others.

3.3 Extracorporeal membrane oxygenation related complications

The complications related to ECMO support are relatively common and associated with increased morbidity and mortality. These complications can be categorized into general complications related to ECMO use, mode specific as well as disease related (**Table 1**). Bleeding is the most common complication; it occurs in almost 10–30% of patients [13]. It occurs more frequently in V-A ECMO patients than in V-V patients. In a cohort study of 158 patients, 37% of V-A ECMO patients required interventions to control the bleeding, while only 17% of the V-V ECMO ones [14]. The most common sites of bleeding are the invasive procedure sites such as the surgical incisions, cannulation sites, thoracostomy tubes, tamponade, or retroperitoneal bleeding. However, bleeding can occur anywhere, such as intracranial hemorrhage, pulmonary hemorrhage, or gastrointestinal bleeding [15]. The risk of bleeding on ECMO is related to the use of systemic anticoagulants, depletion of the coagulation factors, mainly Von Willebrand factor (vWF) by the extracorporeal circuit, platelet activation, and consumption [16]. The management of bleeding relay on stopping anticoagulants, correct coagulopathy, transfuse as needed, and surgical interventions as indicated.

Thromboembolic complications could happen but now with biocompatible devices it is less of an issue. Thrombosis could happen in the patient or the circuit. Micro thrombosis of the oxygenator is common. It is estimated 10–16% of the oxygenator develop thrombi with subsequent decrease in the ECMO efficiency [17]. Air embolism can happen if there is a break in the negative side of the circuit or with excessive drainage and subsequent air cavitation. There thrombotic event can lead to devastating neurological or systemic complications. Hence the routine use of systemic anticoagulation is adopted by most ECMO centers. A challenging scenario is heparin induced thrombocytopenia (HIT). Despite being a rare complication, it carries significant morbidity and mortality. So early recognition and utilization of direct thrombin inhibitors are advised [18].

Another common complication for patients on ECMO is secondary infection. In a retrospective cohort analysis of 145 patients on ECMO, 44.8% developed sepsis [19]. The risks for infection in patients with ECMO are related to the severity of illness, the immunocompromised status related to the underlying medical condition, the presence of invasive devices. Diagnosis of infection requires a high index of suspicion. The presence of hypo or hyperthermia, hemodynamic instability, increased oxygen requirement with desaturation, respiratory secretions, frank pyuria or worsening of renal or liver function, alteration in sensorium, coagulopathy, and new skin lesions [20]. White blood cell count might not a reliable marker for infection [21]. Other markers of inflammation like C-reactive protein (CRP) or erythrocyte sedimentation rate (ESR) could be helpful but remain non-specific. In a study of 220 V-A ECMO patients on ECMO, the most common sources of infection were ventilator-associated pneumonia (VAP) (55%), blood-stream infection (18%), cannula infections (10%), and mediastinitis (11%) [22]. Infection control should focus on prevention by

Device-related	**Common Complications and risk factors**	
	Cannula	
		Bleeding
		Vascular Dissection
		Malposition
		Accidental decannulation
	Circuit	
		Rupture
		Air embolism
	Pump failure	
	Oxygenator	
		Thrombosis
		Malfunction
	Heater	
		Sepsis
		Malfunction
		Electrolytes imbalance
Patient-related		
	Bleeding	
		Cannula site
		Mucosal bleeding / ENT
		Gastrointestinal bleeding
		Hemothorax
		Pericardial tamponade
		Respiratory hemorrhage
		Cerebral hemorrhage
	Coagulation abnormalities	
		Consumptive coagulopathy
		Thrombocytopenia
		Altered vWF
		Platelet dysfunction
		Decrease anti-thrombin III
		Increase D-dimer
		Increase prothrombin fragment
		Increase prothrombin-antithrombin complex
	Thromboembolism	
		Deep venous thrombosis
		Pulmonary embolism
		Ischemic stroke
		Limb ischemia

		Mesenteric ischemia
		Myocardial infarction
	Secondary infections	
		Ventilator associated pneumonia
		Blood stream infection
		Cannula related infection
		Mediastinitis
	Neurological complications	
		Ischemic stroke
		Intra-cranial hemorrhage
		Hypoxic encephalopathy
		Spinal cord injury
Mode-specific		
	V-A ECMO	
		Differential oxygenation
		Limb ischemia
	V-V ECMO	
		Recirculation
		Venous thromboembolism

ENT = ear, nose, and throat; V-A ECMO = venoarterial extracorporeal membrane oxygenation; and V-V ECMO = venovenous extracorporeal membrane oxygenation.

Table 1.
Common complications during extracorporeal membrane oxygenation (ECMO) support.

adherence to the universal hand hygiene and sterile techniques during the insertion. There is no evidence to support the use of prophylactic antibiotics in ECMO patients. For treating a suspected infection, the choice of antibiotics should be made based on the index of suspicion and the local antibiogram recommendations for each institution.

Neurological complications rates vary based on the patient characteristics, underlying medical conditions, and the mode of ECMO support. In a retrospective analysis of single-center experience, 13.3% of ECMO patients experienced neurological complications [23]. Most commonly ischemic stroke (7.0%), intracerebral hemorrhage (3.4%), hypoxic ischemic encephalopathy (3.6%), and spinal cord injury (1.2%). Neurological complications were more common in V-A ECMO (18%) rather than V-V ECMO (4.6%). ECMO especially V-A increases the risk of stroke through thromboembolism, differential oxygenation, and the associate coagulopathy. It is imperative to monitor the patient neurological examination and conduct frequent neurological assessment to recognize early neurological complications and to provide the appropriate interventions.

Vascular complications are more common in the V-A ECMO patients as well. Vascular complications are major cause of mortality. In a study, the vascular complications led to increase the mortality from 18 to 49% [24]. Acute limb ischemia affects 10–70% of the V-A ECMO patients [25, 26]. Other forms of vascular complications are dissection, pseudoaneurysm, and retroperitoneal hematomas. The risk of vascular complications is higher in women, small patients, difficult cannulation, and patients without distal perfusion cannulas. Early identification is by physical examination that shows signs of malperfusion, near infrared spectrometer (NIRS), and Doppler ultrasound. These conditions require emergent vascular surgery assessment and intervention.

V-A ECMO specific complications are differential oxygenation, left-ventricular distension, and cardiac and systemic thromboembolism. The retrograde arterial flow, particularly in peripheral V-A ECMO, increases the left ventricular afterload and impairs its drainage. As a result, cause left ventricular distension, stagnation of the blood, and backflow into the lungs. The left ventricular distension cause increase of the wall stress and could hinder left ventricular recovery [27]. The stasis of the blood can cause intra and extra-cardiac thrombi. In a retrospective analysis, the authors showed that 4% of patients on femoral V-A ECMO developed intra and extra-cardiac thrombosis despite adequate anticoagulation [28]. Another potential complication with V-A ECMO is the North-South syndrome or the Harlequin syndrome. It is characterized by lower oxygen saturation in the upper right extremity, cerebral, and coronary blood supply in comparison to the lower part of the body. It is best monitored by examining the blood from the right upper extremity or cerebral NIRS [29].

3.4 Prevention of complications

The staffing model adopted by different institutions has the most impact on the ECMO patients' outcome and plays a major role in prevention of complications. ECMO specialist has the knowledge to understand the patient-circuit interaction, conduct frequent surveillance to prevent complications, and equipped to manage circuit emergencies. There is institutional variation in the staffing model due to the available resources and staffing capabilities. In an international survey of 177 ECMO centers, most institutions adopt 24/7 ECMO nurse specialist at 1:1 ratio with backup from perfusionists [30]. The ECMO specialist works collaboratively with the bedside nurse to ensure safe care for the critically ill patients with multiple organ dysfunction.

Usually, patients supported by ECMO do not require sedation during the ECMO run. There are multiple benefits associated with being awake while on ECMO support. For instance, ability to communicate, engaged in decision making, participate in active physical activity, and elimination of side effects of sedatives with delirium being the most prominent one [31]. We understand it might not be feasible for some patient populations, however having a timeline to achieve these goals is important. Patients might need to be sedated immediately after ECMO initiation, to ensure hemodynamic stability and proper gas exchange. Afterwards, gradual weaning of sedation is advised [32].

4. Emerging indications for extracorporeal membrane oxygenation

There are many operative indications for ECMO that can be categorized based on the required support and modality (**Table 2**).

4.1 Anticipated difficult airway

ECMO can be used in patients with anatomically difficult airways, especially at or below the level of glottis, such as in patients with near complete tracheal

Organ—system	Indications
Airway	
	Anticipated difficult airway
	Complex airway surgery
Thoracic	
	General thoracic surgery
	Peri-lung transplantation
	Trauma—lung contusion
	Massive pulmonary embolism
	Surgical embolectomy for massive pulmonary embolism
	Acute respiratory distress syndrome—bacterial pneumonia
	Acute respiratory distress syndrome—viral pneumonia
	Acute respiratory distress syndrome—Aspiration
	Acute asthma exacerbation
	Chronic obstructive pulmonary disease (COPD) exacerbation
	Interstitial lung disease as bridge to lung transplant
	Inhalation lung injury
	Acute eosinophilic pneumonia
	Diffuse alveolar hemorrhage or pulmonary hemorrhage
	Large bronchopleural fistula
Heart	
	Post-cardiotomy shock
	Ventricular tachycardia ablation
	High-risk percutaneous coronary intervention (PCI).
	Transcatheter aortic valve implantation (TAVI)
	Pulmonary hypertension
	Cardiogenic shock—acute on chronic heart failure
	Cardiogenic shock—myocardial infarction
	Cardiogenic shock—myocarditis
	Cardiogenic shock—structural heart disease
	Cardiogenic shock—congenital heart disease
	Refractory ventricular tachycardia
	Heart transplantation—primary graft dysfunction or rejection
	Isolated right ventricular failure
High-risk pregnancy	
	Severe acute respiratory distress syndrome
	Peripartum cardiogenic shock
	Massive pulmonary embolism
	Amniotic fluid embolism

Organ—system	Indications
	Cardiac arrest
Liver transplantation	
Cardiac arrest	
Hypothermia	
Cardio-toxins / medications overdose	

Table 2.
Some of the indications for extracorporeal membrane oxygenation (ECMO) in the operative setting.

obstruction [33]. Induction of general anesthesia leads to the loss of the respiratory muscle tone and collapse of the airway [34]. In some situations, bag mask ventilation and positive end expiratory pressure (PEEP) are ineffective to maintain oxygenation and ventilation. In a systematic review of literature from 1976 to 2017, 45 patients were placed on ECLS for critical airway diseases [35] pre-induction, with 18 patients placed on V-V ECMO, two patients on V-A ECMO, and 24 patients on cardiopulmonary bypass; one patient did not have a support mode not specified. The airway pathologies ranged from tracheal tumors, tracheal stenosis, and head and neck cancers. All patients survived to hospital discharge without significant complications.

4.2 Complex airway surgeries

ECMO facilitates complex tracheobronchial resection surgeries by providing adequate ventilation, hemodynamic support, (in the case of V-A ECMO) and allowing proper surgical exposure. In a single center, retrospective analysis of 10 patients who underwent complex tracheobronchial reconstructions on peripheral V-A ECMO, complete resection was accomplished in 8 patients with no perioperative mortality [36]. Another retrospective analysis highlighted 19 patients supported via V-V ECMO during malignant mass removal requiring rigid bronchoscopy and insertion of tracheal stents. V-V ECMO was weaned successfully in 18 patients, with one patient dying from massive bleeding [37]. Finally, there are multiple case reports that describe utilizing ECLS as an adjunctive intervention in the endoscopic removal of tracheal papillomas and repair of tracheobronchial fistulas [38, 39]. Use of ECMO to prevent any instrumentation of the airways without need for intubation is also described.

4.3 General thoracic surgeries

ECMO is a reasonable alternative for selective lung ventilation when it is difficult or not possible. Selective lung ventilation is usually required in tracheobronchial surgeries or single-lung surgery. In a retrospective questionnaire of 34 centers in France from 2009 to 2012, 36 patients required ECMO support during surgery (16 V-A and 20 V-V ECMO) [40]. Patients were divided into three groups (complete respiratory support, partial support, and patients with ARDS on ECMO preoperatively). The survival at 30-days were 7%, 40%, and 67% respectively. The authors concluded that ECMO is a valid alternative for in-field ventilation, with the outcome depending on preoperative respiratory status of the patient. In addition, there have been many reports regarding the use of ECMO in lung volume reduction surgeries [41]. These reports must be interpreted in the context of the outcome for such surgeries.

4.4 Lung transplantation

ECMO is used at various stages in patients who require lung transplantation (bridge to transplant, intra-operatively, and post-transplantation in the case of primary graft dysfunction). The primary aim for ECMO as a bridge to transplant is to provide adequate gas exchange while maintaining the patient's functional status, with dual-lumen cannula V-V ECMO ideal for that goal. The presence of pulmonary hypertension can require assessment for other configurations such as V-PA or V-A ECMO to offload from the dysfunctional right ventricle. In a single-center study of 72 patients receiving ECMO as a bridge to lung transplantation, 42 patients received lung transplant from which 92.5% survived to hospital discharge and 84% survived at 2-years post-transplantation [42].

Intra-operatively, V-A ECMO is preferred over conventional cardiopulmonary bypass (CPB). V-A ECMO use is associated with a lower incidence of acute renal failure requiring dialysis post-transplantation, lower risk of bleeding, less requirement for blood transfusion, less incidence of primary graft dysfunction, shorter intensive care unit (ICU) and hospital length of stay [43, 44]. Post-lung transplantation, ECMO is used for primary graft dysfunction. The choice of which modality depends on the presence of associated pulmonary hypertension. In absence of pulmonary hypertension, V-V ECMO can provide the required support and the configuration is subject to the anticipated patient needs. However, if the patient has pulmonary hypertension, those patients are better served with V-A ECMO, V-PA, or hybrid configuration. In a single-center study of 58 patients required ECMO support for primary graft dysfunction, the survival rate was 58% at 30-days. There was no difference between V-V and V-A ECMO outcomes [45].

4.5 Severe trauma victims

There are multiple indications for ECMO in chest trauma patients. V-A ECMO can be used in patients with cardiopulmonary failure such as myocardial contusion, myocarditis, cardiac ischemia, and massive pulmonary embolism. On the other hand, V-V ECMO is used in lung contusions, or severe ARDS [46]. In a systematic review of 58 articles analyzing a total of 548 trauma patients who required ECMO support [47] the overall in-hospital mortality was 30.3%. Most of those patients (71.3%) received V-V ECMO and 24.5% were supported through V-A ECMO. Only 60% of the patients received systemic anticoagulation, 22.9% had hemorrhagic complications, and 19% experienced thrombotic events.

4.6 Liver transplantation

ECMO has been used in the setting of orthotopic liver transplantation. Patients with liver failure are at risk for ARDS either before or after liver transplantation. The successful use of V-V ECMO in the pre-transplant setting has been described in the literature but it is unclear if it is a contraindication for liver transplantation [48], considering that the presence of mechanical ventilation and moderate ARDS is associated with poor outcomes in this patient population [49]. One of the major challenges with these patients is anticoagulation management since they are coagulopathic due to the underlying liver dysfunction and ECMO-related coagulopathy is an added layer of risk and complexity. More commonly, ECMO has been used after liver transplantation in the form of V-V ECMO to overcome hepato-pulmonary syndrome or pulmonary infection; additionally, liver transplantation induces pulmonary remodeling, causing ventilation/perfusion mismatch that may require V-V ECMO support. Some patients post transplantation may also be supported with V-A ECMO, such as when they develop hemodynamic compromise in the setting of pulmonary embolism or right ventricular failure [50, 51]. Also, because liver transplantation patients are predisposed to right ventricular failure which could cause hepatic congestion and impair the freshly transplanted liver, V-A ECMO can facilitate decompression of the right ventricle, supporting the transplanted organ. In a recent case series of eight liver transplantation patients requiring ECMO support, 38% survived to hospital discharge [52]. However, utilization of ECMO in liver transplantation patients remains a challenge given the hematological, hemodynamic, and the immunological profile of this patient population.

4.7 Massive pulmonary embolism

Massive pulmonary embolism is associated with poor survival because of its association with obstructive shock, end-organ dysfunction, and cardiac arrest. High-risk pulmonary embolism is defined as persistent hypotension (systolic blood pressure less than 90 mmHg, drop in systolic blood pressure more than 40 mmHg, and the need for vasopressors for more than 15 min) despite resuscitation [53, 54]. Systemic thrombolysis and anticoagulation remain the first line therapy for high-risk pulmonary embolism. However, this can be associated with increased risk of bleeding including intracranial hemorrhage especially in the elderly patients with multiple co-morbidities [55]. When systemic thrombolysis is contraindicated, V-A ECMO can provide perfusion to the end-organs. Also, the use of systemic anticoagulation can mitigate the need for systemic thrombolysis by allowing time for endogenous thrombolytics to act [56]. V-A ECMO can also be used in scenarios when thrombolytics fail, for hemodynamic support before intervention, refractory cardiogenic shock, or cardiac arrest [57]. In a study of 59 patients with massive pulmonary embolism, 29 patients were treated by surgical embolectomy and 27 patients were placed on V-A ECMO with systemic anticoagulation with or without subsequent surgical embolectomy. One year survival was significantly higher in the ECMO group (96%) versus the control group (73%) [58].

4.8 Extracorporeal cardiopulmonary resuscitation (ECPR)

ECPR is defined as the initiation of ECMO when CPR is ongoing (i.e., the patient does not achieve return of spontaneous circulation prior to going on ECMO). There are multiple patient populations that could benefit from ECPR, such as patients who arrest from cardiomyopathy, right ventricular dysfunction, and massive pulmonary embolism. Induction of anesthesia and intubation place those patients at higher risk of cardiac arrest. The best predictors for favorable neurological outcome in these patients, like patients who sustain a cardiac arrest, include witnessed cardiac arrest, immediate initiation of chest compressions, shockable rhythm, cardiac arrest due to a reversible etiology, and low flow time of less than 60 min [59, 60]. The longer the time to ECMO, the less the benefit of ECPR [61]. In a retrospective comparison of ECPR for in-hospital cardiac arrest to conventional CPR, ECPR led to favorable neurological outcome at 3 months [62]. Use of ECPR in out of hospital arrest is also becoming of increasing use and descriptions of both on-site ECPR implementation and that using a specific algorithm to apply emergently once the patient arrives to the hospital have shown some success [63, 64].

4.9 ECMO during pregnancy

The increased use of ECMO in pregnant patients is attributed to increasing rates of cardiogenic shock in the peripartum period [65]. The presence of cardiogenic shock is associated with 18.81% of maternal mortality and usually leads to adverse events such as cardiac arrest and intrauterine fetal death. Similarly, the presence of severe ARDS in this patient population is associated with increased maternal mortality and fetal asphyxia [66]. V-A ECMO successfully provides the necessary circulatory support until the heart recovers. Also, it has been used as rescue intervention in pregnant patients with a massive pulmonary embolism, amniotic fluid embolism and maternal pulmonary hypertension [67]. V-V ECMO in patients with severe ARDS provides the necessary gas exchange when the patient's native lungs are inadequate due to increased intra-abdominal pressures in pregnancy [68]; further, it allows using ultra-protective lung settings, reducing ventilator induced lung injury.

In an analysis of the ELSO data between 1997 and 2017, the overall survival for pregnant patients who are supported on ECMO was 70%. There was no difference in the outcome between both V-V and V-A ECMO [69]. Pregnant patients who required ECPR had the same survival rate that is comparable to non-pregnant ones (54.8% versus 58%) [70].

4.10 High-risk cardiac procedures

Refractory ventricular tachycardia (VT) is associated with hemodynamic instability in the form of progressive cardiogenic shock, and even cardiac arrest [71]. Urgent VT ablation is required if the patient fails to respond to antiarrhythmics, intubation, heavy sedation, and neuromuscular blockade. Performing VT ablation on a hemodynamically unstable patient is challenging; additionally, VT ablation can exacerbate the underlying instability and worsen outcomes [72]. V-A ECMO can provide the required circulatory support before and during a VT ablation procedure. In terms of outcomes, one study, which was a systematic review of all patients that were placed on V-A ECMO for periprocedural VT ablation, showed short-term mortality of 15% and all-cause mortality at longest follow-up at 25% [73]. The most common causes of death were refractory VT, cardiac arrest, and acute heart failure. The duration of V-A ECMO support ranged from 140 min to 6 days. This study, among others, highlighted the role of V-A ECMO in refractory VT patients, and described that further data is needed on appropriate patient selection, outcomes, and procedural optimization. For patients with refractory arrhythmia, implementation of ECMO may improve myocardial oxygenation and normal rhythm may result.

Another use for V-A ECMO is in high-risk percutaneous coronary intervention (PCI). High-risk PCI carries an increased incidence of morbidity and mortality during and after the procedure. There are multiple risk factors for high-risk PCI, which include patient characteristics such as age, diabetes mellitus, chronic kidney disease, prior myocardial infarction, peripheral vascular disease, signs of heart failure and left ventricular function [74]. Other risk factors include the presence of multi-vessel disease, left main disease, and a saphenous vein graft lesion. PCI can induce transient myocardial ischemia that is not well-tolerated in the high-risk patients. V-A ECMO has the advantage of providing adequate biventricular support that can reach more than 5 LPM. In addition, it can be quickly deployed at bedside in the event of significant hemodynamic compromise or cardiac arrest. In certain circumstances, it can be initiated prior to high-risk PCI; in a case series of a single center experience, five patients were placed on ECMO in preparation for high-risk PCI. All patients tolerated their procedure and four of them were weaned off ECMO in less than 24 hours [75].

4.11 Extracorporeal membrane oxygenation during coronavirus 2019 pandemic

The role of extracorporeal membrane oxygenation (ECMO) in Coronavirus 2019 (COVID-19) associated severe acute respiratory distress syndrome (ARDS) has been a subject of debate because of the early negative results [76, 77]. Despite that ECMO has been recommended as supportive intervention by multiple societies [78, 79]. However, subsequent studies from the extracorporeal life support organization (ELSO) showed that the use of V-V ECMO in COVID-19 is associated with an in-hospital mortality of 36.9–51.9% at 90 days [80, 81]. Similarly, in a French retrospective single healthcare system analysis, the estimated probability of death at 60 days post-ECMO initiation was 31% [82]. Most recently, in a comparative analysis of COVID Critical Care Consortium, the use of V-V ECMO in comparison to mechanical ventilation only was associated with a significantly reduced mortality especially in patients less than 65 years old and with a $PaO_2/FiO_2 < 80$ mm Hg or with driving pressures >15 cmH2O during the first 10 days of mechanical ventilation [83].

5. Transportation of patients on extracorporeal membrane oxygenation (ECMO)

While the transportation of patients on ECMO is usually minimized, it commonly must occur—for instance, when the patient is placed on ECMO in the Operating Room, the Emergency Department, or a different center, and requires transportation back to the ICU, or specific imaging or catheterization is required for the patient. Thus, establishing a systematic approach and becoming comfortable with the transport of patients on ECMO is an important component in any ECMO center. Some studies report the rate of complications associated with ECMO transport close to 30% [76], with most of the complications being patient related. Having a dedicated multi-disciplinary team with assigned roles and responsibilities is the first step in the process [77] to achieving safer transports. The team usually includes the ECMO specialist, with their primary focus being on the equipment function and connection, the critical care nurses who manage infusions and monitor patient vitals, the respiratory therapist who is responsible for the mechanical ventilation, and the physician who focuses on the continuous monitoring of the patient/their vitals. The roles of different team members may appear isolated but is mutual and overlapping. Transport teams which do not require as many team members, especially if the patient is already cannulated, can also be successful if experienced. Physician physical presence can also be provided remotely but medical oversight to the team should be provided. Clear, closed loop communication is an important aspect throughout. The best method to train the transport team is by conducting simulation scenarios to address the most common complications that could arise [78]. ECMO centers are highly encouraged to develop ECMO transport checklists aimed at minimizing the near misses and reduce human-factor error. The literature and ELSO guidelines have many examples that could be adopted by different institutions [77, 79]. Both hospitals based and private ECMO transport teams exist.

6. Weaning of extracorporeal membrane oxygenation

Readiness for discontinuation of ECMO is determined by the degree of heart and lung recovery. In V-V ECMO, the resolution of the lung pathology as evident by improvement of lung compliance, resolution of the lung pathology on chest imaging, and adequate gas exchange without ECMO support [80]. The adequacy of gas-exchange is usually assessed by turning of the sweep gas for at least 24-hours. If adequate oxygenation (PaO_2/FiO_2 ratio > 150), and ventilation is maintained with acceptable patient respiratory effort, V-V ECMO can be removed. In the V-A ECMO, cardiac recovery is assessed by stable hemodynamics and vasoactive medication doses on decreasing the V-A ECMO flow [81]. Echocardiography is crucial part of assessing the heart right and left ventricular function before decannulation of the V-A ECMO, which can be done in the operating room or bedside based on the institution experience.

7. Discussion

Our review highlighted some of the indications for ECMO in acute care setting. These indications represent the expansion and familiarity by the ECMO advanced technology. Barbaro et al. demonstrated that the annual extracorporeal membrane oxygenation (ECMO) patient volume has a potential impact on case-mix–adjusted hospital mortality rate for patients supported by ECMO [3]. However, a recent paper challenged this observation and did not show an associated between the hospital volume and the ECMO outcome [82]. ECMO is resource intensive technology and that might limit its use [83]. To overcome these limitations, it is important to establish an organization of ECMO centers internally and externally (in the same region or country) to optimize the cost-effectiveness. Internal organization, based on the importance of establishing protocols, investing in the technology and education. Also, having multi-disciplinary team that actively participate in decision making, reviewing the patient outcomes based on preidentified quality indicators. External organization is based on coordination of care among the ECMO centers in the same region to refer patients based on specific center expertise and resource availability [84].

Despite the expansion of ECMO use, there are variation in the selection of patients who will benefit the most of this technology. Most of the selection criteria are based on the anticipated duration of support and the likelihood of weaning of ECMO support. Hence the decision is based mostly on the local institution experience, especially in the light of absence of rigorous clinical evidence. Utilization of mortality prediction score such as Survival after Veno-Arterial ECMO (SAVE) score and Respiratory ECMO Survival Prediction (RESP) score, could be helpful in decision making and informing the caregivers regarding the potential clinical outcomes [85, 86].

8. Conclusion

In conclusion, the expansion of ECMO use and technology has created new opportunities for its utilization beyond the conventional indications for ECMO. The robust evidence for each indication is still lacking. However, the early deployment of ECMO in high-risk cases for cardiac and respiratory failure is important before the patient experiences a massive complication such as cardiac arrest. Similarly, this advanced supportive technology is associated with known complications and requires extensive expertise to manage patients on ECMO. Hence the need for expanding the clinical and scientific knowledge to delineate the best patient's population with might benefit from ECMO, in context of the best structure and staffing of the ECMO programs. The decision to place a patient on ECMO must be discussed with a multi-disciplinary team weighing the risks and the benefits.

Author details

Akram M. Zaaqoq[1*], Mariam Gabrial[2] and Heidi J. Dalton[2]

1 Department of Critical Care Medicine, MedStar Washington Hospital Center, Georgetown University, Washington, DC, USA

2 Department of Pediatrics, Inova Fairfax Hospital, Falls Church, VA, USA

*Address all correspondence to: akramzaaqoq@gmail.com

IntechOpen

© 2022 The Author(s). Licensee IntechOpen. This chapter is distributed under the terms of the Creative Commons Attribution License (http://creativecommons.org/licenses/by/3.0), which permits unrestricted use, distribution, and reproduction in any medium, provided the original work is properly cited.

References

[1] Hill JD, O'Brien TG, Murray JJ, Dontigny L, Bramson ML, Osborn JJ, et al. Prolonged extracorporeal oxygenation for acute post-traumatic respiratory failure (shock-lung syndrome). Use of the Bramson membrane lung. The New England Journal of Medicine. 1972;**286**(12):629-634

[2] Stentz MJ, Kelley ME, Jabaley CS, O'Reilly-Shah V, Groff RF, Moll V, et al. Trends in extracorporeal membrane oxygenation growth in the United States, 2011-2014. ASAIO Journal. 2019;**65**(7):712-717

[3] Barbaro RP, Odetola FO, Kidwell KM, Paden ML, Bartlett RH, Davis MM, et al. Association of hospital-level volume of extracorporeal membrane oxygenation cases and mortality. Analysis of the extracorporeal life support organization registry. American Journal of Respiratory and Critical Care Medicine. 2015;**191**(8):894-901

[4] Stokes JW, Katsis JM, Gannon WD, Rice TW, Lentz RJ, Rickman OB, et al. Venovenous extracorporeal membrane oxygenation during high-risk airway interventions. Interactive CardioVascular and Thoracic Surgery. 2021;**33**(6):913-920

[5] Lehle K, Philipp A, Gleich O, Holzamer A, Müller T, Bein T, et al. Efficiency in extracorporeal membrane oxygenation-cellular deposits on polymethylpentene membranes increase resistance to blood flow and reduce gas exchange capacity. ASAIO Journal (American Society for Artificial Internal Organs : 1992). 2008;**54**(6):612-617

[6] Strunina S, Hozman J, Ostadal P. The peripheral cannulas in extracorporeal life support. Biomedizinische Technik Biomedical Engineering. 2019;**64**(2):127-133

[7] Donker DW, Brodie D, Henriques JPS, Broomé M. Left ventricular unloading during Veno-arterial ECMO: A simulation study. ASAIO Journal. 2019;**65**(1):11-20

[8] Loftsgard TO, Newcome MD, Hanneman MR, Patch RK 3rd, Seelhammer TG. Management of Neurogenic Pulmonary Edema and Differential Hypoxemia in an adult supported on Venoarterial extracorporeal membrane oxygenation. Journal of Cardiothoracic and Vascular Anesthesia. 2017;**31**(6):2170-2174

[9] Ius F, Sommer W, Tudorache I, Avsar M, Siemeni T, Salman J, et al. Veno-veno-arterial extracorporeal membrane oxygenation for respiratory failure with severe haemodynamic impairment: Technique and early outcomes. Interactive Cardiovascular and Thoracic Surgery. 2015;**20**(6):761-767

[10] Brasseur A, Scolletta S, Lorusso R, Taccone FS. Hybrid extracorporeal membrane oxygenation. Journal of Thoracic Disease. 2018;**10**(Suppl 5): S707-Ss15

[11] Lawler PR, Silver DA, Scirica BM, Couper GS, Weinhouse GL, Camp PC Jr. Extracorporeal membrane oxygenation in adults with cardiogenic shock. Circulation. 2015;**131**(7):676-680

[12] Schmidt M, Pham T, Arcadipane A, Agerstrand C, Ohshimo S, Pellegrino V, et al. Mechanical ventilation management during extracorporeal membrane oxygenation for acute respiratory distress syndrome. An international multicenter

prospective cohort. American Journal of Respiratory and Critical Care Medicine. 2019;**200**(8):1002-1012

[13] Bartlett RH, Gattinoni L. Current status of extracorporeal life support (ECMO) for cardiopulmonary failure. Minerva Anestesiologica. 2010;**76**(7):534-540

[14] Aubron C, Cheng AC, Pilcher D, Leong T, Magrin G, Cooper DJ, et al. Factors associated with outcomes of patients on extracorporeal membrane oxygenation support: A 5-year cohort study. Critical Care (London, England). 2013;**17**(2):R73

[15] Makdisi G, Wang IW. Extra corporeal membrane oxygenation (ECMO) review of a lifesaving technology. Journal of Thoracic Disease. 2015;7(7):E166-E176

[16] Cartwright B, Bruce HM, Kershaw G, Cai N, Othman J, Gattas D, et al. Hemostasis, coagulation and thrombin in venoarterial and venovenous extracorporeal membrane oxygenation: The HECTIC study. Scientific Reports. 2021;**11**(1):7975

[17] Doyle AJ, Hunt BJ. Current understanding of how extracorporeal membrane oxygenators activate Haemostasis and other blood components. Frontiers in Medicine. 2018;**5**:352

[18] Zaaqoq AM, Brammer RC, Chan CM, Shorr AF. Heparin-induced thrombocytopenia in extra-corporeal membrane oxygenation: Epidemiology, outcomes, and diagnostic challenges. Journal of Thrombosis and Thrombolysis. 2022;**53**(2):499-505

[19] Allyn J, Ferdynus C, Lo Pinto H, Bouchet B, Persichini R, Vandroux D, et al. Complication patterns in patients undergoing venoarterial extracorporeal membrane oxygenation in intensive care unit: Multiple correspondence analysis and hierarchical ascendant classification. PLoS One. 2018;**13**(9):e0203643

[20] Gopalakrishnan R, Vashisht R. Sepsis and ECMO. Indian Journal of Thoracic and Cardiovascular Surgery. 2021;**37**(Suppl. 2):267-274

[21] Pieri M, Greco T, De Bonis M, Maj G, Fumagalli L, Zangrillo A, et al. Diagnosis of infection in patients undergoing extracorporeal membrane oxygenation: A case-control study. The Journal of Thoracic and Cardiovascular Surgery. 2012;**143**(6):1411-1416

[22] Schmidt M, Bréchot N, Hariri S, Guiguet M, Luyt CE, Makri R, et al. Nosocomial infections in adult cardiogenic shock patients supported by venoarterial extracorporeal membrane oxygenation. Clinical Infectious Diseases : An Official Publication of the Infectious Diseases Society of America. 2012;**55**(12):1633-1641

[23] Chapman JT, Breeding J, Kerr SJ, Bajic M, Nair P, Buscher H. CNS complications in adult patients treated with extracorporeal membrane oxygenation. Critical Care Medicine. 2021;**49**(2):282-291

[24] Tanaka D, Hirose H, Cavarocchi N, Entwistle JW. The impact of vascular complications on survival of patients on Venoarterial extracorporeal membrane oxygenation. The Annals of Thoracic Surgery. 2016;**101**(5):1729-1734

[25] Bisdas T, Beutel G, Warnecke G, Hoeper MM, Kuehn C, Haverich A, et al. Vascular complications in patients undergoing femoral cannulation for extracorporeal membrane oxygenation support. The Annals of Thoracic Surgery. 2011;**92**(2):626-631

[26] Foley PJ, Morris RJ, Woo EY, Acker MA, Wang GJ, Fairman RM, et al. Limb ischemia during femoral cannulation for cardiopulmonary support. Journal of Vascular Surgery. 2010;**52**(4):850-853

[27] Werdan K, Gielen S, Ebelt H, Hochman JS. Mechanical circulatory support in cardiogenic shock. European Heart Journal. 2014;**35**(3):156-167

[28] Weber C, Deppe AC, Sabashnikov A, Slottosch I, Kuhn E, Eghbalzadeh K, et al. Left ventricular thrombus formation in patients undergoing femoral veno-arterial extracorporeal membrane oxygenation. Perfusion. 2018;**33**(4):283-288

[29] Lo Coco V, Lorusso R, Raffa GM, Malvindi PG, Pilato M, Martucci G, et al. Clinical complications during veno-arterial extracorporeal membrane oxigenation in post-cardiotomy and non post-cardiotomy shock: Still the achille's heel. Journal of Thoracic Disease. 2018;**10**(12):6993-7004

[30] Daly KJ, Camporota L, Barrett NA. An international survey: The role of specialist nurses in adult respiratory extracorporeal membrane oxygenation. Nursing in Critical Care. 2017;**22**(5):305-311

[31] Abrams D, Garan AR, Brodie D. Awake and fully mobile patients on cardiac extracorporeal life support. Annals of Cardiothoracic Surgery. 2019;**8**(1):44-53

[32] Haji JY, Mehra S, Doraiswamy P. Awake ECMO and mobilizing patients on ECMO. Indian Journal of Thoracic and Cardiovascular Surgery. 2021;**37**(Suppl. 2):309-318

[33] McRae K, de Perrot M. Principles and indications of extracorporeal life support in general thoracic surgery. Journal of Thoracic Disease. 2018;**10**(Suppl. 8): S931-Ss46

[34] Hedenstierna G. Alveolar collapse and closure of airways: Regular effects of anaesthesia. Clinical Physiology and Functional Imaging. 2003;**23**(3):123-129

[35] Chakalov I, Harnisch LO, Meyer AC, Moerer O. Preemptive veno-venous ECMO support in a patient with anticipated difficult airway: A case report. Respiratory Medicine Case Reports. 2020;**30**:101130

[36] Lang G, Ghanim B, Hötzenecker K, Klikovits T, Matilla JR, Aigner C, et al. Extracorporeal membrane oxygenation support for complex tracheo-bronchial procedures†. European journal of cardio-thoracic surgery. Official Journal of the European Association for Cardio-Thoracic Surgery. 2015;**47**(2):250-255; discussion 6

[37] Hong Y, Jo KW, Lyu J, Huh JW, Hong SB, Jung SH, et al. Use of venovenous extracorporeal membrane oxygenation in central airway obstruction to facilitate interventions leading to definitive airway security. Journal of critical care. 2013;**28**(5):669-674

[38] Smith IJ, Sidebotham DA, McGeorge AD, Dorman EB, Wilsher ML, Kolbe J. Use of extracorporeal membrane oxygenation during resection of tracheal papillomatosis. Anesthesiology. 2009;**110**(2):427-429

[39] Walles T, Steger V, Wurst H, Schmidt KD, Friedel G. Pumpless extracorporeal gas exchange aiding central airway surgery. The Journal of Thoracic and Cardiovascular Surgery. 2008;**136**(5):1372-1374

[40] Rinieri P, Peillon C, Bessou J-P, Veber B, Falcoz P-E, Melki J, et al.

National review of use of extracorporeal membrane oxygenation as respiratory support in thoracic surgery excluding lung transplantation†. European Journal of Cardio-Thoracic Surgery. 2014;**47**(1):87-94

[41] Oey IF, Peek GJ, Firmin RK, Waller DA. Post-pneumonectomy video-assisted thoracoscopic bullectomy using extra-corporeal membrane oxygenation. European Journal of Cardio-Thoracic Surgery : Official Journal of the European Association for Cardio-Thoracic Surgery. 2001;**20**(4):874-876

[42] Biscotti M, Gannon WD, Agerstrand C, Abrams D, Sonett J, Brodie D, et al. Awake extracorporeal membrane oxygenation as bridge to lung transplantation: A 9-year experience. The Annals of Thoracic Surgery. 2017;**104**(2):412-419

[43] Biscotti M, Yang J, Sonett J, Bacchetta M. Comparison of extracorporeal membrane oxygenation versus cardiopulmonary bypass for lung transplantation. The Journal of Thoracic and Cardiovascular Surgery. 2014;**148**(5):2410-2415

[44] Machuca TN, Collaud S, Mercier O, Cheung M, Cunningham V, Kim SJ, et al. Outcomes of intraoperative extracorporeal membrane oxygenation versus cardiopulmonary bypass for lung transplantation. The Journal of Thoracic and Cardiovascular Surgery. 2015;**149**(4):1152-1157

[45] Bermudez CA, Adusumilli PS, McCurry KR, Zaldonis D, Crespo MM, Pilewski JM, et al. Extracorporeal membrane oxygenation for primary graft dysfunction after lung transplantation: Long-term survival. The Annals of Thoracic Surgery. 2009;**87**(3):854-860

[46] Swol J, Cannon JW, Barbaro RP, Fanning JJ, Zonies D. Extracorporeal membrane oxygenation in trauma. ASAIO Journal. 2022;**68**(4):e62-ee3

[47] Wang C, Zhang L, Qin T, Xi Z, Sun L, Wu H, et al. Extracorporeal membrane oxygenation in trauma patients: A systematic review. World Journal of Emergency Surgery : WJES. 2020;**15**(1):51

[48] Monsel A, Mal H, Brisson H, Luo R, Eyraud D, Vézinet C, et al. Extracorporeal membrane oxygenation as a bridge to liver transplantation for acute respiratory distress syndrome-induced life-threatening hypoxaemia aggravated by hepatopulmonary syndrome. Critical Care (London, England). 2011;**15**(5):R234

[49] Sundaram V, Jalan R, Wu T, Volk ML, Asrani SK, Klein AS, et al. Factors associated with survival of patients with severe acute-on-chronic liver failure before and after liver transplantation. Gastroenterology. 2019;**156**(5):1381-91.e3

[50] Belohlavek J, Rohn V, Jansa P, Tosovsky J, Kunstyr J, Semrad M, et al. Veno-arterial ECMO in severe acute right ventricular failure with pulmonary obstructive hemodynamic pattern. The Journal of Invasive Cardiology. 2010;**22**(8):365-369

[51] Nayyar D, Man HS, Granton J, Gupta S. Defining and characterizing severe hypoxemia after liver transplantation in hepatopulmonary syndrome. Liver Transplantation : Official Publication of the American Association for the Study of Liver Diseases and the International Liver Transplantation Society. 2014;**20**(2):182-190

[52] Braun HJ, Pulcrano ME, Weber DJ, Padilla BE, Ascher NL. The utility

of ECMO after liver transplantation: Experience at a high-volume transplant center and review of the literature. Transplantation. 2019;**103**(8):1568-1573

[53] Kearon C, Akl EA, Ornelas J, Blaivas A, Jimenez D, Bounameaux H, et al. Antithrombotic therapy for VTE disease: CHEST guideline and expert panel report. Chest. 2016;**149**(2):315-352

[54] Konstantinides SV, Meyer G, Becattini C, Bueno H, Geersing GJ, Harjola VP, et al. 2019 ESC guidelines for the diagnosis and management of acute pulmonary embolism developed in collaboration with the European Respiratory Society (ERS): The task force for the diagnosis and management of acute pulmonary embolism of the European Society of Cardiology (ESC). European Heart Journal. 21 Jan 2020;**41**(4):543-603

[55] Mikkola KM, Patel SR, Parker JA, Grodstein F, Goldhaber SZ. Increasing age is a major risk factor for hemorrhagic complications after pulmonary embolism thrombolysis. American Heart Journal. 1997;**134**(1):69-72

[56] Moon D, Lee SN, Yoo KD, Jo MS. Extracorporeal membrane oxygenation improved survival in patients with massive pulmonary embolism. Annals of Saudi Medicine. 2018;**38**(3):174-180

[57] Wu MY, Liu YC, Tseng YH, Chang YS, Lin PJ, Wu TI. Pulmonary embolectomy in high-risk acute pulmonary embolism: The effectiveness of a comprehensive therapeutic algorithm including extracorporeal life support. Resuscitation. 2013;**84**(10):1365-1370

[58] Pasrija C, Shah A, George P, Kronfli A, Raithel M, Boulos F, et al. Triage and optimization: A new paradigm in the treatment of massive pulmonary embolism. The Journal of Thoracic and Cardiovascular Surgery. 2018;**156**(2):672-681

[59] Richardson AC, Tonna JE, Nanjayya V, Nixon P, Abrams DC, Raman L, et al. Extracorporeal cardiopulmonary resuscitation in adults. Interim guideline consensus statement from the extracorporeal life support organization. ASAIO Journal. 2021;**67**(3):221-228

[60] Tonna JE, Selzman CH, Girotra S, Presson AP, Thiagarajan RR, Becker LB, et al. Resuscitation using ECPR during In-hospital cardiac arrest (RESCUE-IHCA) mortality prediction score and external validation. JACC: Cardiovascular Interventions. 2022;**15**(3):237-247

[61] Yu HY, Wang CH, Chi NH, Huang SC, Chou HW, Chou NK, et al. Effect of interplay between age and low-flow duration on neurologic outcomes of extracorporeal cardiopulmonary resuscitation. Intensive Care Medicine. 2019;**45**(1):44-54

[62] Patricio D, Peluso L, Brasseur A, Lheureux O, Belliato M, Vincent JL, et al. Comparison of extracorporeal and conventional cardiopulmonary resuscitation: A retrospective propensity score matched study. Critical Care (London, England). 2019;**23**(1):27

[63] Belohlavek J, Smalcova J, Rob D, Franek O, Smid O, Pokorna M, et al. Effect of intra-arrest transport, extracorporeal cardiopulmonary resuscitation, and immediate invasive assessment and treatment on functional neurologic outcome in refractory out-of-hospital cardiac arrest: A randomized clinical trial. Journal of the American Medical Association. 2022;**327**(8):737-747

[64] Yannopoulos D, Bartos J, Raveendran G, Walser E, Connett J,

Murray TA, et al. Advanced reperfusion strategies for patients with out-of-hospital cardiac arrest and refractory ventricular fibrillation (ARREST): A phase 2, single Centre, open-label, randomised controlled trial. Lancet (London, England). 2020;**396**(10265):1807-1816

[65] Banayan J, Rana S, Mueller A, Tung A, Ramadan H, Arany Z, et al. Cardiogenic shock in pregnancy: Analysis from the National Inpatient Sample. Hypertension in Pregnancy. 2017;**36**(2):117-123

[66] Critical illness due to. A/H1N1 influenza in pregnant and postpartum women: Population based cohort study. BMJ (Clinical Research ed). 2009;**2010**(340):c1279

[67] Moore SA, Dietl CA, Coleman DM. Extracorporeal life support during pregnancy. The Journal of Thoracic and Cardiovascular Surgery. 2016;**151**(4):1154-1160

[68] Fuchs F, Bruyere M, Senat MV, Purenne E, Benhamou D, Fernandez H. Are standard intra-abdominal pressure values different during pregnancy? PLoS One. 2013;**8**(10):e77324

[69] Ramanathan K, Tan CS, Rycus P, Anders M, Lorusso R, Zhang JJY, et al. Extracorporeal membrane oxygenation in pregnancy: An analysis of the extracorporeal life support organization registry. Critical Care Medicine. 2020;**48**(5):696-703

[70] Beckett VA, Knight M, Sharpe P. The CAPS study: Incidence, management and outcomes of cardiac arrest in pregnancy in the UK: A prospective, descriptive study. BJOG : An International Journal of Obstetrics and Gynaecology. 2017;**124**(9):1374-1381

[71] Hendel RC, Berman DS, Di Carli MF, Heidenreich PA, Henkin RE, Pellikka PA, et al. ACCF/ASNC/ACR/AHA/ASE/SCCT/SCMR/SNM 2009 appropriate use criteria for cardiac radionuclide imaging: A report of the American College of Cardiology Foundation appropriate use criteria task force, the American Society of Nuclear Cardiology, the American College of Radiology, the American Heart Association, the American Society of Echocardiography, the Society of Cardiovascular Computed Tomography, the Society for Cardiovascular Magnetic Resonance, and the Society of Nuclear Medicine. Journal of the American College of Cardiology. 2009;**53**(23):2201-2229

[72] Virk SA, Keren A, John RM, Santageli P, Eslick A, Kumar S. Mechanical circulatory support during catheter ablation of ventricular tachycardia: Indications and options. Heart, Lung & Circulation. 2019;**28**(1):134-145

[73] Vallabhajosyula S, Vallabhajosyula S, Vaidya VR, Patlolla SH, Desai V, Mulpuru SK, et al. Venoarterial extracorporeal membrane oxygenation support for ventricular tachycardia ablation: A systematic review. ASAIO Journal (American Society for Artificial Internal Organs : 1992). 2020;**66**(9):980-985

[74] Rihal CS, Naidu SS, Givertz MM, Szeto WY, Burke JA, Kapur NK, et al. 2015 SCAI/ACC/HFSA/STS clinical expert consensus statement on the use of percutaneous mechanical circulatory support devices in cardiovascular care: Endorsed by the American Heart Association, the Cardiological Society of India, and Sociedad Latino Americana de Cardiología Intervencionista; affirmation of value by the Canadian Association of Interventional Cardiology-Association Canadienne de

Cardiologie d'intervention. Journal of the American College of Cardiology. 2015;**65**(19):2140-2141

[75] Shaukat A, Hryniewicz-Czeneszew K, Sun B, Mudy K, Wilson K, Tajti P, et al. Outcomes of extracorporeal membrane oxygenation support for complex high-risk elective percutaneous coronary interventions: A single-center experience and review of the literature. The Journal of Invasive Cardiology. 2018;**30**(12):456-460

[76] Ericsson A, Frenckner B, Broman LM. Adverse events during inter-hospital transports on extracorporeal membrane oxygenation. Prehospital Emergency Care : Official Journal of the National Association of EMS Physicians and the National Association of State EMS Directors. 2017;**21**(4):448-455

[77] Broman LM. Interhospital transport on extracorporeal membrane oxygenation of neonates—Perspective for the future. Frontiers in Pediatrics. 6 Aug 2019;**7**:329

[78] Labib A, August E, Agerstrand C, Frenckner B, Laufenberg D, Lavandosky G, et al. Extracorporeal life support organization guideline for transport and retrieval of adult and pediatric patients with ECMO support. ASAIO Journal (American Society for Artificial Internal Organs : 1992). 2022;**68**(4):447-455

[79] Labib A, Alinier G. Transport and retrieval on extracorporeal membrane oxygenation (ECMO): Setup and activities of an immersive transport and retrieval on ECMO workshop. Journal of Cardiothoracic and Vascular Anesthesia. 2021;**35**(6):1603-1610

[80] Vasques F, Romitti F, Gattinoni L, Camporota L. How I wean patients from veno-venous extra-corporeal membrane oxygenation. Critical Care. 2019;**23**(1):316

[81] Fried JA, Masoumi A, Takeda K, Brodie D. How I approach weaning from venoarterial ECMO. Critical Care. 2020;**24**(1):307

[82] Ng PY, Ip A, Fang S, Lin JCR, Ling L, Chan KM, et al. Effect of hospital case volume on clinical outcomes of patients requiring extracorporeal membrane oxygenation: A territory-wide longitudinal observational study. Journal of Thoracic Disease. 2022;**14**(6):1802-1814

[83] Combes A, Brodie D, Chen YS, Fan E, Henriques JPS, Hodgson C, et al. The ICM research agenda on extracorporeal life support. Intensive Care Medicine. 2017;**43**(9):1306-1318

[84] Abrams D, Garan AR, Abdelbary A, Bacchetta M, Bartlett RH, Beck J, et al. Position paper for the organization of ECMO programs for cardiac failure in adults. Intensive Care Medicine. 2018;**44**(6):717-729

[85] Schmidt M, Bailey M, Sheldrake J, Hodgson C, Aubron C, Rycus PT, et al. Predicting survival after extracorporeal membrane oxygenation for severe acute respiratory failure. The respiratory extracorporeal membrane oxygenation survival prediction (RESP) score. American Journal of Respiratory and Critical Care Medicine. 2014;**189**(11):1374-1382

[86] Schmidt M, Burrell A, Roberts L, Bailey M, Sheldrake J, Rycus PT, et al. Predicting survival after ECMO for refractory cardiogenic shock: The survival after veno-arterial-ECMO (SAVE)-score. European Heart Journal. 2015;**36**(33):2246-2256

Chapter 6

Anesthesia for Non-Cardiac Surgery for the LVAD Patient

Kathryn Foster and Steven S. Silvonek

Abstract

Heart failure is poorly tolerated and end stage heart failure (classified as New York Heart Association (NYHA) class IV) has a two-year survival with medical therapy that approaches 0%. Innovation in this sphere has yielded mechanical therapies, principally the left ventricular assist device (LVAD). In the last decade one-year survival rates of Left ventricular assist device patients have increased from 52–83%. As this therapy is more commonly used to treat advanced heart failure, coupled with the increase in patient survival after implantation, patients are increasingly encountered in the peri-operative arena requiring anesthesia for non-cardiac surgeries. The goal of this chapter is to provide the non-cardiac trained anesthesia provider a primer on what an LVAD is, how it functions, the physiological changes that occur with implantation, and considerations for administering anesthesia to patients with LVADs for non-cardiac surgery. Review of articles from 2018 to 2022 found from a search on PubMed and Google Scholar using the keywords: "Left Ventricular Assist Device", "LVAD", "anesthesia", "non-cardiac surgery", "Doppler blood pressure measurement", "VAD coordinator". Non-cardiac trained anesthesia providers can safely administer the anesthetics to LVAD patients undergoing non-cardiac surgery as long as appropriate considerations are taken.

Keywords: anesthesia, left ventricular assist device, LVAD, non cardiac surgery, blood pressure measurement

1. Introduction

Cardiovascular disease continues to be the leading cause of death in America. Around six million Americans are diagnosed with heart failure of varying degrees each year [1–5]. Left Ventricular Assist Devices are indicated for patients with advanced stage heart failure. Medical optimization can include renin angiotensin-aldosterone system antagonists, sympathetic nervous system antagonists, beta blockers [1, 4–8]. Cardiac resynchronization therapy is often used in chronic heart failure candidates to stave off final implantation [1, 4–8]. In end-stage heart failure, conventional medical therapies have a mortality at 2 years of almost 100% [9]. These patients are classified NYHA class IV or Stage D by the American College of Cardiology Foundation/American Heart Association. Clinically, they have shortness of breath at rest and their echo shows an ejection fraction (EF) of 40% or less. While cardiac transplant is a definitive treatment for severe advanced heart failure and may be the preferred treatment, this solution is limited by donor availability. The failure

IntechOpen

Bridge to Recovery (BTR)	**VAD is used to support heart until recovered function from shock via ventricular remodeling**
Bridge to transplant (BTT)	VAD is used while patient awaits heart transplant
Destination Therapy (DT)	This is definite treatment for patients who are not transplant eligible
Bridge to decision (BTD)/ Bridge to candidacy (BTC)	Used in patients who are not currently but may become eligible for heart transplant related to recent malignancy or potential for improved end organ function with VAD assistance.

Table 1.
Indications of LVAD therapy [4, 5, 8, 11, 14, 15].

of medical management, the shortage of heart donors, and the realization that these patients were not suitable transplant candidates led to the development of the LVAD [2, 4, 5, 10–12].

The first LVADs were used in the 1960s as bridge to therapy (BTT), or as a bridge to recovery (BTR) [2, 4, 5, 8]. Initially, they were designed to emulate the pulsatile action of the heart, had many moving parts and membranes, and were prone to frequent failure. After improvements in portability and mechanical design, the latest generation of devices are all continuous. By 2010, LVADs were approved for destination therapy (DT). As of 2020 destination therapy accounts for 78% of LVAD implantations in the US [13]. **Table 1** describes indications for LVAD therapy.

The evolution of the LVAD devices is a nascent, growing field and improvement to its models was rapid: In 2009, the one-year survival rate of an LVAD patient was 52%. By 2018, the one-year survival rate after an LVAD implant increased to over 80%; the two-year survival was above 70%; some patients lived 4 years or more [1–5, 7, 16–19]. As patients with these devices live longer, they may experience complications or other medical conditions that require surgical intervention and therefore anesthesia. One early review of Medicare patients found that in 2012, 64 LVAD patients had non-cardiac surgery (NCS) and that number increased in 2017 to 304 LVAD patients [7]. No doubt the number now is far higher in the 2020s. As more patients with these devices present for non-cardiac surgery, it is important for anesthesia providers to understand the hemodynamic and physiologic changes that result from LVAD placement and how our anesthetic techniques and medications affect its function [6, 20].

2. The LVAD

The current LVAD is a rotary continuous pump system that is implanted at the apex of the left ventricle and propels blood into the aorta via an outflow graft, typically to the ascending aorta. **Figure 1** shows a basic silhouette of the Heart Mate III, now the most implanted device of the 2020s [1].

The pump receives energy from a driveline that connects extracorporeally to a battery system through a controller when on battery power [1, 3, 11]. This device is so compact, the functional parts fit completely inside the thoracic cavity. The drive train can also be attached to a wall unit for power and with a larger display screen.

2.1 First generation devices

The first generation of LVADs were pulsatile and large [4, 16]. The Thoratec PVAD was the first LVAD to be approved by the Food and Drug Administration. It was used

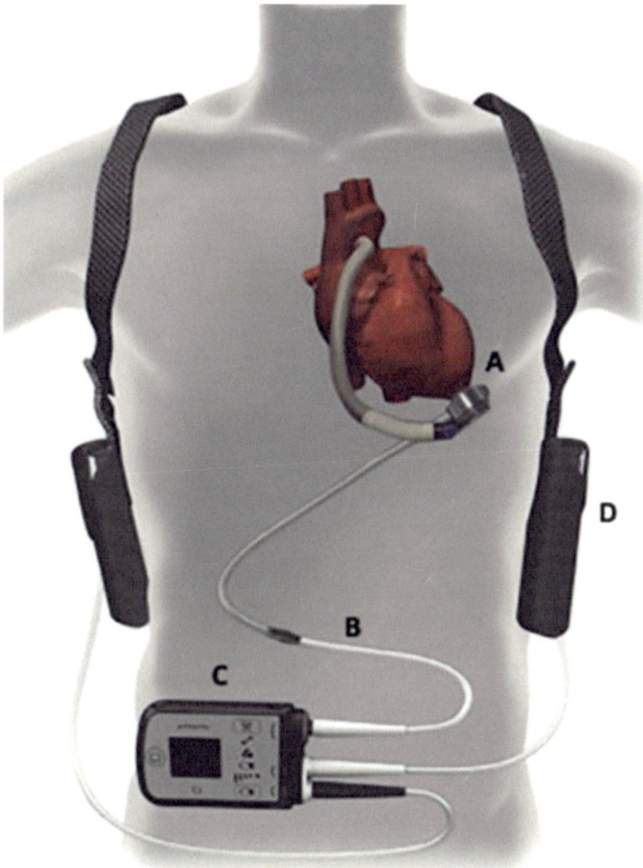

Figure 1.
The silhouette of the heart mate III components, the most implanted device of the 2020s. (a) Centrifugal pump (b) driveline cable (c) controller panel (d) portable battery [1].

in more than four thousand patients as a bridge to transplant [4]. Its pump was not implanted but had to be carried extracorporeally [16].

The Novacor and HeartMate I (HM I) became the first implantable LVADs. **Figure 2** shows an image of a HeartMate I device and its parts. The pumps of these devices were implanted in a preperitoneal pocket under the abdominal muscles. The Novacor had great durability, lasting for 5–6 years. However, the rate of stroke among its users was near 50% [1]. The HM1 device attempted to recreate physiologic pulsatile flow and was used as a BTT and BTR for more than two decades [4, 16]. The HM I had a 52% one-year survival rate, 48% better results than medical management at those times. Unfortunately, it was mechanically complex, was prone to malfunction, and also had high rates of severe adverse events and infection. The device was trialed for Destination Therapy (DT) but ultimately failed, as it was deemed not ideal and its parts wore out at about 18 months [1, 4].

2.2 Second generation devices

The HeartMate II (HM2) device was introduced in 2008 (**Figure 3**) [4]. It is considered a second-generation device because it delivers continuous flow (CF)

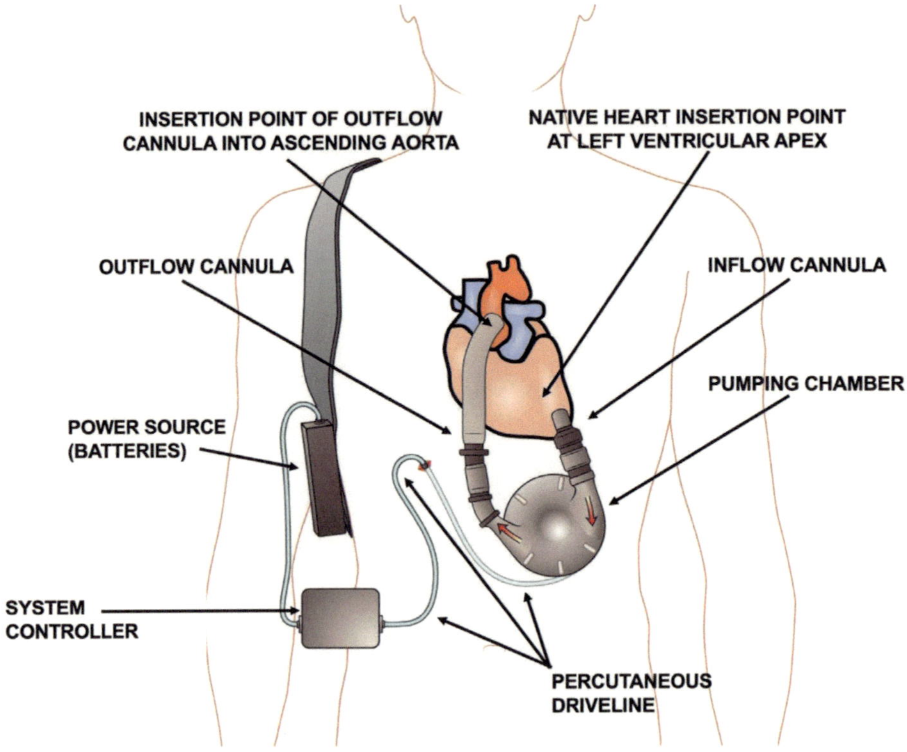

Figure 2.
The HeartMate 1 [3].

powered by an axial flow rotor propeller. The pump of the HM2 is 1/7th the size of the HM I [21], about the size of a D battery but is similarly implanted in a preperitoneal pocket [1, 16]. The HM2 boasted a 68% one-year survival rate with improved quality of life and physical activity noted at 3 months post implantation [4]. It achieved a 58% two-year survival rate compared to the HeartMate I (24%) in the 2010 REMATCH trial.

The HM II was the first device approved for destination therapy (DT) [2, 4, 15, 16, 18]. Rates of stroke, bleeding, infection, and device malfunction were less than its predecessors [1, 4]. With advances in implantation technique, design, and RV support devices, DT patients were approaching a 70% two-year survival rate, with one patient documented to have their HM2 for greater than 8 years [1, 7, 17]. However, the HM2 had its own unique complications related to its continuous axial flow.

Patients with HM2 unfortunately would present with pump thrombus. As a result, use of systemic anticoagulation, such as with warfarin, became a standard for all LVAD patients in 2011 [1]. Acquired von Willebrand deficiency and arteriovenous malformations (AVM) developed related to altered physiology associated with continuous flow LVADs. When combined with prophylactic anticoagulation, the incidence of gastrointestinal bleeding rose [1, 2, 4, 10, 11, 16].

2.3 Third generation devices

Second generation CF devices improved longevity compared to first generation but had multiple moving parts. Third generation CF devices, such as the Heart Mate

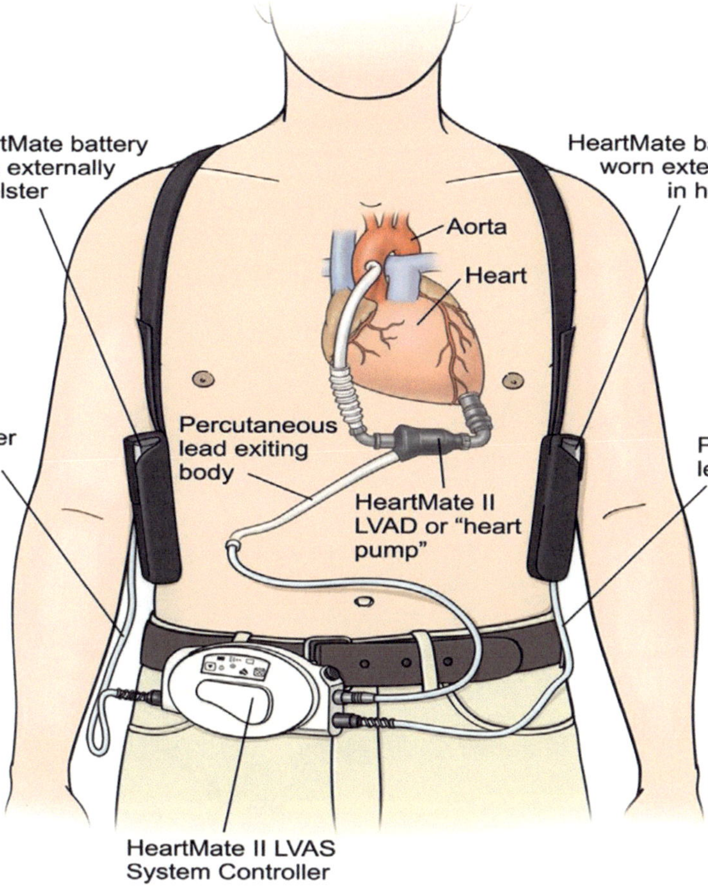

Figure 3.
The heart mate II [4].

III and the HeartWare HVAD, are positioned at the apex of the left ventricle blood pumps blood in a centrifugal manner [1, 4, 16]. Both devices are smaller than their predecessors. They have also shown greater longevity with significantly less need for reimplantation than the HM2 [1, 4, 5].

2.4 HVAD

The Medtronics HeartWare HVAD (**Figure 4**) was approved by FDA in November of 2012 for BTT. It has been implanted in more than 20,000 heart failure patients worldwide, with one HVAD being implanted for greater than 7 years [1, 22]. The HVAD functions via both passive magnetic levitation and a hydrodynamic bearing system [22]. In June of 2021, the sale and implantation of the HVAD was discontinued secondary to technical issues with the device not restarting after planned or accidental power disconnection. The HVAD patients also held a statistically significant incidence of stroke [12, 22]. About 4000 patients worldwide still have HVADs implanted. As a result, Society of Thoracic Surgeons recommends explantation of the HVAD to HM3 only in instances of malfunction, as electively changing devices carries just as much risk as keeping the HVAD [11, 22].

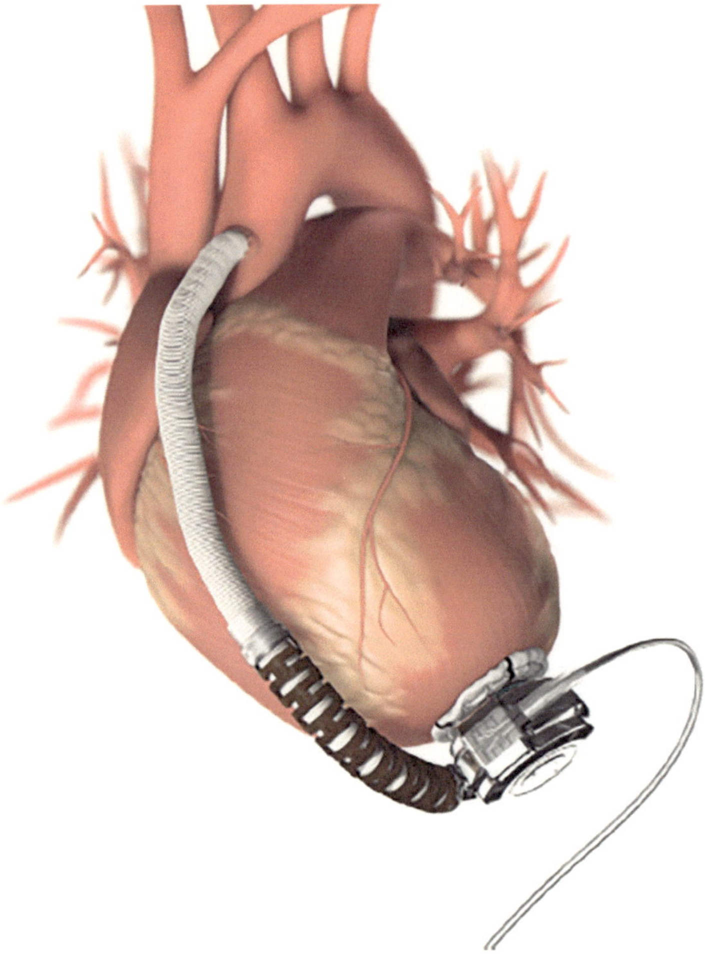

Figure 4.
The internal components of the Heartware HVAD [4].

2.5 HeartMate III

The Abbott HeartMate III system is a completely magnetically levitated centrifugal pump (**Figures 1** and **5**) [1, 4, 16, 22]. The centrifugal flow of the HM3 not only improves longevity of the devices but produces less shear on blood components. This has resulted in milder acquired von Willebrand syndrome. Other adverse events such as pump thrombus, stroke, and GI bleeding are decreased in HM3 compared to HM2 [1, 4, 5, 17, 23]. HM3 patients also spend less days in the hospital 2 years post implant [17]. Unfortunately, rates of right heart failure and infection with third generation devices remain similar to previous generations [1, 4, 17].

2.6 External components of the LVAD

Figure 6 shows an example of a Heartmate III controller. The controller contains a screen that displays four values: pump speed (rotations/minute), pump flow (liters/min), pulsatility index (PI), and pump power (watts) [3, 11, 16]. When in the OR

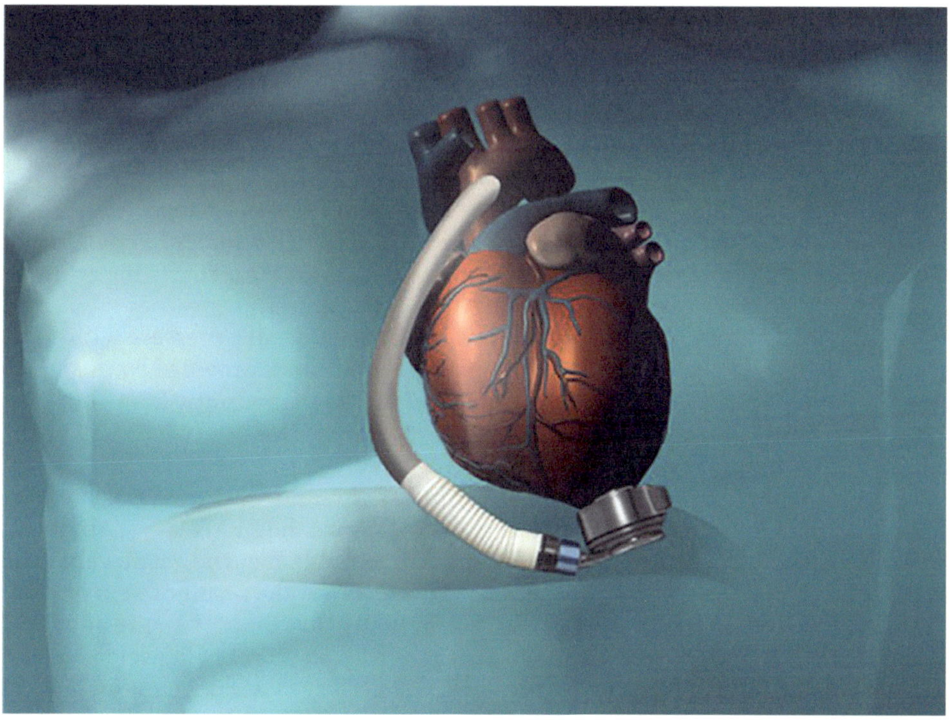

Figure 5.
The internal components of the HeartMate 3 [4].

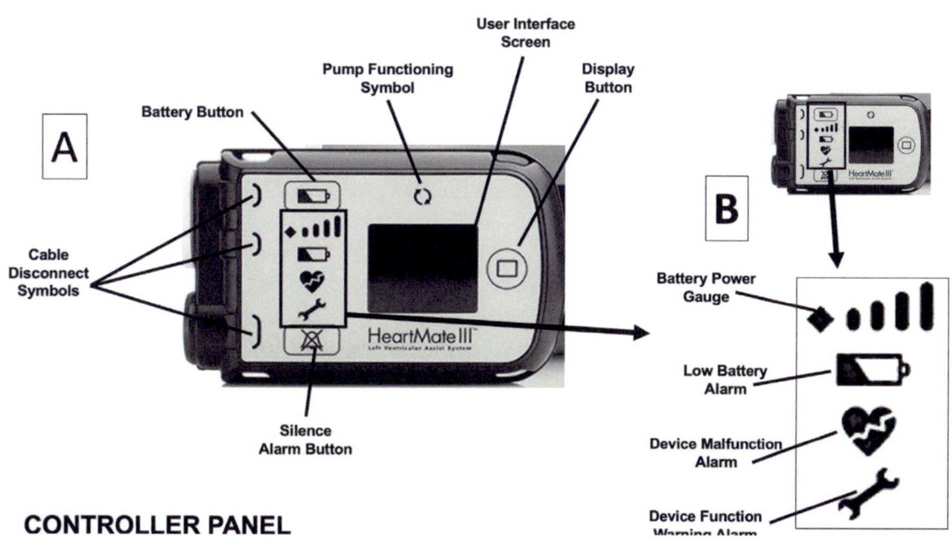

Figure 6.
Controller panel of the HeartMate 3. (A) LVAD controller panel and (B) panel of indicator lights [3].

and connected to wall power, a larger monitor can be fashioned to display all values concurrently.

Pump speed shows how fast the LVAD centrifuge is spinning and is the only directly modifiable value of the LVAD. Pump speed can be adjusted to optimize function under visualizaiton with echocardiogram. Pump flow is analogous to cardiac output and is different for each model; this value is typically a derived number calculated with proprietary formulas [16, 24].

Pump power is indicative of how much power is being required to run the pump at a specific set pump speed. In its normal function, this value varies linearly with systemic vascular resistance.

Pump flow is therefore a calculated value from pump power. Changes and trends of the pump flow value can also indicate complications. For example, any increase in power not related to an increase in actual flow will cause an erroneously high flow to read, such as the presence of a thrombus in the inflow cannula.

The pulsatility index is the difference of systolic and diastolic pressure within the pump system. Its magnitude reflects the amount of assistance provided by the LVAD; when the left ventricle contracts, the PI increases the flow transiently in the LVAD. This value is key to interpreting Doppler blood pressures (DopBP), which will be discussed later in this chapter [16, 19, 25].

Table 2 displays normal values for the three continuous flow LVADs currently in use or available for implantation [3, 11, 18, 24]. Since the LVAD is essentially a conduit bypassing the left ventricle, it is entirely possible that the aortic valve does not routinely open. Any pulsatility that does occur is not the result of ventricular ejection through the aortic valve, per se. It is actually the result of any residual left ventricular function that with each beat provides an increase in preload to the LVAD, resulting in a transiently higher flow. The newest LVAD devices, including the HM III, routinely cycle their RPMs transiently higher and lower than their set value instead of remaining static, thus creating more pulsatility than their predecessors. This decreases the incidence of AVMs which often are responsible for GI bleeding.

Many factors can affect physiologic LVAD pump function, including hypovolemia, anesthetic agents, surgical positioning and technique. **Figure 7** is a flow diagram of changes in pump values that may indicate different physiologic states when the pump flow is increased. Patients with high pump flows and low PI values may be indicative of vasodilation, aortic valve regurgitation, or high pump speed. Of the three, vasodilation is the most likely cause related to anesthesia and should be treated with titration of vasopressors, inotropes, and intravenous fluids. If the pump flow is high and the PI is increased, then the patient may be hypervolemic or have increased myocardial contractility, such as with inotrope usage [3, 12, 24]. **Figure 8** details a flow diagram to help interpret changes when the pump flow is decreased. Low pump flow with high PI can be caused by hypertension, decreased VAD speed, or partial outflow obstruction from the outflow cannula. Of the three, hypertension is the cause most likely associated with an anesthetic. Titrating antihypertensives, administering pain medication, or increasing depth of anesthesia are ways to address these changes. If pump flow and PI are both low, this may indicate partial inflow obstruction or low

VAD	Pump speed (rpm)	Flow Liters/min	Power, Watts	Pulsitility Index
HeartMate 2	8000-10,000	4–8	4–8	4–6
HeartMate 3	5000-6000	3–6	3–7	2–4
HVAD	2400-3200	4–7	3–7	8 peak, 2 troughs

Table 2.
Normal value ranges of LVAD devices for speed (rotations per minute (rpm)), flow, and power [3, 10, 18, 24].

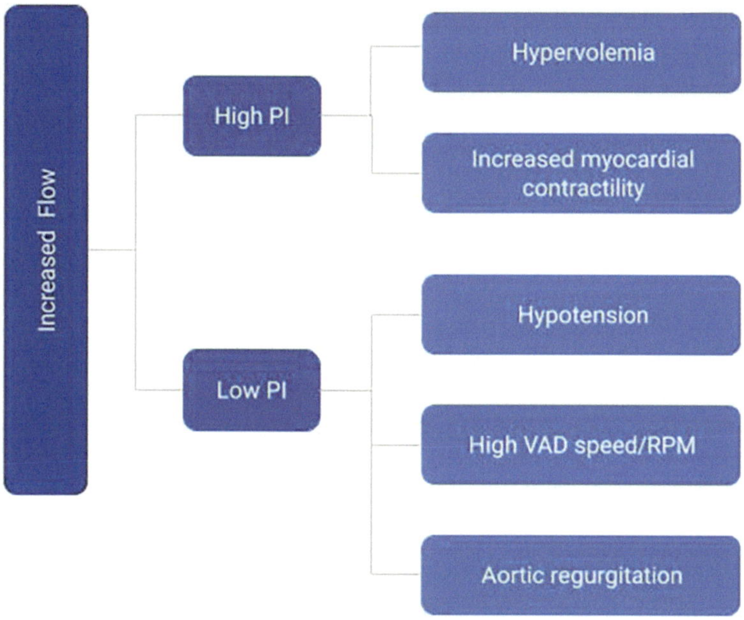

Figure 7.
Flow diagram for interpreting changes in LVAD function with increased flow [12, 24].

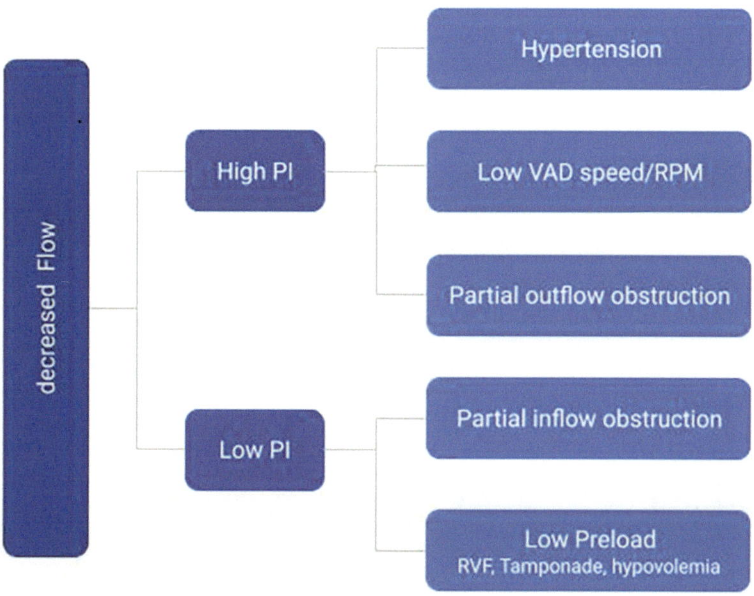

Figure 8.
Flow diagram for interpreting changes in LVAD function decreased flow [12, 24].

preload secondary to hypovolemia, right sided heart failure, or cardiac tamponade. In the setting of an anesthetic, hypovolemia is most likely the cause of this pattern and can be treated with titration of a fluid bolus [3, 12, 24].

3. Complications of LVAD device

The most common complications with continuous flow LVADs are right ventricular (RV) failure, gastrointestinal (GI) bleeding, infection, pump thrombus, stroke, and ventricular arrhythmias [3, 4, 11, 14, 17, 23].

3.1 Right ventricular failure

RV failure is noted in about 35%- 40% of LVAD patients. This may present acutely right after implantation or is a delayed phenomenon attributed to increased preload, septal shift, and less contractility [4, 6, 12, 14, 17]. 10–25% of LVAD patients will require RV support as a poorly functioning RV limits the LVAD system by way of preload [6, 14]. Supportive measures may include a variety of modalities such as lusitropic medications, diuretics, and pulmonary vasodilators [11, 12]. Patients who are refractory to medical management may require a right ventricular assist device (RVAD) or in some cases total artificial heart [4].

3.2 Gastrointestinal bleeding

GI bleeds occur in around 30% of patients with LVADs [2, 8, 16–18]. Upper GI bleeds are more common than lower GI bleeds [3, 11]. The most common source of bleeding is arterial venous malformations, the formation of which is attributed to lack of arterial pulsatility and acquired von.

Willebrand disease [1, 2, 4, 10, 11, 16, 26]. Interestingly, the HM III is thought to partially mitigate this by cycling its RPMs (revolutions per minute), thus creating a partially pulsatile state. Patients with history of gastric ulcers, colon polyps, and hx blood thinner use prior to LVAD placement are at higher risk for developing GI bleeds [4]. The requirement of anti-coagulation, typically with coumadin targeting an INR of 1.5–3, as well as aspirin, also exacerbate the bleeding risk [2, 4, 10, 16]. **Figure 9** provides a visual for how these factors contribute to GI bleeds.

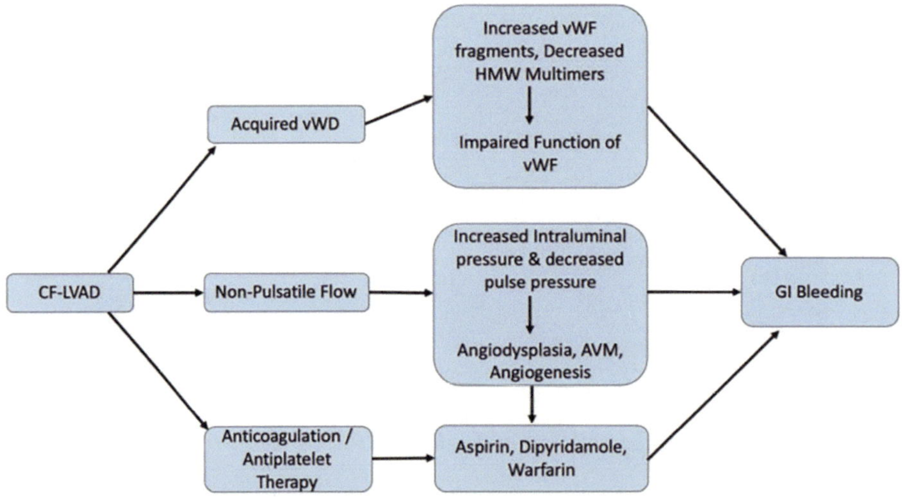

Figure 9.
Factors of continuous flow (CF) LVADs that contribute to GI bleeding [2].

Acute management of GI bleeding will likely include a combination of holding anticoagulation/antiplatelet medications, providing octreotide, and performing an endoscopy exam [2, 11, 12]. Holding anticoagulation has shown to be safe for short periods of time and should be restarted slowly with a lowered INR goal after signs of bleeding have stopped [2, 4, 15, 16]. Octreotide is a somatostatin analog that functions by decreasing gastric secretions that prevent clot formation [12]. Endoscopies require anesthesia and diagnose the source of bleeding in 1/3 of patients. In cases of severe GI bleed, reversal of anticoagulation with vitamin K or fresh frozen plasma may be used. Von Willebrand factor may also be administered [2, 12]. If the source of bleeding is not identified and bleeding continues, angiography may be attempted to identify and embolize source vessels [11]. Maintaining lower doses of anticoagulants may be used as long-term treatment and prevention of GI bleeding [12].

3.3 Infection

Infection can occur at surgical incisions or anywhere along the device system. Driveline infections are the most common, comprising 80% of LVAD associated infections [4, 12]. Any infection in the LVAD patient will be treated with hospital admission and intravenous antibiotics to prevent sepsis [12]. Driveline infections may also require surgical debridement in the operating room [12]. Explantation of the LVAD device with re-implantation is the final treatment if any components of the internal device become infected [4, 10]. Self-care education of LVAD users is key to prevention of infection. Lifelong antibiotic suppressive therapy is an alternative for those who are too high a surgical risk. Using techniques such as anchoring the driveline near the skin and using a silver dressing have shown to decrease infections in a small study [12].

3.4 Pump thrombus

Pump thrombus is a complication unique to continuous flow LVADs. HM3 has the least incidence of suspected pump thrombus; less than 3% at the two-year post implantation mark [4, 12, 17]. Thrombus can occur anywhere within the pump. A thrombus in the inflow and outflow cannula may be seen on CT scan with contrast. Visualization of thrombus anywhere else within the system can only occur with explantation [12]. An elevated pump power with decreased pulsatility index will be noted on the controller screen of the LVAD [4]. Transthoracic or transesophageal echocardiogram may show a dilated left ventricle, mitral regurgitation, and aortic valve opening with systole [12]. Clinically, a palpable pulse may be felt secondary to aortic valve opening [2, 6]. Labs will show an increased lactic dehydrogenase and decreased hemoglobin when suspecting LVAD pump thrombus [12]. In 50% of less severe cases, the patient will successfully be treated with heparin and inotropes [14]. In severe cases where pump thrombus treatment is refractory to medical management, the pump is exchanged as definitive treatment [4, 10]. Strategies such as maintaining INR 2–2.5 with warfarin, daily aspirin, and mid-range pump speeds decrease thrombus rates significantly. The PREVENT study saw a decrease in thrombus rates from 8.9 to 1.9% by implementing the following strategies: coumadin to keep INR 2–2.5, daily aspirin, and pump speeds greater than 9000 RPMs (for HM II) [3, 4, 14].

3.5 Stroke

There is an increased incidence of stroke associated with pump thrombus and mean arterial pressure (MAP) greater than 90 mmHg. For LVAD patients, a MAP greater than 90 mmHg is considered HTN [3, 4, 11]. Data shows that about 9% of patients with an LVAD have a stroke within 34 months of implantation [12]. Favored treatment for ischemic strokes in the LVAD population is endovascular thrombectomy. Intravenous thrombolysis has not yet been tested sufficiently [3, 12]. The histology of clots is different in LVAD patients and clot retrieval devices require more passes of devices are typically required to alleviate ischemic strokes in LVAD patients vs. non-LVAD patients [27]. A decrease in stroke rates by two thirds was noted with adherence to the same regimen that decreased pump thrombus. The protocol includes maintaining mid-range pump speed, anticoagulation with warfarin to keep INR values 2–2.5, and daily aspirin [3, 4]. The newer generation HM3 has less incidence of stroke compared to the HMII [3, 4, 12].

3.6 Ventricular arrhythmias

Ventricular arrhythmias occur in about 15–34% of LVAD patients, with the highest incidence in the first 30 days post implantation. An average of 34% of LVAD patients have an episode of ventricular tachycardia within 1 year of implantation [4, 6, 16]. Many have an ICD implanted prior to LVAD implantation [4, 6, 10, 14, 16]. Ventricular arrhythmias may be caused by so-called "suck down" events: when the left ventricle has a low volume and collapses on itself [4, 6, 11, 16, 28].

Treatment is to slow the VAD speed to allow increased filling of the ventricle, and support with vasopressors [4, 6]. Management of ventricular arrhythmias and suction events will be discussed further in the Intraoperative management section of this chapter.

4. Perioperative considerations for LVAD patients undergoing non-cardiac surgery

As people are living longer with LVADs, other health issues may arise that require surgical intervention and therefore the need for anesthesia [15, 20]. 15–20% of LVAD patients present for non-cardiac surgery (NCS), whether elective or urgent/emergent [7, 18]. In one study held in Europe from 2012 to 2019, within 60% of LVAD patients who had surgical interventions, 39% of procedures were unplanned and 61% were elective [18]. Over half of the patients required general anesthesia, whereas 5% of cases were performed under local [18]. A review of Medicare patients with LVADs in the United states within the same time period shows close to 75% of the non-cardiac surgery cases were unplanned and around 25% reported as elective [7]. Common procedures LVAD patients may undergo include treatment of GI bleeding, surgical debridement of skin infections, ICD generator changes, and emergent orthopedic and cystoscopy cases [7, 18]. Another report described the care of morbidly obese LVAD patients for laparoscopic sleeve gastrectomies, to improve transplant candidacy [29].

Ideally, surgical procedures involving an LVAD patient should take place at a medical center that implants LVADs. It is suggested that for any complex patients or larger surgeries that a cardiac anesthesiologist be the primary anesthetic provider. Many smaller procedures, sedation cases, and well-maintained patients may not necessitate the need for cardiac trained anesthesia providers [15, 16].

4.1 Surgical optimization during the pre admission testing and preoperative period

The typical patient living with an LVAD may be in better physiological condition when compared with patients with severe heart failure not on LVAD therapy. Studies show that around 30–70% of non-cardiac surgery events in LVAD patients are electively scheduled [7, 11, 15, 18]. Efforts should be made to have an LVAD coordinator plan and organize care for these patients [30]. Duties include communicating and coordinating needs of the planned procedure, providing patient education, including anticoagulation management, organizing availability of LVAD staff and anesthesia, and setting up goals for postoperative care [16, 20].

Most elective and many unplanned procedures may not require a cardiac trained anesthesia provider [15, 16, 18]. However, it is suggested that both a CT surgeon and a cardiac anesthesiologist are aware of the patient having a procedure and be available for consultation. For LVAD patients that present with hemodynamic instability, it is recommended that a cardiac anesthesia team be present for surgery [16].

The type of anesthesia required is case dependent. However, ideally and whenever possible, cases should be performed under local, regional, or MAC [16]. Neuraxial anesthesia is not typically thought of an ideal modality for LVAD patients due in part to their requirement of systemic anticoagulation, but most troublesome is the profound vasodilation and subsequent abatement of preload that can rapidly lead to ventricular "suck down" phenomenon if not appropriately anticipated. In normalization of practice, it has been found that an epidural may even be provided to laboring women with LVADs [14]. General anesthesia can safely be administered in a patient with an LVAD, provided once again, one accounts for the frequent shifts in hemodynamics [20]. Discussing the type of anesthesia and the expected patient experience is important [16].

LVAD patients may need to be admitted 24–72 hours prior to scheduled procedure for heparin bridging and fluid optimization [16, 18, 20]. Management of anticoagulants will depend largely on the type of surgery and anticipated blood loss. Warfarin is most commonly stopped and bridged with heparin in hospital. Aspirin may be continued as the antiplatelet therapy has proven to be beneficial perioperatively [18, 20]. Fresh frozen plasma, prothrombin complex concentrate (PCC), and vitamin K can be used in emergent situations to reverse warfarin [3, 16, 18, 20]. In small cases with little to no anticipated blood loss, patients may be instructed to stop or decrease anticoagulation doses within a few days of scheduled procedure. Studies have shown that stopping or decreasing the dose of anticoagulation does not increase risk of adverse events [4, 15, 16].

Also understand that all LVAD patients have acquired von Willebrand's disease related to blood shearing forces that flow through the pump [4, 16]. Perioperative DDAVP may be indicated depending on the type of surgery. Actual use is quite low at 0.3% [26].

Fluid status is important given the dependency of LVAD to function well with adequate preload. A pre-op echocardiogram can be performed to ensure the most complete assessment of the patient's cardiac function, including RV function and to provide opportunities for fluid optimization.

Should a patient have an ICD, it is recommended that the device be interrogated and/or reprogrammed to accommodate surgery, especially in cases where electrocautery will be used [16]. The anesthesia provider should also assess the driveline location and be familiar with individual patients' pump and baseline parameters [16]. In regards to physical examination, LVAD patients should not have a palpable pulse and heart sounds may not be elicited well upon auscultation, secondary to the hum of the.

LVAD device [3, 10, 11, 25]. In fact, a palpable pulse may indicate pump thrombus [3]. Setup and teamwork among the operating room staff members is important for an LVAD patient. The intended procedure should be reviewed, and all positioning and equipment needs considered and verified. Communication among all staff should be emphasized and the surgical team reminded of the sensitive hemodynamic state of an LVAD patient, for instance, during types of positioning or when viscera is manipulated [18]. Some positions may affect positioning of the inflow cannula and impede pump flow. Improper drive line cushioning could lead to pressure injury and tissue necrosis. For laparoscopic procedures, insufflation of abdomen should be increased in a stepwise fashion and need not exceed 10–12 mmhg until hemodynamic stability is assured [16]. Rapid escalation or high insufflation pressures can impede preload and affect flow. LVAD monitoring equipment such as Near Infrared Spectroscopy (NIRS) and Doppler supplies should be present and properly functioning.

The patient's advance directives, such as goals for CPR, should be discussed during the pre op assessment. Two lines of thought arise with the need for cardiac compressions and whether it is safe for the LVAD device. On one spectrum, compressions should never be performed as components of the LVAD may be dislodged. On the other end, no incidences of this have ever been reported in a case study [3, 16]. It is a consensus of many that early defibrillation and optimization of LVAD dynamics should be the preferred method to achieve return of spontaneous circulation (ROSC). It is not uncommon for patients who are in ventricular fibrillation to be conversant and alert.

4.2 Intraoperative phase

Upon entering the OR, it is prudent to connect the drivetrain to wall power using a red outlet (one that would still work with emergency power) [16]. Do keep extra batteries available in case of power failure [26]. The battery life of HM3 is 10–12 hours. When plugged into wall power the monitor is large enough to display all VAD parameters at once [12]. It is very important to remind the staff that the LVAD will be plugged into the wall and to not unplug it or trip over the cord.

When applying standard vital sign monitors, be aware that traditional NIBP may not be obtainable because of the lack of pulsatile blood flow [16]. The pulse oximeter may periodically work due to intermittent pulsatility. In lieu of standard pulse oximetry, NIRS could be used to monitor cerebral blood oxygen content. Cerebral oximeters work by trending venous weighted oxyhemoglobin saturation [26].

Blood pressure and mean arterial pressure (MAP) can be monitored by an arterial line or Doppler device [3, 4, 8, 11, 16, 25]. Arterial lines are the gold standard for an LVAD patient undergoing general anesthesia [16, 19]. The waveform will have a somewhat flat appearance related to low pulse pressure [3]. The use of Doppler devices for blood pressure monitoring are recommended for smaller cases that involve local anesthesia or IV sedation/MAC. It is often necessary to have a dedicated person to measure this as it is a relatively time intensive process. In many institutions, an LVAD nurse accompanies the patient and is charged with this task. The technique uses a Doppler ultrasound at the brachial artery. The cuff is placed on the upper arm and inflated until loss of pulse. The cuff is then slowly deflated and the pressure at the return of signal noted. If the patient has a palpable pulse, the Doppler pressure is associated with systolic pressure. In the absence of a palpable pulse the noted pressure is associated with the mean arterial pressure [19, 25]. The Doppler pressure has been shown to correlate with arterial lines 88% of the time [14]. MAPs should be kept around 70–80 mmHg to prevent pump malfunction while ensuring end organ perfusion [4, 8, 11, 14, 16, 19, 20, 25, 26, 31]. Slow cuff method is another effective technique, but it is not widely available [16, 19]. The slow cuff system deflates more slowly than common non-invasive blood pressure devices (**Figure 10**) [19].

4.3 Induction, maintenance, and emergence phases of anesthesia

Almost any method of induction can be chosen provided hemodynamic purtubations are anticipated. Propofol induction, for example, is not contraindicated but conservative doses are less likely to cause significant hemodynamic swings. An inhalational induction, total, or in part, is also an option.

Using midazolam and ketamine can decrease the amount of other anesthetics. Opioids can decrease sympathetic tone and should be given judiciously. This author uses a balanced technique incorporating small titrated doses of midazolam, ketamine, and propofol to achieve unconsciousness using the minimum dose required. Often, a pre induction fluid bolus is given and a phenylephrine infusion is titrated to the desired mean arterial blood pressure.

Intubation and ventilation can potentially cause changes to VAD function. Airway manipulation can cause sympathetic stimulation and hemodynamic shifts. Although some sources say placement of a double lumen tube should be avoided in favor of a bronchial blocker for thoracic procedures, both have been placed successfully [20]. Positive pressure ventilation and PEEP can affect preload, as can hypercarbia, hypoxia, and acidosis [16, 20]. Valsalva maneuvers may also impede venous return [20, 24].

Generally, the axial flow of an LVAD depends exquisitely on preload and afterload. It pumps the delivered volume and ejects it systemically. The main objectives are therefore to avoid decreased preload, maintenance of afterload, and avoid

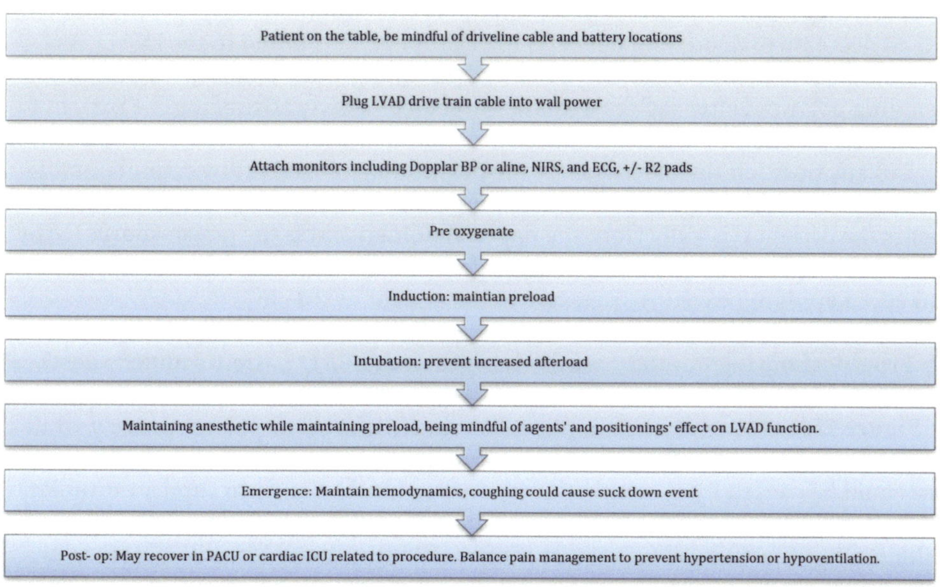

Figure 10.
A flow diagram highlighting key points to consider when managing an LVAD patient in the operating room.

inflow cannula obstruction. Although literature may state to maintain MAPs around 70-80 mmHg to ensure preload and pump function, it is important to pay particularattention to the patient's starting hemodynamics and use them as a target throughout the procedure. Studies have shown that a MAP less than 70 mmHg for greater than 20 minutes is "strongly associated with" acute kidney injury [26]. Avoiding hypovolemia cannot be stressed enough. Often, to optimize preload prior to induction, a judicious amount of fluid is given, and may include 1–2 bottles of 5% albumin [pisanksy]. One must be mindful of blood loss and insensible fluid losses. Arterial blood gas sampling and monitoring of the hematocrit is important. A more liberal transfusion target may be appropriate given ongoing losses. It is important to use irradiated and leukoreduced blood products as many of these patients will be transplant candidates.

It is also important to use inotropes in addition to vasopressors to maintain right heart function in presence of hypotension, particularly if known right heart dysfunction is already present. Chronic LVAD support changes RV geometry and RV dysfunction might exist but not be clinically apparent. Causes of RV failure intro can be due to multiple factors including the inflammatory cascade, blood product administration, hypoxia, hypercarbia, and acidosis, among many. Vasopressin is cited as a pressor of choice related to its lack of effect on the pulmonary vasculature [20, 28]. Milrinone infusion may also be employed to ensure decreased stress on the right ventricle [3, 11]. Lastly, a TEE machine and appropriately trained personnel can provide additional insights if management is difficult or intraoperative adventures are encountered.

4.4 Positioning

Positioning of the patient with an LVAD requires much attention for multiple reasons. For one, patient positioning can affect a patient's preload, pressure or impingement on the drivetrain, and/or access to the patient to obtain Doppler pressures [11, 20]. Positions such as beach chair, reverse Trendelenburg, prone, and lateral will all decrease preload, and hence, impair proper functioning to the LVAD. As some surgical procedures may necessitate these undesirable positions, a discussion involving potential alternatives with the surgeon or slowly advancing the patient to the desired position as hemodynamically tolerated is imperative [16]. Prone positioning and any position that could affect the positioning of the inflow cannula should be readily reversible. Vigilant attention should also be paid to the driveline cable as it exits the patient typically from the upper abdomen and is the power source to the LVAD. When positioning care should be taken to make sure the cable is not pulled, kinked, or applying excessive pressure to the patient's skin [16].

4.5 Troubleshooting hemodynamic changes with LVAD patients under anesthesia

Figure 11 lists some acute complications that might occur perioperatively while the patient is under anesthesia and some immediate actions to take. Acute hypertension could be caused by sympathetic response to intubation or to surgical stimulation. MAPs above 90 mmHg can affect pump function and should be immediately treated by increasing anesthetic depth or titrating small increments of antihypertensives. Currently there is no standardized management of hypertension in LVAD patients [14]. If hypertension should arise and forward LVAD flow becomes impeded, anesthetic depth can be titrated [18]. Hydralazine is noted to be an appropriate and

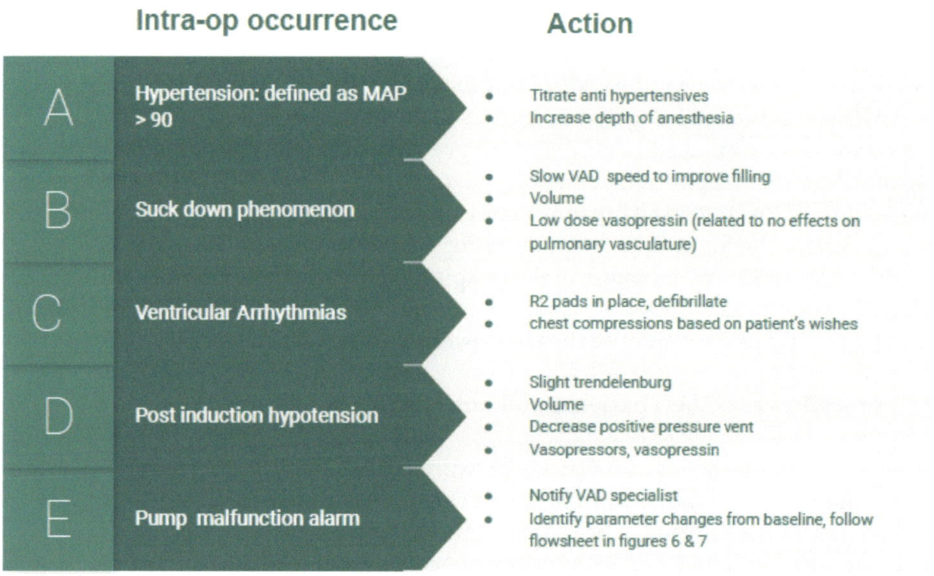

Figure 11.
Intra operative troubleshooting of an LVAD patient under general anesthesia.

effective choice to treat HTN in LVAD patients. Beta blockers are cautioned because of their negative inotropic effect [4, 11].

Suck down phenomenon can occur with decreased left ventricular filling. The VAD will suction onto the septal wall with low volumes [3, 4, 16]. Suction event may be recognized by speed, flow, and power values all being decreased [3] or low left ventricular volumes on the transesophageal echocardiogram [3, 16]. Treatment for suction events is to slow the VAD speed to allow increased filling of the ventricle, support with vasopressin, and increase preload via fluid bolus [4, 16]. Suction events may trigger ventricular tachycardia.

If an LVAD patient presents with ventricular tachycardia (VT), one should consider placing R2 pads prior to induction. R2 pad placement is the same as for non-LVAD patients and shocking with R2 pads does not disrupt LVAD function. Suction events are the most common cause of VT in LVAD supported patients [4, 16]. It is possible that some patients will be hemodynamically stable during episodes of VT as LVAD will continue to function. Additional treatment for VT includes 300 mg IV boluses of amiodarone [11]. A hemodynamically unstable patient may require advanced cardiac life support measures [3].

Post induction hypotension is best prevented by slow thoughtful induction, as described earlier. In the event of hypotension placing the patient in slight Trendelenburg and decreasing positive pressure ventilation, for positive pressure ventilation can put strain on the RV and decrease preload [16]. Small fluid bolus and titration of vasopressors should be used to support blood pressure and maintain preload.

Pump malfunction alarms may indicate the pump is not functioning, power is disrupted, or flow rate has changed. Consult the LVAD specialist. Meanwhile check that all connections are intact, from the wall/battery to the control panel to the driveline. Check the driveline for connections, kinks, or damage. If an alarm is sounding because of low or high flow rates use the diagrams in **Figures** 7 and **8** to recognize a pattern of changes and identify a potential cause.

4.6 Post-operative

Patients can be recovered in PACU but may be recovered in the ICU [11, 16, 20]. The AICD should be interrogated as soon as possible in the immediate postoperative period. It is paramount to take steps to prevent increased preload by way of hypoventilation and hypertension related to pain [16]. Opioid sparing techniques are suggested for pain control to prevent hypoventilation and sequela post operatively [16, 20]. Again, the focus is to maintain pump flow and pre-operative physiology [18]. Post operative readmissions to the hospital are common as patients with LVADs undergoing non cardiac surgery have high rates of bleeding and acute kidney injury. The need for transfusion may be delayed several hours post surgery [7].

4.7 Case studies for LVAD patients and non cardiac surgery

A. A 24-year-old parturient with a heartware HVAD requests an epidural placement for induction of labor and subsequent cesarean section. The patient stopped lovenox 24 hours prior to hospital admission.
Once admitted, invasive BP monitoring, central line and Swan Ganz placement were performed.
Subsequently, an epidural catheter was placed prior to induction of labor.
The patient was permitted a patient-controlled epidural device (PCEA) that dispensed a bupivacaine and fentanyl solution. With the decision to perform cesarean section the epidural was dosed with 2% lidocaine in small increments. Vasopressin and norepinephrine drips were used throughout to maintain MAPs greater than 70 mmHg.
The patient received transverse abdominal plane blocks post operatively for pain control. No complications with the LVAD were noted [28].

B. A 72-year-old female with a HM3 underwent a total knee replacement procedure. Pre operative surgical optimization assessments by orthopedics, cardiology, and anesthesia were performed. Warfarin was discontinued 6 days prior to surgery and was admitted 2 days prior to surgery for heparin bridging.
The patient received a 500 mL intravenous fluid bolus and an abductor canal block for postop pain control in the holding suite. Upon entering the operating room, American society of Anesthesiologists (ASA) standard monitors were placed, as well as an arterial line. The patient then received a spinal of 12 mg of hyperbaric bupivacaine. Her pressures were supported with epinephrine and phenylephrine drips. Sedation was maintained with propofol. The case reported minimal blood loss and no anesthetic complications. The patient was taken to cardiac ICU for recovery on no drips [32].

C. A 68-year-old with a HM3 had a total thyroidectomy procedure under monitored anesthesia care. The patient entered the operating room and after connecting the LVAD to wall power an arterial line was started in addition to ASA standard monitors. The patient received 2 mg of versed and an alfentanil infusion and the surgical team administered a superficial cervical block. This technique was chosen related to minimal potential of shifts in hemodynamics compared to general endotracheal anesthesia. No pressors were required throughout the case and the patient did not have any pain or discomfort throughout. The patient was recovered in the ICU post operatively [31].

D. A 66-year old male with a HMII with prostate cancer present for robotic laparoscopic prostatectomy.

   Prior to the surgical date the patient had a ramp transthoracic echocardiogram to optimize his LVAD function. The patient was admitted the night prior to his procedure for LVAD and ICD interrogation. His warfarin was held the night before surgery. An INR of 3.2 was noted prior to surgical start time, prothrombin complex concentrate was administered; prior to incision INR was 1.4. An arterial line and right internal jugular central venous catheter were placed prior to induction. A rapid sequence induction was performed with 1.5 mcg/kg fentanyl, 1 mg/kg of propofol, and 1.2 mg/kg rocuronium. Anesthesia was maintained with sevoflurane. Post induction the patient became hypotensive and was treated with a 250 mL bolus of albumin. With the start of pneumoperitoneum the patient became hypertensive. This was managed with a bolus of propofol and initiation of dobutamine and nicardipine drips to maintain preload and afterload. As the patient was transitioned into trendelenberg a rise in central venous pressure was noted, but LVAD parameters maintained within the patient's normal range and no action was taken at that time. Approximately 40 minutes after being positioned in trendelenberg the CVP had increased significantly and the PI was decreasing. A cardiac anesthesiologist was consulted for TEE, which showed septal bowing and right ventricular dysfunction. Inhaled epoprostenol was administered as treatment, CVP and PI returned to baseline. During desufflation of the pneumoperitoneum the patient became hypotensive requiring a second albumin bolus and short term epinephrine and phenylephrine drips while the surgical procedure finished. All drips were weaned off; the patient was extubated and taken to the cardiac intermediate care unit to recover. No postoperative complications were noted and the patient was discharged to home 2 days postoperatively [33].

5. Discussion

It is estimated that by 2030, the number of Americans with heart failure will increase to over 8 million [1, 5]. The number of heart transplants per year has been between 2 and 5 thousand and will continue to be limited by the number of donors. Donor availability may soon increase related to hepatitis C no longer disqualifying donation, however, even this breakthrough is not anticipated to fulfill the need for heart transplant patients [5, 23]. Therefore, there is likely to be an increased need for alternative definitive treatment for advanced heart failure, such as LVADs.

There is a campaign to recognize advanced heart failure sooner and to implant an LVAD before patients develop significant end organ disease [4, 23]. The strategy is to standardize criteria across all LVAD centers. One suggestion is to use AI algorithms to evaluate electronic medical records for increased frequency of visits and other criteria indicative of advancing heart failure [23].

Current targets for advancement include development of a completely implantable device and standardization of minimally invasive surgery (MIS) technique for LVAD implantation [23]. MIS technique requires two thoracotomy incisions; one 2 centimeters at the right intercostal space and a second larger (8-10 cm) at the 5-6th intercostal space. These incisions expose the ascending aortic arch and apex of the left ventricle, respectively [34]. In addition to preserving the sternum MIS affords less blood loss, less need for transfusion, and less intrathoracic trauma [22, 23, 34]. One retrospective study also noted patients who underwent MIS placement had significantly shorter time to extubation, less incidence of RV failure, shorter ICU time, and fewer readmissions [34].

The fully implantable device has the potential to significantly decrease incidence of LVAD infections [4]. Three fully implantable devices have been developed and begun trials. The Abicor total artificial heart and the Arrow Lion heart did not achieve long term survival but showed significantly lower infection rates than devices with extracorporeal components [23].

A 2019 paper reported two patients received Jarvik 2000 LVADs designed without any percutaneous parts. The modified devices were produced to trial with a coplanar power system. The coplanar energy transfer system (CETS) wirelessly transfers energy from an external energy source to the internal battery/controller component, which directly powers the LVAD. When fully charged the internal battery system provides up to 6 hours of power. The system also includes a wristwatch monitor to display parameters. Patient A was noted to have an intraoperative neurological complication but pump implantation was successful. This patient developed a pump thrombus, in conjunction with his complicated postoperative course the device was turned off and the patient maintained on inotropes.

Patient B had a successful implantation and was discharged 30 post implantation. No infections or issues with the CETS were noted during either patients' hospital stays. No long term follow up information was available at the time of this publication [35].

A fourth device, the Calon Leviticus fiVAD is under development in Europe. In a preclinical study the fully implantable device completed a promising 6 day trial in sheep. It was paired with the same coplanar power system as the Jarvik trial mentioned above [36].

The technology of the LVAD has improved drastically over the last two to three decades increasing the longevity of these devices and those who benefit from them. Currently 1 year survival is 90% and mid 80% for heart transplant and LVAD respectively [4]. As these devices continue to improve and the common complications are better understood and managed, LVADs have the potential to become the preferred treatment for severe heart failure [4].

6. Conclusion

The LVAD was originally intended to support the patient with heart failure until a donor heart became available. Today they are implanted for a variety of therapeutic intentions and have extended the life span of critical heart failure patients. LVAD implantation changes the physiology of the heart and comes with some related complications. Caring for this patient population takes extra planning, optimization, and coordination. Adjustments to pre op assessment, monitoring devices, and peri operative management will be needed. However, by understanding these devices and related physiological changes, a non-cardiac anesthesia provider can safely administer a variety of anesthetics to a patient with an LVAD presenting for non-cardiac surgery.

Conflict of interest

The authors declare no conflict of interest.

Author details

Kathryn Foster* and Steven S. Silvonek
Department of Anesthesiology, St. Luke's University Health Network, USA

*Address all correspondence to: kafoster1223@gmail.com

IntechOpen

© 2023 The Author(s). Licensee IntechOpen. This chapter is distributed under the terms of the Creative Commons Attribution License (http://creativecommons.org/licenses/by/3.0), which permits unrestricted use, distribution, and reproduction in any medium, provided the original work is properly cited.

References

[1] Stone ME, Pawale A, Ramakrishna H, Weiner MM. Implantable left ventricular assist device therapy-recent advances and outcomes. Journal of Cardiothoracic and Vascular Anesthesia. 2018;**32**(4):2019-2028. DOI: 10.1053/j.jvca.2017.11.003 Epub 2017 Nov 4

[2] Ahsan I, Faraz A, Mehmood A, et al. Clinical approach to manage gastrointestinal bleeding with left ventricular assist device (LVAD). Cureus. 2019;**11**(12):e6341. DOI: 10.7759/cureus.6341

[3] Long B, Robertson J, Koyfman A, Brady W. Left ventricular assist devices and their complications: A review for emergency clinicians. The American Journal of Emergency Medicine. 2019;**37**(8):1562-1570. DOI: 10.1016/j.ajem.2019.04.050 Epub 2019 May 6

[4] Eisen HJ. Left ventricular assist devices (LVADS): History, clinical application and complications. Korean Circulation Journal. 2019;**49**(7):568-585. DOI: 10.4070/kcj.2019.0161

[5] Bowen RES, Graetz TJ, Emmert DA, Avidan MS. Statistics of heart failure and mechanical circulatory support in 2020. Annals of Translational Medicine. 2020;**8**(13):827-827. DOI: 10.21037/atm-20-1127

[6] Bouchez S, Van Belleghem Y, De Somer F, De Pauw M, Stroobandt R, Wouters P. Haemodynamic management of patients with left ventricular assist devices using echocardiography: The essentials. European Heart Journal Cardiovascular Imaging. 2019;**20**(4):373-382. DOI: 10.1093/ehjci/jez003

[7] Mentias A, Briasoulis A, Vaughan Sarrazin MS, Alvarez PA. Trends, perioperative adverse events, and survival of patients with left ventricular assist devices undergoing noncardiac surgery. JAMA Network Open. 2020;**3**(11):e2025118. DOI: 10.1001/jamanetworkopen.2020.25118

[8] Defilippis EM, Nakagawa S, Maurer MS, Topkara VK. Left ventricular assist device therapy in older adults: Addressing common clinical questions. Journal of the American Geriatrics Society. 2019;**67**(11):2410-2419. DOI: 10.1111/jgs.16105 Epub 2019 Aug 10

[9] Rose EA et al. Long-term use of a left ventricular assist device for end-stage heart failure. New England Journal of Medicine. 2001;**345**(20):1435-1443

[10] Kirklin JK, Pagani FD, Goldstein DJ, John R, Rogers JG, Atluri P, et al. American Association for Thoracic Surgery/International Society for Heart and Lung Transplantation guidelines on selected topics in mechanical circulatory support. The Journal of Thoracic and Cardiovascular Surgery. 2020;**159**(3):865-896. DOI: 10.1016/j.jtcvs.2019.12.021 Epub 2020 Jan 23

[11] Ben Gal T, Ben Avraham B, Milicic D, Crespo-Leiro MG, Coats AJS, Rosano G, et al. Guidance on the management of left ventricular assist device (LVAD) supported patients for the non-LVAD specialist healthcare provider: Executive summary. European Journal of Heart Failure. 2021;**23**(10):1597-1609. DOI: 10.1002/ejhf.2327 Epub 2021 Aug 22. Erratum in: Eur J Heart Fail. 2022 Mar 10

[12] Castrodeza J, Ortiz-Bautista C, Fernández-Avilés F. Continuous-flow left ventricular assist device: Current knowledge, complications, and future directions. Cardiology Journal.

2022;**29**(2):293-304. DOI: 10.5603/CJ.a2021.0172 Epub 2021 Dec 30

[13] Shah P et al. Twelfth interagency registry for mechanically assisted circulatory support report: Readmissions after left ventricular assist device. The Annals of Thoracic Surgery. 2022;**113**(3):722-737 - This reference provides latest LVAD numbers implanted (2012-2020)

[14] Lima B, Bansal A, Abraham J, Rich JD, Lee SS, Soleimani B, et al. Evolving mechanical support research group (EMERG). Controversies and challenges of ventricular assist device therapy. The American Journal of Cardiology. 2018;**121**(10):1219-1224. DOI: 10.1016/j.amjcard.2018.01.034 Epub 2018 Feb 13

[15] Briasoulis A, Chehab O, Alvarez P. In-hospital outcomes of left ventricular assist devices (LVAD) patients undergoing noncardiac surgery. ASAIO Journal. 2020;**67**(2):144-148. DOI: 10.1097/mat.0000000000001205

[16] Hwang N-C, Hwang K-Y. Facilitating noncardiac surgery for the patient with left ventricular assist device: A guide for the anesthesiologist. Annals of Cardiac Anaesthesia. 2018;**21**(4):351

[17] Mehra MR, Uriel N, Naka Y, ClevelandJC,YuzefpolskayaM,SalernoCT, et al. A fully magnetically levitated left ventricular assist device — Final report. New England Journal of Medicine. 2019;**380**(17):1618-1627. DOI: 10.1056/nejmoa1900486

[18] Berger R, Nemeth A, Salewski C, Sandoval Boburg R, Acharya M, Weymann A, et al. Is it safe for patients with left ventricular assist devices to undergo non-cardiac surgery? Medicina. 2020;**56**(9):424. DOI: 10.3390/medicina56090424

[19] Lankheet S, Pieterse MM, Rijnhout R, Tuerlings E, Oppelaar AC, van Laake LW, et al. Validity and success rate of noninvasive mean arterial blood pressure measurements in cf-LVAD patients: A technical review. Artificial Organs. 2022;**46**(12):2361-2370. DOI: 10.1111/aor.14367 Epub ahead of print

[20] Sikachi RR, Anca D. Anesthetic considerations in a patient with LVAD and COVID-19 undergoing video-assisted thoracic surgery. Journal of Cardiothoracic and Vascular Anesthesia. 2021;**35**(10):3035-3038. DOI: 10.1053/j.jvca.2020.12.019 Epub 2020 Dec 17

[21] Han J, Trumble DR. Cardiac assist devices: Early concepts, current technologies, and future innovations. Bioengineering. 2019;**6**(1):18

[22] Salerno CT, Hayward C, Hall S, Goldstein D, Saeed D, Schmitto J, et al. Heart ware HVAD system to heart mate 3 left ventricular assist system device exchange advisory group. HVAD to heart mate 3 left ventricular assist device exchange: Best practices recommendations. The Journal of Thoracic and Cardiovascular Surgery. 2022;**163**(6):2120-2127.e5. DOI: 10.1016/j.jtcvs.2021.11.085 Epub 2022 Mar 24

[23] Shaffer A, Cogswell R, John R. Future developments in left ventricular assist device therapy. The Journal of Thoracic and Cardiovascular Surgery. 2021;**162**(2):605-611. DOI: 10.1016/j.jtcvs.2020.07.125 Epub 2020 Sep 16

[24] Tchoukina I, Smallfield MC, Shah KB. Device management and flow optimization on left ventricular assist device support. Critical Care Clinics. 2018;**34**(3):453-463. DOI: 10.1016/j.ccc.2018.03.002

[25] Rangasamy S, Madan S, Saeed O, Goldstein DJ, Jorde UP, Negassa A, et al.

Noninvasive measures of Pulsatility and blood pressure during continuous-flow left ventricular assist device support. ASAIO Journal. 2019;**65**(3):241-246. DOI: 10.1097/mat.0000000000000805

[26] Chung, Mabel MD. Perioperative Management of the Patient with a left ventricular assist device for noncardiac surgery. Anesthesia & Analgesia 2018;**126**(6):1839-1850|DOI:10.1213/ANE.

[27] Kitano T, Sakaguchi M, Yamagami H, Ishikawa T, Ishibashi-Ueda H, Tanaka K, et al. Mechanical thrombectomy in acute ischemic stroke patients with left ventricular assist device. Journal of the Neurological Sciences. 2020;**15**(418):117142. DOI: 10.1016/j.jns.2020.117142 Epub 2020 Sep 17

[28] Gayam S, Staab J, Shih G, Stoops S. Cesarean delivery in a parturient with a left ventricular assist device. International Journal of Obstetric Anesthesia. 2020;**44**:53-55. DOI: 10.1016/j.ijoa.2020.07.007 Epub 2020 Jul 18

[29] Punchai S, Nor Hanipah Z, Sharma G, Aminian A, Steckner K, Cywinski J, et al. Laparoscopic sleeve gastrectomy in heart failure patients with left ventricular assist device. Obesity Surgery. 2019;**29**:1122-1129

[30] Schroeder SE, Boschi S, Schlöglhofer T. The role of the ventricular assist device coordinator: Quo vadis? Annals of Cardiothoracic Surgery. 2021;**10**(3):386-388. DOI: 10.21037/acs-2020-cfmcs-17

[31] Sharma A, Trigo-Blanco P, Oprea AD. Perioperative considerations for a patient with a left ventricular assist device undergoing thyroidectomy. Cureus. 2020;**12**(2):e7132. DOI: 10.7759/cureus.7132

[32] Fegley MW, Gupta RG, Elkassabany N, Augoustides JG, Werlhof H, Gutsche JT, et al. Elective Total knee replacement in a patient with a left ventricular assist device-navigating the challenges with spinal anesthesia. Journal of Cardiothoracic and Vascular Anesthesia. 2021;**35**(2):662-669. DOI: 10.1053/j.jvca.2020.10.012 Epub 2020 Oct 13

[33] Pisansky AJB, Burbano-Vera N, Stopfkuchen-Evans MF. Anesthetic management of a patient with left ventricular assist device undergoing robotic laparoscopic prostatectomy: A case report. JA Clinical Reports. 2020;**6**:57. DOI: 10.1186/s40981-020-00364-1

[34] Gosev I, Wood K, Ayers B, Barrus B, Knight P, Alexis J, et al. Implantation of a fully magnetically levitated left ventricular assist device using a sternal-sparing surgical technique. The Journal of Heart and Lung Transplantation. 2020;**39**(1):37-44

[35] Pya Y, Maly J, Bekbossynova M, Salov R, Schueler S, Meyns B, et al. First human use of a wireless coplanar energy transfer coupled with a continuous-flow left ventricular assist device. The Journal of Heart and Lung Transplantation. 2019;**38**(4):339-343

[36] Trendlines. "Breakthrough in device therapy for patients with late-stage heart disease". 11 January 2022. Available from: https://www.trendlines.com/news/breakthrough-in-device-therapy-for-patients-with-late-stage-heart-disease/

Section 4

Thoracic Anesthesia

Chapter 7

Updates to Thoracic Procedures: Perioperative Care and Anesthetic Considerations

James Pellechi, Sean DuBois and Meredith Harrison

Abstract

Thoracic surgery is a rapidly evolving field, as is the perioperative and anesthetic care of patients undergoing major thoracic surgery. As surgical techniques continue to evolve, new guidelines are needed to help standardize patient care. To this end, Enhanced Recovery After Surgery (ERAS) protocols were created and have seen increasingly widespread adoption within the field of thoracic surgery. Despite their name, the scope of these protocols includes not only the postoperative period, but also helps guide care in the preoperative and intraoperative periods. Thus, ERAS pathways are relevant to both thoracic surgeons and anesthesiologists. This chapter aims to summarize current guidelines for managing patients undergoing thoracic surgery (from the preoperative period all the way through to postoperative care) by discussing recent updates within the field as well as some more well established tenets that remain relevant to the topic.

Keywords: thoracic surgery, anesthesia, enhanced recovery after surgery (ERAS), enhanced recovery after thoracic surgery (ERATS), one-lung ventilation, regional anesthesia

1. Introduction

Within the field of thoracic surgery, recent emphasis has been placed on the creation of standardized enhanced recovery after surgery (ERAS) pathways for patients undergoing intrathoracic procedures. These multidisciplinary pathways are designed to span all temporal aspects of perioperative care — preoperative, intraoperative, and postoperative [1]. Through standardization, such protocols aim to improve provider efficiency, increase patient throughput, and, ultimately, to diminish patient morbidity and mortality after surgery. Although this chapter will address each of these phases, particular attention will be paid to intraoperative ventilatory management and perioperative pain control given their importance within thoracic-specific ERAS protocols.

2. Methods

Literature review was performed using Google Scholar and PubMed databases. Search topics included "thoracic anesthesia", "enhanced recovery after thoracic surgery", "one-lung ventilation", and "thoracic regional anesthesia". Reference lists of eligible articles were crosschecked for other relevant material. Literature from the past five years (2017–2022) was prioritized wherever possible; however, less contemporary sources (1997–2016) were also utilized when more recent data was not available.

3. Enhanced recovery after thoracic surgery

The concept of ERAS protocols was first described with regards to colorectal surgery in 1997 by Kehlet [2], and this protocolized approach was soon adapted to various other surgical specialties, including thoracic surgery [3]. The aim of such protocols is to minimize the stress response to major surgery and thereby expedite postoperative return to homeostasis. enhanced recovery after thoracic surgery (ERATS) protocols, in comparison to other surgical specialties, places a heavier emphasis on the quality rather than the speed of patient recovery [4]. They have been shown to improve patient outcomes after surgery, minimize fluid overload, and reduce the rates of pulmonary and cardiac complications [5]. They have the additional benefit of minimizing not only individual practitioner variability, but also analgesic practices associated with greater negative side effect profiles such as schedule II opioids [6, 7]. Furthermore, with regards to operative strategy (i.e., video-assisted thoracoscopic surgery [VATS] versus thoracotomy], the implementation of ERATS protocols may help minimize the differences in outcome conferred by surgical incision [8].

And while improving the quality of patient recovery remains the focus, the speed and efficiency of postoperative recovery is also improved with ERATS pathways, as demonstrated by a statistically significant decrease in postoperative time to removal of chest drains, time to enteral nutrition, and time to ambulation [9]. The net result of these improvements is a reduction in hospital and ICU length of stay as well as an overall decrease in hospital costs [10, 11]. For patients undergoing pulmonary resections for malignancy, this quicker return to baseline also means a quicker return to intended oncologic treatments, positively affecting the ability of those patients to initiate and complete adjuvant chemotherapy and radiation [4].

In 2018, the ERAS® Society and the European Society of Thoracic Surgeons (ESTS) released recommendations for enhanced recovery after lung surgery [5]. However, ERATS protocols remain largely institution specific in the United States [11].

4. Preoperative phase

4.1 Screening and optimization

The main goals of preoperative care are to identify high-risk patients, address modifiable risk factors, and optimize organ function (**Table 1**) [1].

Preoperative care often begins with preoperative counseling. This can take the form of verbalized education, leaflets, and/or multimedia information. Such counseling helps to address patient concerns and set realistic expectations. It has been suggested that psychological counseling may help improve postoperative pain, behavioral recovery, and length of stay after surgery [12].

Routine preoperative lab work should be collected on patients undergoing thoracic surgery. It is important to identify and correct preoperative anemia, as it is associated with increased postoperative morbidity and mortality [13]. Underlying

Risk Factor	Criteria
Anemia	Hemoglobin <12 g/dL (females) or < 13 g/dL (males)
Dysnatremia	Serum sodium <135 mEq/L or > 145 mEq/L
Malnutrition	10–15% weight loss within 6 months, BMI <18.5 kg/m^2, serum albumin <3.0 g/dL
Hyperglycemia	Elevated HbA1c (for patients with diabetes mellitus)
Renal impairment	High serum creatinine or low GFR
Alcohol dependency	Alcohol use within 4 weeks of surgery (for patients with chronic alcohol abuse)
Active smoking	Ongoing smoking within 4 weeks of surgery
Poor lung function	FEV1 or DLCO <40% of expected
Impaired functional capacity	$VO2_{max}$ < 15 mL/kg/min

BMI (body mass index), HbA1c (glycosylated hemoglobin A), GFR (glomerular filtration rate), FEV1 (forced expiratory volume in 1 second), DLCO (diffusing capacity for carbon monoxide), $VO2_{max}$ (maximal oxygen consumption).

Table 1.
Preoperative considerations for patients participating in ERATS.

causes should be addressed, and iron therapy should be initiated when appropriate. Correction of even mild anemia (hemoglobin <12 g/dL in females and < 13 g/dL in males) can reduce the need for perioperative blood transfusion [14]. Preoperative blood transfusion should be avoided whenever possible, as perioperative transfusion has been associated with worse outcomes in cancer patients [15]. Dysnatremia (serum sodium <135 mEq/L or > 145 mEq/L) should similarly be identified and correctly, as it has also been shown to be an independent risk factor for perioperative mortality in patients with lung cancer [13].

Nutrition is another preoperative consideration, as malnutrition is an important modifiable risk factor. Up to 28% of patients with operable lung cancer are at severe nutritional risk [14], and routine preoperative nutrition screening can help identify malnourished patients who may be at increased risk for postoperative complications. Patients with weight loss of 10–15% within six months, BMI <18.5 kg/m^2, and/or serum albumin <3.0 g/dL should receive nutritional support for 10–14 days prior to surgery, and it may be beneficial to delay surgery to allow for this support [1, 14]. Although the traditional methodology has been to keep patient NPO after midnight on the day of surgery, it has been shown that these restrictions are needlessly prohibitive. Instead, it is recommended to allow intake of clear liquids up to two hours prior to surgery and solid foods up to 6 hours prior to surgery for patients without conditions associated with gastric outlet obstruction [5]. Preoperative carbohydrate loading—often in the form of carbohydrate drinks—can decrease postoperative insulin resistance and, although this has not been thoroughly investigated in diabetic patients, is generally believed to be safe in patients with well-controlled diabetes [5]. It may also serve to decrease postoperative nausea and vomiting (PONV).

Glycemic management is an important factor to consider in patients undergoing thoracic surgery. This is true not only of patients with known history of diabetes mellitus, but also those without. A glycosylated hemoglobin A (HbA1c) may be checked preoperatively in order to assess overall glycemic control. A higher HbA1c is associated with high levels of intraoperative insulin resistance, and intraoperative hyperglycemia has been shown to be an independent predictor of postoperative complications and mortality in patients with and without diabetes [16, 17]. Patients with uncontrolled preoperative glucose levels should therefore be referred to either their primary care physician or endocrinologist for optimization prior to surgery.

Alcohol dependency is associated with increased postoperative pulmonary complications (PPCs) and mortality in patients undergoing surgery for lung cancer [5]. The chronic effects of alcohol abuse are known to have deleterious effects on cardiac function as well as coagulation and immune functions, thereby leading to increased morbidity. Patients with alcohol dependency should therefore completely abstain from alcohol intake prior to undergoing thoracic surgery; while this may reduce the incidence of PPCs, it has not been shown to significantly reduce mortality or LOS [5]. It should be noted that this recommendation only applies to patients with alcohol use disorder rather than all patients who consume alcohol.

Smoking cessation should be strongly encouraged in all patients undergoing thoracic surgery. Active smoking is associated with high risk for post-operative complications, and its risks are slowly mitigated by complete preoperative cessation [18]. Not only does it confer an elevated risk of myocardial infarction, cerebrovascular accident, and likelihood of death within 30 days of surgery [1], but patients who smoke are twice as likely to experience PPCs than never smokers or, importantly, those who had quit smoking for at least four weeks [5]. Furthermore, ongoing smoking at the time of surgery is associated with poor postoperative quality of life, increased fatigue, and reduced long-term survival [19]. The deleterious effects of smoking on pulmonary function have been shown to improve within four weeks of cessation, and, when feasible, it may be reasonable to delay surgery for up to four weeks to allow for smoking cessation [20]. Various smoking cessation interventions such as behavioral support, pharmacotherapy, and nicotine replacement may be used, although there is no strong evidence to suggest that these specific methods actively decrease postoperative morbidity [5].

Poor preoperative lung function and physical inactivity are also among the biggest risk factors for poor outcomes after thoracic surgery [1]. The most common preoperative assessments of lung function include exercise testing in conjunction with pulmonary function tests. Thus, preoperative optimization of pulmonary function ("pulmonary prehabilitation") is another tenet of ERATS protocols. Although there are no current consensus guidelines regarding the exact nature and duration of pulmonary prehabilitation, patients who underwent moderate to high intensity preoperative training programs for a median duration of four weeks with a frequency of five sessions per week were demonstrated to have a significant improvement in lung function [21], as well as improved postoperative outcomes and quality of life [1]. Patients with untreated chronic obstructive pulmonary disease (COPD) are at increased risk for PPCs and therefore stand to benefit significantly from preoperative pulmonary optimization. Such patients should be started on a long-acting bronchodilator to improve respiratory symptoms and pulmonary function; additionally, inhaled corticosteroids may help to improve postoperative outcomes in these patients [14].

4.2 High-risk patients and procedures

It is important to note, however, that ERATS protocols are designed with most, but not all patients in mind. Patient selection and safety are paramount, and protocol should never be allowed to supersede surgical decision making. High-risk surgical candidates should be identified through routine preoperative screening. Risk factors for poor outcomes after thoracic surgery include age, obesity, poor preoperative lung function (forced expiratory volume in 1 second [FEV1] or diffusing capacity for carbon monoxide [DLCO] <40% of expected), impaired functional capacity (maximal oxygen consumption [$VO2_{max}$] <15 mL/kg/min), higher ASA physical status, ongoing alcohol abuse, active smoking, insulin-dependent diabetes mellitus, chronic kidney disease, and regular preoperative analgesic use [14]. Providers may wish to exclude such high-risk patients from ERATS pathways. Special consideration should also be given to patients undergoing particularly high-risk procedures (e.g., esophagectomy or pneumonectomy), as there are no current guidelines specific to such procedures [7], although traditional ERATS pathways may still be of benefit [22]. As the adoption of ERATS protocols continues to rise, perhaps high-risk procedure-specific recommendations will be made.

5. Intraoperative phase

5.1 Pulmonary physiology

At the most basic level, the pulmonary system exists to facilitate gas exchange from the environmental air we breathe in to the blood in the circulatory system. Respiratory tract organs include the nose, throat, larynx, trachea, bronchi, and lungs, the right lung having three lobes and the left lung having two lobes. The lobes of the lung are made up of small sacks of air called alveoli, and it is at the surface of these alveoli where oxygen exchange occurs via diffusion from the air into pulmonary arterioles. Clinically this is important because an improperly functioning pulmonary system will manifest as hypoxia in the thoracic patient. Hypoxia can have many different etiologies. Hypoventilation occurs when ventilation of the alveoli is decreased. Ventilation-perfusion (V/Q) mismatch occurs when there is an imbalance between available ventilation and arteriolar perfusion, either related to anatomical regions of the lung or various disease states. Right-to-left shunting occurs when deoxygenated blood from the right side of the heart is allowed to bypass the lungs and instead move to the left side of the heart, either anatomical or physiological, and results in a pathological alternate pathway of circulation. Diffusion limitation occurs when oxygen cannot efficiently move from alveoli to pulmonary arterioles, usually related to chronic disease states [23].

Understanding these basic principles is important in understanding the pathophysiologic mechanisms that underlie the creation of acute lung injury (ALI) during and after one-lung ventilation (OLV) in the thoracic surgery patient [24]. Injury to the ventilated lung is primarily through hyperperfusion and ventilator-induced injury. High tidal volumes produce end-inspiratory lung overdistention and result in alveolar damage, increased alveolar-capillary permeability, and gross pulmonary edema [24]. Hyperperfusion, when the ventilated lung is exposed to high pulmonary blood flow, can result in capillary shear stress and disruption of the capillary endothelium. Injury to the non-ventilated, collapsed lung is primarily through ischemia–reperfusion injury, as well as shear stress on reventilation. Lung re-expansion from the atelectatic state exposes the alveolar units to significant mechanical stress and creates high shear forces affecting the adjacent alveoli [24]. Hypoperfusion and ischemia in the collapsed lung can result in microvascular permeability, capillary leak, and lung edema, while reperfusion injury is similar to hyperperfusion injury in the ventilated lung. Systemic factors affecting both lungs include the release of proinflammatory cytokines and reactive oxygen species (ROS), resulting in damage to the endothelial glycocalyx and a leaky alveolar-capillary membrane [24]. Surgical trauma and manipulation alone can cause alveolar damage. It is important to realize that OLV in any form is nonphysiologic and will result in some degree of lung injury, but protective OLV can be implemented to reduce the risk and severity of ALI in this specific patient population.

5.2 One-lung ventilation

The idea of isolated lung ventilation can be dated back as early as the late 19th century, and its birth and development have allowed for facilitation of complex thoracic surgical procedures, as well as extension of use into esophageal, mediastinal, orthopedic, and neurosurgical procedures [25]. OLV in its most basic form allows the anesthesiologist to control ventilation to each lung, deflating the operative (nondependent) lung and preferentially ventilating the non-operative (dependent) lung. OLV facilitates good surgical exposure of the collapsed lung in the thoracic patient, while ensuring adequate gas exchange of the ventilated lung and protecting it from contamination with surgical debris, pus, or secretions from the operative lung [26, 27]. OLV is not an all-or-nothing phenomenon, as the extent of lung deflation differentiates lung separation (adequate deflation) from lung isolation (complete deflation) [27]. Common indications include pulmonary resection, video-assisted thoracoscopic surgeries, biopsies of the lungs or lymph nodes, thoracic aortic surgery, esophageal surgery, mediastinal surgery, among many others.

5.3 Anesthesia equipment

OLV is typically achieved using either a double-lumen endobronchial tube (DLT) (**Figure 1**), or an endobronchial blocker (BBs) (**Figure 2**), although DLTs are the predominant technique utilized. Recent surveys conducted by the European Association of Cardiothoracic Anesthesiologists suggest that DLTs are preferred by a large majority (>90%) of thoracic anesthesiologists, with many of these experts (up to 30%) stating they never use BBs [26]. Despite the predominance of DLTs, users should still be familiar with and possess basic knowledge of BBs, as well as SLTs, to ensure safe management of OLV and ensure safety of the thoracic patient while on the operation table. Both DLTs and BBs can be used safely in most thoracic procedures, and choice of device is typically guided by patient-specific factors, operator preference and experience, etc.

Single-lumen endobronchial tubes (SLTs) are another alternative, possessing a single lumen with a distal bronchial cuff and a proximal tracheal cuff. Both lungs can be ventilated when the proximal cuff is inflated and the tip of the SLT remains within the trachea, or the SLT can be advanced into one of the mainstem bronchi and OLV achieved with inflation of the distal cuff (proximal cuff remains deflated) [27]. These have fallen out of favor for reasons such as inability to aspirate secretions from the operative lung. Their use is mainly reserved for emergency situations intraoperatively (such as an initially unrecognized difficult airway) where securing the airway is the main priority, as this is performed quickest and easiest with a SLT; they can also be used in pediatric populations. Additionally, in situations where a patient has known anatomical abnormalities of the airway (e.g., after laryngeal or pharyngeal surgery, tracheostomy), the patient has a predicted or recognized difficult airway, or are at risk for vocal cord injury, use of SLTs would be a suitable option [27].

DLTs remain the gold standard technique for OLV in many thoracic surgical procedures, and their design is thanks to Frank Robertshaw in the mid-20th century,

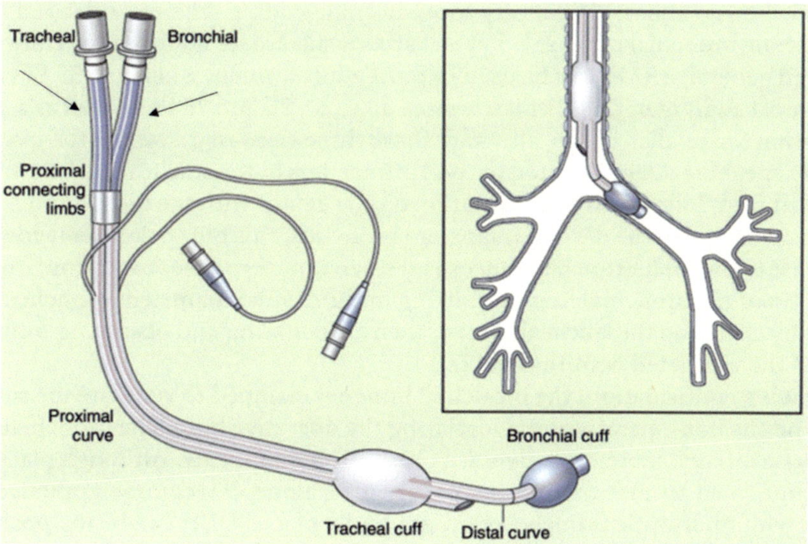

Figure 1.
Typical double lumen tube (DLT) and appropriate positioning within the trachea and mainstem bronchi. Arrows indicating where to clamp each of the tracheal and bronchial lumens as detailed in section 4.3.

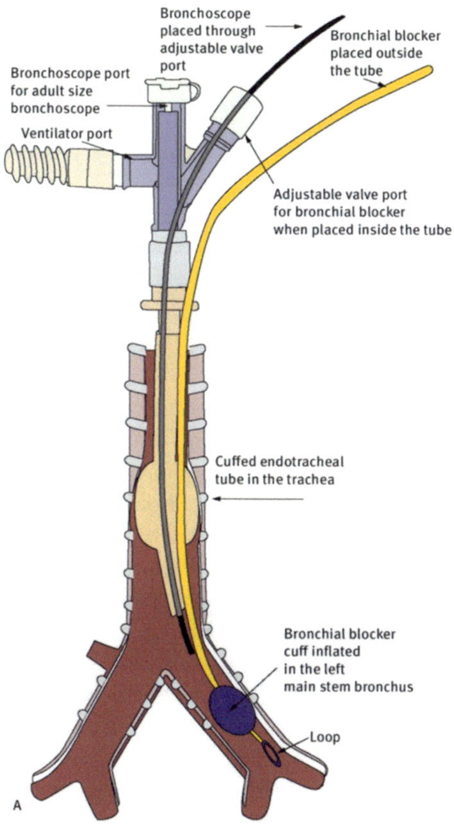

Figure 2.
Bronchial blocker and appropriate positioning within the trachea and main stem bronchi.

who settled on an almost universally adopted color-coding scheme with a red tracheal cuff and blue bronchial cuff [25]. Typical sizes available for adults range from 35 to 41 French; in general, a 37 Fr can be used in most adult women, whereas a 39 Fr can be used in most adult men [27]. Pediatric sizes do exist, 26 and 28 Fr, as well as a smaller 32 Fr option for smaller adults, although these three sizes are newer on the market relatively speaking. Once inserted to the optimal depth, the tracheal cuff should be inflated first, followed by confirmation of placement with the distal bronchial component sitting in the desired mainstem bronchus, this blue color easily identified in contrast to the pink bronchial mucosa by fiber-optic bronchoscopy. Confirmation that the tip of the bronchial lumen is sitting in the desired mainstem bronchus can be done by clamping the tracheal lumen, then auscultating and observing unilateral ascent of the ventilated hemithorax [27].

Following confirmation, the bronchial lumen is clamped to ventilate the tracheal lumen and the non-operative lung, deflating the operative lung. The bronchial cuff can then be inflated incrementally until the air leak disappears. Although placement can be confirmed by auscultation and observation alone, it is common practice confirm with fiber-optic bronchoscopy, as blindly placed DLTs can be malpositioned upwards of 50% of the time. Importantly, the margin of error for positioning a right-sided DLT is much less compared to a left-sided DLT, given the distance from the carina to the splitting of the upper lobe bronchus on the right (~2.5 cm) compared to the left (~5 cm) [27]. One challenge of DLT use is the lack of objective data and guidance for selection of appropriate size and optimal depth; chest x-ray, computed tomography, and ultrasound have all been suggested to measure tracheal diameter, factoring in patient sex and height to predict DLT size and depth [26, 27]. Undersized tubes can lead to auto positive end-expiratory pressure (PEEP) and pulmonary hyperinflation, failed lung collapse, or tube malposition, while oversized cuffs could potentially lead to serious airway complications such as trachea-bronchial rupture, although the incidence is <1% [26].

Advantages of DLTs include their wide applicability including bronchopulmonary lavage, rapid lung deflation-reinflation times, allowing for bronchoscopy of the non-ventilated lung, and their suitability for operation on both lungs even sequentially in the same surgery. They are inexpensive and easily disposable, allowing for safe, quick and accurate placement. Disadvantages include the higher risk of airway trauma and other adverse events, and occasional need for multiple tube exchanges in settings such as post-operative ventilation and in patients already intubated with a SLT.

Bronchial blockers allow for blocking of one main stem or lobar bronchus and resulting collapse of the lung or lobe distal to that blockage. These are better suited for patients with difficult airway anatomy, pediatric populations, or presence of a tracheostomy. BBs can be used in both nasal and oral intubations, can deflate selective lobes or segments, and can be removed at the conclusion of surgery without the need for tube exchange. Interestingly, transient post-operative symptoms such as sore throat, hoarseness, and irritating cough have been less reported with the use of BBs when compared to DLTs [27]. Disadvantages include limited options for adequate suctioning relative to DLTs, increased risk of balloon displacement, impossibility of differential lung ventilation, high price, and more limited availability.

5.4 Ventilatory protective strategies during one-lung ventilation

Despite being advantageous and useful for the surgeon, OLV subjects the patient to some degree of barotrauma, volutrauma, atelectatrauma, and oxygen toxicity, all of these contributing to ventilator-induced lung injury [28]. Acute ventilatory-induced lung injury and the PPCs that can result will have a strong effect on the morbidity and mortality of the thoracic patient. Ventilatory protective strategies are implemented to mitigate the risks of lung injury and reduce PPCs, usually encompassing the combination of positive-end expiratory pressures (PEEP), tidal volumes (TV), and alveolar recruitment maneuvers (ARMs). Only recently has the idea of individualized PEEP gained popularity, as it was historically set at fixed values, either high or low, with no verdict as to which was better to prevent PPCs. Individualized PEEP can prevent alveolar collapse in the dependent lung, increase the residual volume, improve the V/Q ratio and respiratory compliance, and reduce the shear stress damage caused by periodic opening and closing of the alveoli [28]. This allows for reduced PPCs, such as atelectasis, and better perioperative oxygenation when using an individualized PEEP. Fixed-setting PEEP, on the other hand, may lead to either over-distended or under-ventilated lungs.

Low, rather than high, tidal volumes during OLV have been shown in the clinical setting to decrease the expression of proinflammatory cytokines and their resulting alveolar damage and reduce the risk of postoperative respiratory failure [29]. Large tidal volumes >8–10 mL/kg are typically where you start to see increased inflammatory response, injury to the lungs, and increases in postoperative complications [30]. Lower tidal volumes around 4–6 mL/kg can be used to reduce airway pressures, maintaining driving pressures <25 cmH2O. Lower tidal volumes are associated with preserved gas exchange after OLV, as well as lower incidences of pulmonary infiltration and acute respiratory distress syndrome (ARDS) [30].

5.5 Management of Hypoxia

Thanks to improvements in lung isolation devices, patient positioning techniques, and newer anesthetic agents, the incidence of hypoxemia during OLV has significantly decreased since its early use, approximately 4–10% today compared to 25% in the 1970s [27, 31]. Although less frequent, it is still important to be able to properly manage hypoxemia intra-operatively and understand why it occurs in the first place. When the operative lung is deflated and excluded from ventilation, it becomes atelectatic but continues to be perfused by the pulmonary vasculature, creating a large ventilation-to-perfusion (V/Q) mismatch, and resulting obligatory pulmonary shunt. Hypoxemia results when SpO2 drops below 85–90%, or partial pressure of oxygen (PaO2) drops below 60 mmHg. The pulmonary vasculature detects these changes and responds with vasoconstriction, termed hypoxic pulmonary vasoconstriction (HPV), redirecting blood flow from the poorly ventilated regions of the operative lung to the well-ventilated regions of the non-operative, in an attempt to decrease the pulmonary shunt that was created. HPV is believed to reach its peak within 20–30 minutes of OLV, and the shunt fraction is estimated to be upwards of 35% by 30 minutes of OLV [27, 30]. It is intuitive, then, that any factors inhibiting HPV will worsen the V/Q mismatch and result in hypoxemia.

Risk factors for the development of hypoxemia during OLV can be separated into two categories: patient specific and surgery specific (**Table 2**). As is the case with many other operations and procedures, individuals with other comorbidities including cardiovascular, cerebrovascular, or pulmonary disease are at increased risk of hypoxemia and hypoxemia-induced complications. These patient factors include high BMI (>30 kg/m^2), history of lung surgery on the contralateral side, low baseline PaO2, and normal preoperative spirometry (interestingly, COPD

Risk factors for the development of hypoxemia during OLV
Patient-specific
Cardiovascular, cerebrovascular, or pulmonary disease
BMI > 30 kg/m^2
History of contralateral lung surgery
Low baseline PaO_2
Normal preoperative spirometry
Surgery-specific
Supine positioning
Right-sided laterality for surgery

BMI (body mass index), PaO_2 (partial pressure of oxygen in the arterial blood).

Table 2.
Risk factors for the development of hypoxemia during OLV.

decreases the risk of hypoxemia). Surgery specific factors that increase the risk of hypoxemia during OLV include positioning (supine position) and side of the surgery (right-sided surgery with right lung collapse and left-sided ventilation). Generally speaking, healthy individuals (i.e., normal preoperative spirometry, age < 50 years, BMI <30 kg/m^2, non-smoker, absence of COPD or other major comorbidities) with normal cardiopulmonary function will tolerate transient episodes of desaturation and hypoxemia well without systemic acidosis or circulatory impairment [30]. That said, it is still important to recognize risk factors, recognize when it occurs, and address it appropriately.

Given the risk for hypoxemia during OLV, anesthesia providers should be familiar with the various techniques to identify and correct the cause (**Figure 3**). It is standard to pause from any nonurgent portion of the surgical procedure, restore two-lung ventilation, and increase the fraction of inspired oxygen (FiO2) to 100%. It is important to assess for common causes of hypoxemia such as malpositioning of the lung isolation device. This can be done using fiberoptic bronchoscopy to confirm visually the DLT/BB in optimal position. Fiberoptic bronchoscopy can also be used to inspect all ventilated bronchi and ensure the airway is clear of secretions [30]. After hypoxemia is treated and corrected, OLV can be re-established, and the surgery can move forward. Because persistently high FiO2 has been shown to cause lung injury secondary to its induction of an inflammatory response, oxidative stress, and lung edema, it is important to be judicious in the delivery of oxygen. The goal is to maintain adequate oxygenation while minimizing these deleterious effects of high FiO2, with most sources agreeing on trying to keep FiO2 at or below 60% when possible.

Some pharmacologic interventions have been suggested for the treatment of hypoxemia intraoperatively, although not yet widely adopted. Theoretically, inhaled nitric oxide (iNO) should improve V/Q mismatch via pulmonary artery dilation and increased blood flow to the ventilated lung, however this benefit has not been consistently shown and its routine use is therefore not recommended [30]. Inhaled anesthetics are known to inhibit HPV and worsen V/Q mismatch compared to intravenous anesthetics, so one would think using intravenous anesthetics to maintain general anesthesia would improve oxygenation. This has not consistently been shown to be the case, although volatile anesthetics such as sevoflurane have been shown to

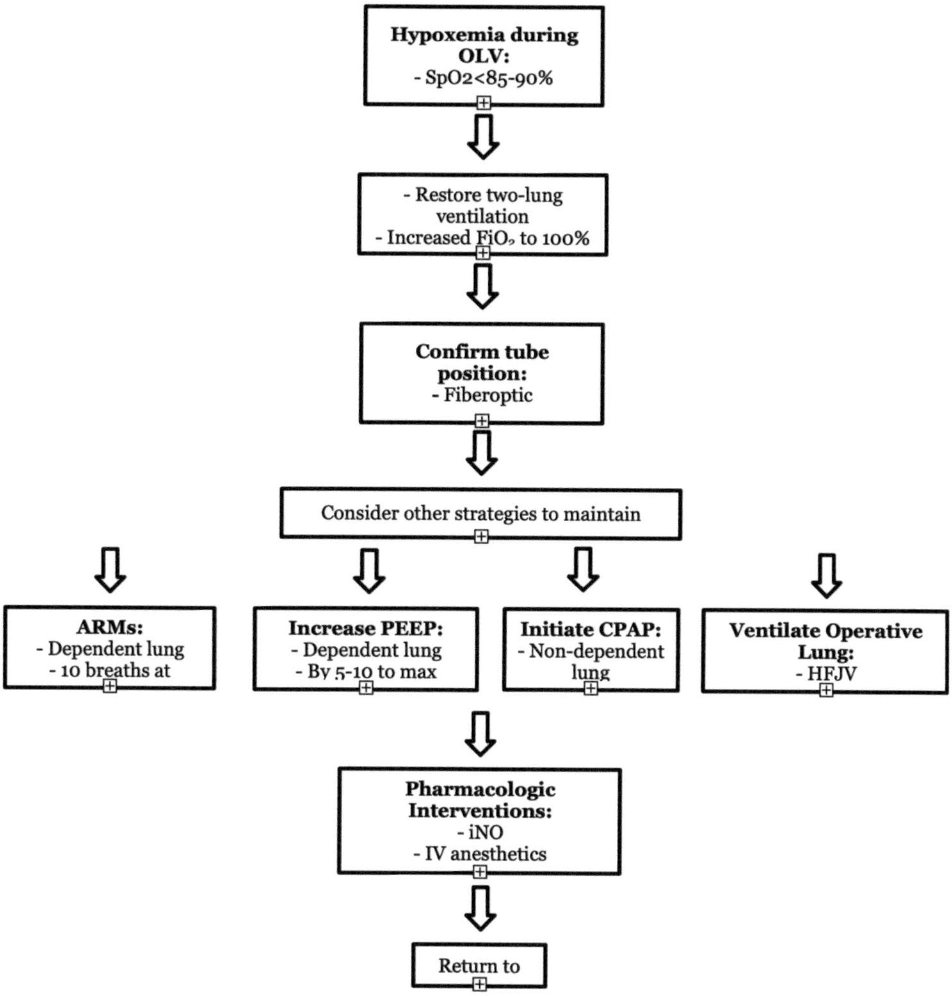

Figure 3.
Strategies for the management of hypoxemia during OLV. HFJV (high-frequency jet ventilation).

attenuate the inflammatory response in the lung and protect the endothelial glycocalyx, without worsening hypoxemia [27].

Alveolar recruitment maneuvers (ARM) before OLV initiation or shortly thereafter have been shown to improve arterial oxygenation and decrease pulmonary shunting as well as dead space, so it is conceivable that ARMs can also treat hypoxemia after it occurs [30]. This typically consists of ten consecutive breaths at a plateau pressure of 40 mmHg. This serves to reserve atelectasis through brief, controlled increases in airway pressure [30]. Incremental increases in PEEP of the non-operative lung, usually levels of 5–10 to a maximum of 20 cmH2O of PEEP, can also improve hypoxemia by opening atelectatic alveoli. It is well accepted that application of PEEP should be individualized to the patient during surgery, rather than generally aiming for high or low PEEP. Continuous positive airway pressure (CPAP) can also be applied to the nondependent, operative lung to improve oxygenation through passive mechanisms, usually starting at 5 cmH2O [27, 30].

5.6 Fluid management

The main goal of fluid management during the intra- and peri-operative periods of thoracic surgery is to minimize end-organ injury while also reducing and preventing postoperative ALI. This is done with targeted fluid administration, where euvolemia, rather than liberal fluid administration, is the goal in surgeries such as lung resection and esophagectomy, to achieve an ideal lung water state [27]. Practice over time has shifted away from the historical standard of liberal fluid administration, as the deleterious effects this can cause have been more documented and understood. Postoperative complications such as pulmonary edema, ARDS, pneumonia, reintubation, prolonged hospital and/or ICU stay, and generally increased morbidity and mortality, can all result from excessive fluid administration in the intra- and peri-operative periods [27]. On the other hand, aggressive fluid restriction can result in postoperative acute kidney injury (AKI), which is associated with increased morbidity. A universally accepted protocol or rule on ideal fluid management strategy has yet to be developed, and the topic remains controversial among surgeons in the field. Goal-directed fluid therapy (GDFT) is gaining favor most recently, using hemodynamic parameters such as pulse pressure variation and stroke volume variation to target fluid administration [27]. GDFT is not applicable to all surgical settings and procedures, however, and further progress needs to be made in fluid management strategies and protocol.

5.7 Regional Anesthesia

Thoracic epidural analgesia (TEA) has traditionally been considered the "gold standard" for postoperative pain control after thoracic surgery. TEA is not without significant risks, however, including hypotension, postoperative urinary retention, and muscle weakness [5]. Regional anesthesia was therefore developed as an alternative to TEA, and a multitude of thoracic wall fascial plane blocks have since been developed. There is evidence to suggest that many of these techniques are equivalent analgesia to TEA [32]. Furthermore, the widespread adoption of ultrasound has revolutionized regional anesthesia. Ultrasound has been instrumental in the development of fascial plane blocks, which rely on the passive spread of local anesthetic (LA) to target nerves, as its use can both guide and confirm needle placement and fascial spread of LA [33].

Regional anesthesia provides pain relief via unilateral afferent nerve blockade, affecting both the somatic and sympathetic nervous systems, thereby downregulating the stress response through decreased activation of the neuroendocrine system [34]. TEA also acts through similar neural mechanisms; however, the bilateral sympathetic blockade produced by TEA is significantly more likely to result in hypotension than is the unilateral effect of regional anesthesia [35]. This phenomenon makes regional blocks an especially attractive option in higher-risk cardiac patients with other comorbid conditions.

Other benefits of regional anesthesia include relative ease of performance and its safety when compared to TEA. The targets for injection are relatively distant from critical structures, resulting in minimal risk of spinal cord injury, epidural hematoma, major vascular injury, and lung or pleural damage [33]. There is the additional benefit that injections sites tend to be superficial and easily compressible, limiting the likelihood of expansile hematomas [36]. As such, thoracic wall blocks may also be considered in patients with coagulopathy, albeit with careful consideration of the risks and benefits. When compared to opioid-based postoperative pain regimens, regional anesthesia is associated with less sedation, less PONV, and less constipation, and thus encourages both earlier postoperative mobilization and earlier initiation of enteral nutrition [37, 38].

While the benefits of regional anesthesia are many, there are several drawbacks associated with fascial plane blocks. Epidural spread of local anesthetic is possible (such as with retrolaminar or erector spinae plane blocks), thus there is a potential concern for resultant hypotension, although the risk is far lower than with TEA [33]. The extent and intensity of pain blockade can be variable due to injection technique as well as several anatomic factors, such as contralateral and/or overlapping innervation [33]. Perhaps the most notable risk of fascial plane blocks is the risk of local

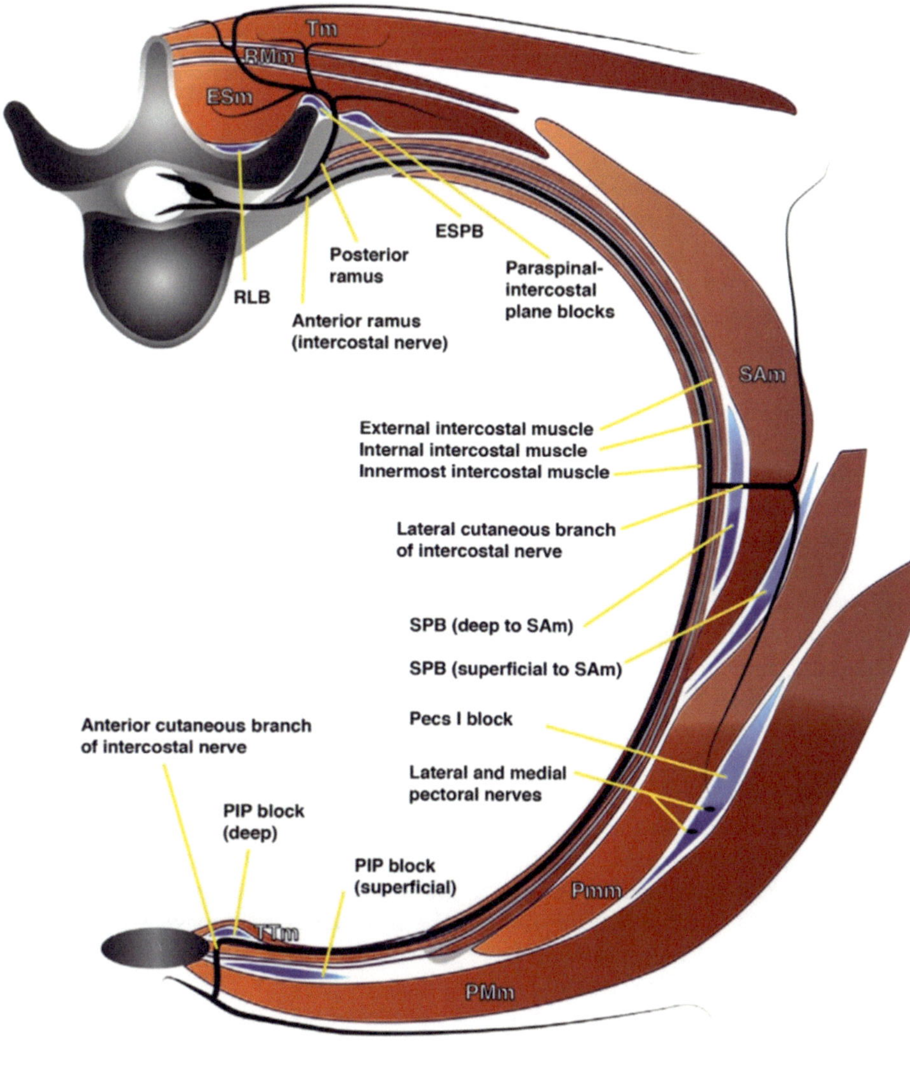

Figure 4.
Thoracic wall fascial plane blocks. PIP (parasternal-intercostal plane), SPB (serratus plane block), ESPB (erector spinae plane block), RLB (retrolaminar block), Tm (trapezius muscle), RMm (rhomboid major muscle), ESm (erector spinae muscle), SAm (serratus anterior muscle), Pmm (pectoralis minor muscle), TTm (transversus thoracis muscle).

anesthetic systemic toxicity (LAST), as relatively large volumes of LA into well-vascularized tissues where the systemic absorption is high thirty). The risk of LAST can be minimized by remaining within the maximum recommended weight-based LA dose limits, adding epinephrine to reduce the systemic absorption of LA, and closely monitoring patients for at least thirty minutes following LA injection with easy accessibility of LAST rescue medications [33].

There are numerous types of thoracic wall and fascial plane blocks available, and providers can tailor specific blocks to expected areas of postoperative pain for each procedure (**Figure 4**). A thorough description of each block is beyond the scope of this chapter; however, a brief review is useful to demonstrate the uses of more commonly used blocks. Included among this list are the intercostal nerve block (ICNB), the paravertebral block (PVB), the erector spinae plane block (ESPB), and the serratus anterior plane block (SAPB). Newer alternatives to the PVB include the retrolaminar block and the mid-point transverse process to pleura block (MTPB).

The ICNB is perhaps one of the most widely utilized blocks given its effectiveness and relative ease of performance. It is most commonly performed intraoperatively by the surgeon prior to chest closure by sequential LA injection into the relevant intercostal spaces, thus interrupting the transmission of afferent pain signals [34]. Its attractiveness has been greatly enhanced by the introduction of liposomal bupivacaine, which allows for up to 96 hours of drug diffusion following a single injection [39]. Studies have shown that ICNB can provide equivalent analgesia to that of TEA [40], and its use has been demonstrated to decrease the risk of major pulmonary complications [41]. As previously noted, there is a risk of LAST with ICNB, as well as bleeding due to the proximity of the intercostal nerves to the associated intercostal arteries.

The PVB is another frequently used form of regional anesthesia in patients undergoing thoracic surgeries. It is performed on the side of surgery either by single injection or catheter placement for continuous infusion [34]. Both methods have been shown to lower postoperative pain scores, postoperative opioid consumption, and rates of PONV; however, continuous PVB can provide a longer duration of analgesia compared to the single injection technique [37]. It provides unilateral somatic and sympathetic analgesia via blockade of both the dorsal and ventral rami as well as the sympathetic chain [35]. It is thus safer to use than TEA given its diminished risk for causing hypotension. Notably, it may provide more intense and longer lasting analgesia compared to interpleural blocks [35].

Newer alternatives to the PVB include the retrolaminar block and MTPB. The retrolaminar block was developed as a simpler landmark-guided alternative to PVB, and entails injection of LA into the fascial plane that lies between the posterior surface of the thoracic lamina and the transversospinalis muscles [33]. Thus, this technique avoids the need to enter the true paravertebral space by forgoing the need to pierce the superior costotransverse ligament. The MTPB is similar to the retrolaminar block but involves LA injection just beyond the posterior aspect of the thoracic transverse processes while still remaining superficial to the superior costotransverse ligament [33]. The advantages of these two approaches are conferring a similar level of analgesia to PVB while carrying less risk of pleural puncture [33].

The ESPB involves injection of LA into the fascial plane between the thoracic transverse processes and the longissimus thoracis muscle [35]. This results in LA spread to the paravertebral and epidural spaces, as well as to the lateral cutaneous branches of the intercostal nerves [33]. Performance of ESPB confers lower postoperative active and passive pain scores, less PONV, and faster time to postoperative mobilization, and it has been shown to be non-inferior to PVB [37]. Additionally, it may be more specifically indicated if damage to the parietal pleural leaflet has occurred, which would preclude the use of PVB with catheter [37].

The SAPB is a relatively quick and easily performed technique and may be performed either superficial to or deep within the serratus anterior muscle [33]. Both techniques primarily target the lateral cutaneous branches of the intercostal nerves, although may also target the long thoracic nerve and/or thoracodorsal nerve as well depending on injection site and amount of LA infiltrated [35]. It can be performed anywhere between the anterior and posterior axillary lines between the second and seventh ribs. It has limited side-effects, although has been associated with slightly higher levels of opioid consumption when compared to PVB [37].

It is worth noting that these methods of regional anesthesia do little to alleviate the postoperative shoulder pain that stems from diaphragmatic irritation transmitted along the phrenic nerve. This commonly encountered symptom may be addressed anesthetizing the phrenic nerve intraoperatively via LA infiltration of the periphrenic fat pad above and below the hilum [34, 42]. Performance of phrenic nerve infiltration, however, should be contingent the absence of any respiratory contraindication and requires close postoperative monitoring [43].

In 2022, new PROSPECT (PROcedure-SPEcific Postoperative Pain ManagemenT) guidelines were released detailing recommendations for VATS. Either PVB or ESPB is recommended for all patients undergoing VATS, and SAPB may be used as a second-line choice; TEA is not recommended for any VATS procedures [37]. Whereas previous PROSPECT guidelines had recommended TEA when performing thoracotomy, PVB is now recommended for open thoracic surgeries as well [44].

6. Postoperative phase

6.1 Postoperative pain control

Postoperative pain can have a significant effect on patient outcomes following thoracic surgery. Acute pain alters pulmonary mechanics, such as diminished vital capacity and poor pulmonary toilet [45]. Such deleterious effects can lead to the development of atelectasis and pneumonia [1]. The long-term effects of inadequate analgesia are also important to consider, as circulating humoral inflammatory factors can induce central sensitization [32]. Consequently, poorly controlled postoperative pain has been linked to the development of chronic postoperative pain (CPOP), such as post-thoracotomy pain syndrome [7, 46]. As surgery on the chest is often considered among the most painful surgical procedures, adequate perioperative pain control is critically important, not only due to ethical considerations and patient satisfaction, but also for improving patient outcomes after thoracic surgery.

ERATS protocols are focused on attenuating the stress response and homeostatic disruptions that accompany major surgery [5, 7]. Tissue damage from surgery activates a systemic inflammatory response, thereby causing changes in the neuroendocrine, metabolic, and immune systems [47]. This pro-inflammatory immune imbalance can lead to organ dysfunction and, ultimately, higher rates of postoperative complication. Poorly-controlled postoperative pain can worsen this immune imbalance through further modulation of the neuroendocrine axis, thereby increasing the body's stress response to surgery [32]. It is logical, therefore, that attenuation of pain perception with adequate analgesia has been shown to decrease levels of proinflammatory cytokines [34].

Multimodal analgesia is the cornerstone of postoperative pain control after thoracic surgery and is a major component of ERATS protocols. The combination of opioid and non-opioid analgesics, when used in conjunction with perioperative regional anesthesia, provides both a central and peripheral pain block, and has been shown to improve patient outcomes and decrease HLOS [32]. Multimodal pain control stems from the concept that several analgesic agents with different mechanisms of action may have synergistic effects in both the prevention and the treatment of acute postoperative pain [7]. Ideally, this also allows for the minimization of side effects of each individual anesthetic agent as well [5]. By utilizing non-opioid adjuncts, there is the additional benefit of reducing opioid-related side effects, such as constipation, PONV, and sedation.

The use of oral acetaminophen for postoperative analgesia is well established, and it is a vital component of ERATS pathways. At clinical doses, acetaminophen has few adverse effects or contraindications, and it can additionally be used safely in patients with renal failure [5]. Intravenous acetaminophen, having been approved by the United States Food and Drug Administration in 2010, has also been increasingly utilized for thoracic surgery [32].

Non-steroidal anti-inflammatory drugs (NSAIDs) are another frequently used adjunct in postoperative pain control. The combination of NSAIDs with acetaminophen has been shown to be more effective than either drug when used alone [48]. Intravenous ketorolac has powerful analgesic effects; however, the risks and benefits should be carefully weighed prior to administering, as its use has been shown to increase the volume of blood in thoracic drains [49]. Cyclooxygenase-2 inhibitors such as celecoxib are sometimes preferred in the postoperative setting due to their lessened effect on platelet function. There is a risk of renal failure with NSAID use, especially in patients with advanced age, hypovolemia, or pre-existing renal failure, and these risk factors may be present in patients undergoing thoracic surgery [5]. There is also the theoretical concern that the anti-inflammatory properties of NSAIDs may reduce the efficacy of surgical pleurodesis, although this phenomenon has yet to be proven in human studies. Animal studies, however, have demonstrated a significant reduction in the quality of pleural adhesions with NSAID use [50].

The use of N-methyl-D-aspartate (NMDA) antagonists has become increasingly popular given their analgesic properties. Ketamine should be considered for use in some postoperative patients; it is an especially attractive option for patients with a history of chronic opioid use [5]. The addition of low-dose ketamine to morphine in patient-controlled analgesia (PCA) was shown to reduce morphine use and improve early postoperative lung function in patients who had undergone thoracic surgery [51]. Although the NMDA receptor is known to play a role in central sensitization and neuropathic pain, studies have unfortunately failed to show a reduction in the incidence of CPOP with NMDA antagonist use [32].

Gamma-aminobutyric acid (GABA) analogs such a gabapentin and pregabalin, target neuropathic pain pathways, and while they have demonstrated efficacy in multiple neuropathic pain conditions, multiple studies have failed to show that these agents reduce either acute or chronic postoperative pain following thoracic surgery [5, 11, 32, 37]. Furthermore, it was not shown to alleviate the ipsilateral shoulder pain commonly seen in patients receiving TEA [5]. Therefore, neither PROSPECT nor ERAS/ESTS guidelines recommended postoperative gabapentinoid use.

Glucocorticoids have multiple actions, several of which (e.g., analgesic, antiemetic, antipyretic, anti-inflammatory) may be beneficial for patients having recently undergone surgery. However, the adverse effects of glucocorticoid use are also wide ranging, including gastric irritation, poor wound healing, sodium retention, and, notably, impaired glucose homeostasis leading to hyperglycemia [5]. There is no current consensus regarding the optimal dose that balances these advantages and disadvantages. And while the use of steroids such as dexamethasone and methylprednisolone has been shown to produce opioid-sparing effects and reduced pain scores in other surgical settings, there is limited procedure-specific evidence for their use in VATS [37]. Therefore, routine use of glucocorticoids is not recommended for patients undergoing thoracic surgery.

Postoperative opioid use, including PCA, should be minimized or, if feasible, avoided altogether [5]. When opioids are utilized, their benefits (such as analgesia and prevention of splinting) should be very carefully weighed against their multiple detrimental effects (including constipation, PONV, sedation, and ventilatory suppression). If opioids are necessary to achieve adequate levels of pain control, their use should be limited to rescue analgesia in cases of breakthrough pain.

6.2 Postoperative pulmonary complications

Postoperative pulmonary complications may lead to longer HLOS, worsen outcomes, and even increased mortality in patients undergoing thoracic surgery [52]. Thoracic procedures have a higher incidence of PPCs than non-thoracic surgical procedures. This is likely due to the nature of the operation and the patient characteristics, but also the result of interventions done in the intraoperative period. It is for this reason that ventilatory protective strategies are becoming more widely accepted, in attempts to decrease the incidence of such complications. The overall incidence of PPCs in the thoracic surgery patient population has been shown to be as high as 45.7% [53]. These complications range on a spectrum from more minor complications such postoperative supplemental oxygen and hypotension, to more severe complications such as respiratory failure and ARDS, unplanned invasive or non-invasive mechanical ventilation, pneumonia, unplanned ICU admission, increased HLOS, and hospital mortality (**Table 3**) [53]. Predictably, patients deemed moderate to high risk had a higher incidence of PPCs than those deemed low risk, this included increased age, higher BMI, the presence of COPD and other comorbidities, and male gender. Patients with higher preoperative ASA and

Postoperative Pulmonary Complications
Severe
Respiratory failure
Acute respiratory distress syndrome
Invasive ventilation
Non-invasive ventilation
Pneumonia
Unplanned ICU admission
Increased hospital length of stay
Hospital mortality
Minor
Supplemental oxygen
Hypotension
Transient arrythmias

Table 3.
Summary of postoperative pulmonary complications by severity.

ARISCAT scores also had higher incidences of PPCs. Interestingly, there seems to be no difference in incidence of PPCs when comparing OLV to two-lung ventilation (TLV), or when comparing open and endoscopic procedures [53]. It is important to understand the relationship between thoracic surgical procedures, the characteristics of this patient population, and the ensuing PPCs, so that we can develop scores and other strategies of risk prediction specific to this population and optimize the allocation of resources to minimize the incidence of such complications [53].

7. Conclusion

As ERATS protocols continue to gain widespread adoption, they will continue to have a significant impact on how providers manage patients undergoing thoracic procedures. As more research into the efficacies of ERATS protocols emerges, these pathways will inexorably change in response, as they have already done since their inception. So too do advances in surgical and anesthetic techniques affect the course of ERATS protocols. The rise of minimally invasive thoracic surgery over the past three decades has revolutionized the field of thoracic surgery, mandating significant changes in evidence-based guidelines and new standards of care. More recently, the use of robotic surgery has risen and may well continue to gain traction, which may lead to updated guidelines in the future. Already, many of the components of ERATS are now received by a majority of patients undergoing thoracic surgery, such that some aspects may be considered "standard" rather than "enhanced" care [3]. As such, it is possible that we are moving towards a "post-ERATS" era, although this is more a distinction in nomenclature than in actual concept. As new standards of care are adopted, new methods for enhanced care will certainly emerge, although it is difficult to accurately predict the direction this will take. Regardless of the direction they take, such protocols are aimed at providing the best possible outcome for the thoracic surgery patient, and, although practices continue to evolve, providing safe and effective perioperative care for those undergoing thoracic surgeries will always remain at the forefront.

Conflict of interest

The authors declare no conflict of interest.

Author details

James Pellechi*, Sean DuBois and Meredith Harrison
St. Luke's University Health Network, Bethlehem, Pennsylvania, USA

*Address all correspondence to: james.pellechi@sluhn.org

IntechOpen

© 2022 The Author(s). Licensee IntechOpen. This chapter is distributed under the terms of the Creative Commons Attribution License (http://creativecommons.org/licenses/by/3.0), which permits unrestricted use, distribution, and reproduction in any medium, provided the original work is properly cited.

References

[1] Dinic VD, Stojanovic MD, Markovic D, Cvetanovic V, Vukovic AZ, Jankovic RJ. Enhanced recovery in thoracic surgery: A review. Frontiers in Medicine. 2018;**5**:14. Published 2018 Feb 5. DOI: 10.3389/fmed.2018.00014

[2] Kehlet H. Multimodal approach to control postoperative pathophysiology and rehabilitation. British Journal of Anaesthesia. 1997;**78**(5):606-617. DOI: 10.1093/bja/78.5.606

[3] Brunelli A. Enhanced recovery after surgery in thoracic surgery: The past, the present and the future. Video-Assisted Thoracic Surgery. 2017;**2**(7). DOI: 10.21037/vats.2017.07.02

[4] Haywood N, Nickel I, Zhang A, et al. Enhanced recovery after thoracic surgery. Thoracic Surgery Clinics. 2020;**30**(3):259-267. DOI: 10.1016/j.thorsurg.2020.04.005

[5] Batchelor TJP, Rasburn NJ, Abdelnour-Berchtold E, et al. Guidelines for enhanced recovery after lung surgery: Recommendations of the enhanced recovery after surgery (ERAS®) society and the European Society of Thoracic Surgeons (ESTS). European Journal of Cardio-Thoracic Surgery. 2019;**55**(1): 91-115. DOI: 10.1093/ejcts/ezy301

[6] Kodia K, Stephens-McDonnough JA, Alnajar A, Villamizar NR, Nguyen DM. Implementation of an enhanced recovery after thoracic surgery care pathway for thoracotomy patients-achieving better pain control with less (schedule II) opioid utilization. Journal of Thoracic Disease. 2021;**13**(7):3948-3959. DOI: 10.21037/jtd-21-552

[7] Thompson C, French DG, Costache I. Pain management within an enhanced recovery program after thoracic surgery. Journal of Thoracic Disease. 2018;**10**(Suppl. 32):S3773-S3780. DOI: 10.21037/jtd.2018.09.112

[8] Krebs ED, Mehaffey JH, Sarosiek BM, Blank RS, Lau CL, Martin LW. Is less really more? Reexamining video-assisted thoracoscopic versus open lobectomy in the setting of an enhanced recovery protocol. The Journal of Thoracic and Cardiovascular Surgery. 2019;**159**(1):S0022-5223(19)31771-4. DOI: 10.1016/j.jtcvs.2019.08.036

[9] Tahiri M, Goudie E, Jouquan A, Martin J, Ferraro P, Liberman M. Enhanced recovery after video-assisted thoracoscopic surgery lobectomy: A prospective, historically controlled, propensity-matched clinical study. Canadian Journal of Surgery. 2020;**63**(3):E233-E240. Published 2020 May 8. DOI: 10.1503/cjs.001919

[10] Draeger TB, Gibson VR, Fernandez G, Andaz SK. Enhanced recovery after thoracic surgery (ERATS). Heart, Lung & Circulation. 2021;**30**(8):1251-1255. DOI: 10.1016/j.hlc.2021.01.014

[11] Peng T, Shemanski KA, Ding L, et al. Enhanced recovery after surgery protocol minimizes intensive care unit utilization and improves outcomes following pulmonary resection. World Journal of Surgery. 2021;**45**(10):2955-2963. DOI: 10.1007/s00268-021-06259-1

[12] Powell R, Scott NW, Manyande A, et al. Psychological preparation and postoperative outcomes for adults undergoing surgery under general anaesthesia. Cochrane Database of Systematic Reviews. 2016; **2016**(5):CD008646. Published 2016 May

26. DOI: 10.1002/14651858.CD008646.pub2

[13] Jean RA, DeLuzio MR, Kraev AI, et al. Analyzing risk factors for morbidity and mortality after lung resection for lung Cancer using the NSQIP database. Journal of the American College of Surgeons. 2016;**222**(6):992-1000.e1. DOI: 10.1016/j.jamcollsurg.2016.02.020

[14] Jones NL, Edmonds L, Ghosh S, Klein AA. A review of enhanced recovery for thoracic anaesthesia and surgery. Anaesthesia. 2013;**68**(2):179-189. DOI: 10.1111/anae.12067

[15] Luan H, Ye F, Wu L, Zhou Y, Jiang J. Perioperative blood transfusion adversely affects prognosis after resection of lung cancer: A systematic review and a meta-analysis. BMC Surgery. 2014;**14**:34. Published 2014 May 23. DOI: 10.1186/1471-2482-14-34

[16] Lazar HL, McDonnell M, Chipkin SR, et al. The Society of Thoracic Surgeons practice guideline series: Blood glucose management during adult cardiac surgery. The Annals of Thoracic Surgery. 2009;**87**(2):663-669. DOI: 10.1016/j.athoracsur.2008.11.011

[17] Sato H, Carvalho G, Sato T, Lattermann R, Matsukawa T, Schricker T. The association of preoperative glycemic control, intraoperative insulin sensitivity, and outcomes after cardiac surgery. The Journal of Clinical Endocrinology and Metabolism. 2010;**95**(9):4338-4344. DOI: 10.1210/jc.2010-0135

[18] Mason DP, Subramanian S, Nowicki ER, et al. Impact of smoking cessation before resection of lung cancer: A Society of Thoracic Surgeons general thoracic surgery database study. The Annals of Thoracic Surgery. 2009;**88**(2):362-371. DOI: 10.1016/j.athoracsur.2009.04.035

[19] Balduyck B, Sardari Nia P, Cogen A, et al. The effect of smoking cessation on quality of life after lung cancer surgery. European Journal of Cardio-Thoracic Surgery. 2011;**40**(6):1432-1438. DOI: 10.1016/j.ejcts.2011.03.004

[20] Sørensen LT. Wound healing and infection in surgery. The clinical impact of smoking and smoking cessation: A systematic review and meta-analysis. Archives of Surgery. 2012;**147**(4):373-383. DOI: 10.1001/archsurg.2012.5

[21] Sebio Garcia R, Yáñez Brage MI, Giménez Moolhuyzen E, Granger CL, Denehy L. Functional and postoperative outcomes after preoperative exercise training in patients with lung cancer: A systematic review and meta-analysis. Interactive Cardiovascular and Thoracic Surgery. 2016;**23**(3):486-497. DOI: 10.1093/icvts/ivw152

[22] Low DE, Allum W, De Manzoni G, et al. Guidelines for perioperative Care in Esophagectomy: Enhanced recovery after surgery (ERAS®) society recommendations. World Journal of Surgery. 2019;**43**(2):299-330. DOI: 10.1007/s00268-018-4786-4

[23] Brinkman JE, Sharma S. Physiology, Pulmonary. [Updated 2021 Jul 22]. In: StatPearls [Internet]. Treasure Island (FL): StatPearls Publishing; 2022 Available from: https://www.ncbi.nlm.nih.gov/books/NBK482426/

[24] Lohser J, Slinger P. Lung injury after one-lung ventilation: A review of the pathophysiologic mechanisms affecting the ventilated and the collapsed lung. Anesthesia and Analgesia. 2015;**121**(2):302-318. DOI: 10.1213/ANE.0000000000000808

[25] McGrath B, Tennuci C, Lee G. The history of one-lung Anesthesia and the double-lumen tube. Journal of

Anesthesia History. 2017;**3**(3):76-86. DOI: 10.1016/j.janh.2017.05.002

[26] Huybrechts I, Tuna T, Szegedi LL. Lung separation in adult thoracic anesthesia. Saudi Journal of Anaesthesia. 2021;**15**(3):272-279. DOI: 10.4103/sja.sja_78_21

[27] Shoni M, Rodriguez G. Intraoperative Anesthetic Management of the Thoracic Patient. Thoracic Surgery Clinics. 2020;**30**(3):279-291. DOI: 10.1016/j.thorsurg.2020.04.011

[28] Li P, Kang X, Miao M, Zhang J. Individualized positive end-expiratory pressure (PEEP) during one-lung ventilation for prevention of postoperative pulmonary complications in patients undergoing thoracic surgery: A meta-analysis. Medicine (Baltimore). 2021;**100**(28):e26638. DOI: 10.1097/MD.0000000000026638

[29] Kozian A, Schilling T, Schütze H, Senturk M, Hachenberg T, Hedenstierna G. Ventilatory protective strategies during thoracic surgery: Effects of alveolar recruitment maneuver and low-tidal volume ventilation on lung density distribution. Anesthesiology. 2011;**114**(5):1025-1035. DOI: 10.1097/ALN.0b013e3182164356

[30] Campos JH, Feider A. Hypoxia during one-lung ventilation-a review and update. Journal of Cardiothoracic and Vascular Anesthesia. 2018;**32**(5):2330-2338. DOI: 10.1053/j.jvca.2017.12.026

[31] Lohser J. Managing hypoxemia during minimally invasive thoracic surgery. Anesthesiology Clinics. 2012;**30**(4):683-697. DOI: 10.1016/j.anclin.2012.08.006

[32] Maxwell C, Nicoara A. New developments in the treatment of acute pain after thoracic surgery. Current Opinion in Anaesthesiology. 2014;**27**(1):6-11. DOI: 10.1097/ACO.0000000000000029

[33] Chin KJ. Thoracic wall blocks: From paravertebral to retrolaminar to serratus to erector spinae and back again - a review of evidence. Best Practice & Research. Clinical Anaesthesiology. 2019;**33**(1):67-77. DOI: 10.1016/j.bpa.2019.02.003

[34] Novak-Jankovič V, Markovič-Božič J. Regional Anesthesia in thoracic and abdominal surgery. Acta Clinica Croatica. 2019;**58**(Suppl 1):96-100. DOI: 10.20471/acc.2019.58.s1.14

[35] Helander EM, Webb MP, Kendrick J, et al. PECS, serratus plane, erector spinae, and paravertebral blocks: A comprehensive review. Best Practice & Research. Clinical Anaesthesiology. 2019;**33**(4):573-581. DOI: 10.1016/j.bpa.2019.07.003

[36] Jack JM, McLellan E, Versyck B, Englesakis MF, Chin KJ. The role of serratus anterior plane and pectoral nerves blocks in cardiac surgery, thoracic surgery and trauma: A qualitative systematic review. Anaesthesia. 2020;**75**(10):1372-1385. DOI: 10.1111/anae.15000

[37] Feray S, Lubach J, Joshi GP, Bonnet F, Van de Velde M, PROSPECT Working Group of the European Society of Regional Anaesthesia and Pain Therapy. PROSPECT guidelines for video-assisted thoracoscopic surgery: A systematic review and procedure-specific postoperative pain management recommendations. Anaesthesia. 2022;**77**(3):311-325. DOI: 10.1111/anae.15609

[38] Marshall K, McLaughlin K. Pain Management in Thoracic Surgery. Thoracic Surgery Clinics. 2020;**30**(3):339-346. DOI: 10.1016/j.thorsurg.2020.03.001

[39] Mehran RJ, Walsh GL, Zalpour A, et al. Intercostal nerve blocks with liposomal bupivacaine: Demonstration of safety, and potential benefits. Seminars in Thoracic and Cardiovascular Surgery. 2017;**29**(4):531-537. DOI: 10.1053/j.semtcvs.2017.06.004

[40] Rice DC, Cata JP, Mena GE, Rodriguez-Restrepo A, Correa AM, Mehran RJ. Posterior intercostal nerve block with liposomal bupivacaine: An alternative to thoracic epidural analgesia. The Annals of Thoracic Surgery. 2015;**99**(6):1953-1960. DOI: 10.1016/j.athoracsur.2015.02.074

[41] Corsini EM, Mitchell KG, Zhou N, et al. Liposomal bupivacaine intercostal block is important for reduction of pulmonary complications. The Annals of Thoracic Surgery. 2021;**112**(2):423-429. DOI: 10.1016/j.athoracsur.2020.09.017

[42] Martinez-Barenys C, Busquets J, de Castro PE, et al. Randomized double-blind comparison of phrenic nerve infiltration and suprascapular nerve block for ipsilateral shoulder pain after thoracic surgery. European Journal of Cardio-Thoracic Surgery. 2011;**40**(1):106-112. DOI: 10.1016/j.ejcts.2010.10.025

[43] Zhang Y, Duan F, Ma W. Ultrasound-guided phrenic nerve block for intraoperative persistent hiccups: A case report. BMC Anesthesiology. 2018;**18**(1):123. DOI: 10.1186/s12871-018-0589-2

[44] Joshi G, Bonnet F, Shah R, Wilkinson R, Camu F, Fischer B, et al. A Systematic review of randomized trials evaluating regional techniques for postthoracotomy analgesia. Anesthesia & Analgesia. 2008;**107**(3):1026-1040. DOI: 10.1213/01.ane.0000333274.63501.ff

[45] Gerner P. Postthoracotomy pain management problems. Anesthesiology Clinics. 2008;**26**(2):355-vii. DOI: 10.1016/j.anclin.2008.01.007

[46] Reuben SS, Yalavarthy L. Preventing the development of chronic pain after thoracic surgery. Journal of Cardiothoracic and Vascular Anesthesia. 2008;**22**(6):890-903. DOI: 10.1053/j.jvca.2008.02.016

[47] Scholl R, Bekker A, Babu R. Neuroendocrine and immune responses to surgery. The Internet Journal of Anesthesiology. 2012;**30**(3). DOI: 10.5580/2b9a

[48] Ong CK, Seymour RA, Lirk P, Merry AF. Combining paracetamol (acetaminophen) with nonsteroidal antiinflammatory drugs: A qualitative systematic review of analgesic efficacy for acute postoperative pain. Anesthesia and Analgesia. 2010;**110**(4):1170-1179. DOI: 10.1213/ANE.0b013e3181cf9281

[49] Jahangiri Fard A, Farzanegan B, Khalili A, et al. Paracetamol instead of ketorolac in post-video-assisted thoracic surgery pain management: A randomized trial. Anesthesia and Pain Medicine. 2016;**6**(6):e39175. DOI: 10.5812/aapm.39175

[50] Lardinois D, Vogt P, Yang L, Hegyi I, Baslam M, Weder W. Non-steroidal anti-inflammatory drugs decrease the quality of pleurodesis after mechanical pleural abrasion. European Journal of Cardio-Thoracic Surgery. 2004;**25**(5):865-871. DOI: 10.1016/j.ejcts.2004.01.028

[51] Michelet P, Guervilly C, Hélaine A, et al. Adding ketamine to morphine for patient-controlled analgesia after thoracic surgery: Influence on morphine consumption, respiratory function, and nocturnal desaturation. British Journal

of Anaesthesia. 2007;**99**(3):396-403. DOI: 10.1093/bja/aem168

[52] Kiss T, Wittenstein J, Becker C, et al. Protective ventilation with high versus low positive end-expiratory pressure during one-lung ventilation for thoracic surgery (PROTHOR): Study protocol for a randomized controlled trial. Trials. 2019;**20**(1):213. DOI: 10.1186/s13063-019-3208-8

[53] Uhlig C, Neto AS, van der Woude M, et al. Intraoperative mechanical ventilation practice in thoracic surgery patients and its association with postoperative pulmonary complications: Results of a multicenter prospective observational study. BMC Anesthesiology. 2020;**20**(1):179. DOI: 10.1186/s12871-020-01098-4

Section 5

Regional Anesthesia

Chapter 8

Cardiac Arrest Following Central Neuraxial Block

Sadhana S. Kulkarni and Savani S. Futane

Abstract

Central neuraxial blocks (CNB) are used worldwide in anesthesia practice. They are safe, however, not devoid of untoward complications. Cardiac arrest (CA) is one of the major devastating complications. The anesthesiologists are concerned about CA as it can occur unexpectedly and suddenly even in a young ASA grade I patient, undergoing elective surgery, at any time during and after administration of CNB in spite of continuous vigilance. A better understanding of the physiology of CNB, availability of monitoring devices, and safer local anesthetic drugs contribute to reduced mortality, yet cases of CA are reported even recently. These case reports provide information relevant to particular incidents and may be inadequate to provide comprehensive information to explain the overall clinically important aspects related to CA following CNB. This chapter would provide a summary and analysis of the current recommendations about etiology, predisposing factors, preventive measures, and various measures tried for the treatment of cardiac arrest, although the exact etiology and predisposing factors are still not known. The comprehensive information would be helpful for anesthesiologists during day-to-day practice and to increase the safety of patients undergoing CNB. Proper patient selection, pre-/co-loading of fluids, the modifying technique of CNB as per patient's need, early use of epinephrine during bradycardia refractory to atropine, continuous monitoring, vigilance during intra- and postoperative period would help in prevention, early detection, and prompt treatment of CA. Challenges faced by anesthesiologists during CNB practice and newer modalities used for the treatment of refractory CA are also discussed. The mystery of sudden unexpected CA is yet to be solved and research in this direction is warranted. Electronic medical record keeping and reporting untoward incidence to the national board will also help to improve patient safety in the future.

Keywords: anesthesia, epidural, anesthesia, spinal, anesthetic technique, central neuraxial block, complications, bradycardia, cardiac arrest, hypotension

1. Introduction

Central neural blocks (CNB) are commonly used in the perioperative period and are an integral part of anesthetic practice because of well-known reasons [1]. The low rate of complications is one of the reasons for their popularity particularly in regions with the limited health care resources.

The techniques are considered safe but major adverse events such as neurological complications and cardiac arrest (CA) are reported at times, and the techniques are not without risks [1, 2]. It is evident from reports of studies that cardiac arrest following CNB is not rare [3–6]. CA under CNB is a major concern as it is reported in ASA grade I young patients, undergoing elective surgery, and can occur suddenly without warning signs [4, 7]. CA following spinal anesthesia is reported since 1940, yet the exact etiology is not known [1, 8]. Even though the outcome of patients developing CA has improved in the last two decades, the possibility of tragic events does exist despite adequate and timely resuscitation [9]. These case reports provide information relevant to particular incidents and may be inadequate to provide comprehensive information to explain the overall clinically important aspects related to CA following CNB. This chapter would provide a comprehensive view of etiology, predisposing factors, preventive measures, and treatment of cardiac arrest. The information would help to increase patient safety during spinal and epidural anesthesia. The anesthesiologists can make use of this information for proper selection of patients, preoperative optimization of patients, modifying anesthetic technique as well as monitoring as per patient need, to implement measures to prevent severe bradycardia, hypotension, use of different modalities during refractory cardiac arrest and for postoperative care of patients receiving CNB. The importance of vigilance and monitoring during intraoperative as well as in the postoperative period is reinforced as unexpected CA can occur at any time [2, 10]. The chapter would also make the anesthesiologists aware of where the research stands on this critical issue of CNB and in what direction future research is needed.

This chapter is intended to serve as a pragmatic review for use in daily anesthesia practice of CNB (spinal, epidural, and combined spinal-epidural) in adult patients. The manuscript is structured in a way that may help the anesthesiologists to quickly find the most important information about CA relating to the current information and underlying evidence. We did not carry out a systematic literature review. To present a holistic overview of this clinically important subject, a comprehensive literature search was performed in January–April 2022 in MEDLINE, PubMed, and Google Scholar to retrieve articles pertaining to a cardiac arrest related to CNB. The keywords used in various combinations included "Central neuraxial blocks and cardiac arrest"; spinal anesthesia and cardiac arrest; epidural anesthesia and cardiac arrest; local anesthesia systemic toxicity; hypotension and spinal anesthesia. A systematic review would result in a larger and more detailed manuscript that could be difficult to use as a quick clinical reference, even though it would decrease the probability of excluding relevant publications [11].

Incidence of cardiac arrest: The exact incidence of CA is not known [1]. The real incidence of CA related to CNB is heterogeneous and has a wide range from 0.07 to 49 per 10,000 patients [2, 4, 5, 10, 12]. In 2002, the incidence of CA following CNB was 10:10,000 [13]. A better understanding of physiological changes following CNB, availability of safer local anesthetic drugs, and improved monitoring have contributed to the reduction in the incidence of CNB [14]. However, even recent reports confirm that CA under spinal anesthesia is not rare [5, 8, 10].

In 2002, the incidence of CA following spinal anesthesia was more as compared to that following epidural, 2.5/10,000 and 0–0.5/10000, respectively [15, 16]. Incremental doses and slower onset of epidural contribute to a lower incidence of CA as compared with spinal anesthesia [3]. However, Cook et al. observed a higher incidence of permanent neurological damage including death following epidural and combined spinal epidural than spinal, 18.2 and 2.8 per 100,000, respectively [2].

Biboulet et al. reported that the incidence of CA was more following spinal than general anesthesia [17]. However, according to the majority of investigators, the incidence is more during general anesthesia [8, 14, 18]. It may be because the more complicated surgeries and high-risk patients are conducted under general anesthesia.

2. Etiology

The real etiology of CA is still not known, even though CA following spinal was reported in 1940. Etiology of CA following spinal and epidural is multifactorial. Due to inconsistent reporting, risk factors leading to bradycardia and CA under spinal anesthesia remain uncertain and contradictory [19]. Etiology of CA is summarized in **Table 1**.

1. **Respiratory etiology**: In 1988, Caplan postulated after analysis of 14 cases, that CA during spinal anesthesia was related to hypoxemia secondary to excessive sedation and/or sensory level above the T4 segment [7]. However, peak block height had the weakest correlation to bradycardia and there were no changes in tidal volume and the diaphragmatic function was unaffected by mid-thoracic levels of the spinal blockade [20]. As the pulse-oximeter was available, several authors reported that hypoxia was not the primary cause of CA and many of the patients did not receive sedative drugs [9, 21].

2. Cardiocirculatory etiology (Reduction in preload and blockade of cardio-accelerator fibers):

   The most likely etiology of CA during spinal/epidural anesthesia is mainly peripheral vasodilatation and reduction of preload resulting from sympathetic blockade. The level of sympathetic blockade extends two to six dermatomes

Spinal anesthesia	Epidural anesthesia
Reduction in preload and blockade of cardio-accelerator fibers)	Reduction in preload. Cardio-accelerator fibers are blocked in thoracic epidural
Parasympathetic over activity	Parasympathetic over activity
Intrinsic cardiac reflexes	Intrinsic cardiac reflexes
Inhibition of catecholamine release	Inhibition of catecholamine release
Inherent vagotonia	Inherent vagotonia
Sudden bradycardia & cardiac arrest	Sudden bradycardia & cardiac arrest
Myocardial ischemia	Myocardial ischemia
Total spinal following repeat spinal anesthesia	Accidental total spinal
	LAST* due to intravascular injection or overdose toxicity while using mixture of local anesthetics
	Absorbed local anesthetic can add to bradycardia

**LAST—Local anesthetic systemic toxicity.*

Table 1.
Causes of cardiac arrest.

above the sensory blockade [3, 22]. Cardio-accelerator fibers (T1-T4) can be blocked when a sensory level is at T4 and their blockade produces negative chronotropic, inotropic, and dromotropic effects. Nevertheless, it is not uncommon to see high-sensory blockade levels without hemodynamic changes, particularly in young patients. Reduction in right atrial pressure is likely in 36% of the patients, when the level block is less than T4 dermatome and in 53% of patients when it is above that [13, 23]. Anesthesiologists generally test the level initially till the desired level is achieved for surgical procedure. Higher levels achieved subsequently (due to patient position, baricity, type of local anesthetic, and other factors) may remain unnoticed.

3. Exacerbation of the parasympathetic nervous system

Sympathetic blockade results in significant bradycardia and even asystole. The final pathway is the absolute or relative increase in activity of the parasympathetic nervous system [23]. CA is more common in young individuals as they have a greater vagal tone. The parasympathetic response following spinal anesthesia, traction on viscera, pain, etc., is further exaggerated in these patients [3]. Cardiac arrest during needle insertion is reported particularly in the anxious patients [6]. CA was preceded by bradycardia in many studies [9, 16].

4. Intrinsic cardiac reflexes

   A decrease in preload may initiate reflexes leading to severe bradycardia [24] (**Figure 1**).

   a. Reflexes involving the pacemaker stretch: The rate of firing of cells of the pacemaker within the myocardium is proportional to the degree of stretch. Decreased venous return to the right atrium results in the decreased stretch and a slower heart rate.

   b. The reflex from low-pressure baroreceptors in the right atrium and vena cava.

   c. Reflexes arise from inhibitory mechano-receptors in the left ventricle. Decrease in ventricular volume would normally decrease receptor activity leading to tachycardia. However, a rapid decrease in left ventricular volume may trigger a paradoxical increase in the activity of these receptors, which could be due to forceful ventricular contraction around an almost empty chamber. This reflex slowing should allow time for a more complete filling of the heart [25].

Ecoffey et al. studied the effect of sympathetic blockade with echocardiography in unpremeditated volunteers and observed that two out of eight volunteers developed bradycardia and hypotension along with a reduction in left ventricular diameter, with epidural anesthetic levels of T8 and T9. Changes reverted by head-down positioning and rapid infusion of I.V. fluids. The increased levels of human pancreatic polypeptide, a marker of parasympathetic function, associated with these episodes of bradycardia suggest vagal activation. Bradycardia due to an increase in vasopressin levels without changes in catecholamine levels is observed after the head-up tilt in the presence of sympathetic blockade [26]. Pregnant patients undergoing spinal

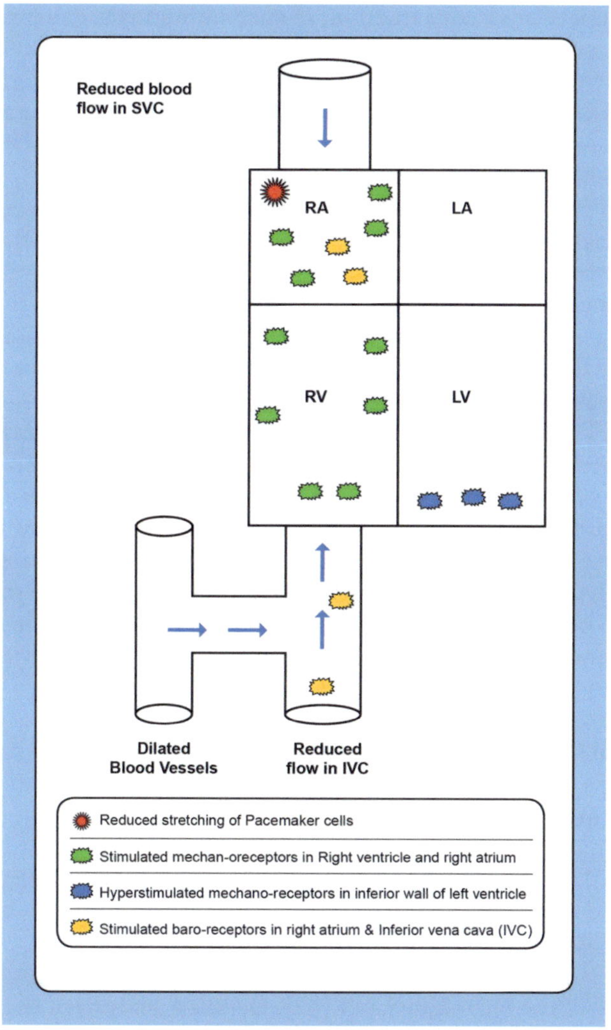

Figure 1.
Receptors in heart responsible for cardiac arrest following CNB.

anesthesia are at increased risk for hypotension and bradycardia due to aortocaval compression and a higher level of spinal block [27].

5. **Inhibition of** catecholamine **release:** Suprarenal glands are innervated from nerve fibers emerging between T8 and L1. There is inhibition of catecholamine release during the spinal.

6. **Inherent vagotonia and autonomic hyper reflexia:** 7% of the population has a sympathetic and parasympathetic imbalance. "Vagotonia" describes the clinical situation of resting bradycardia, atrioventricular (AV) block, or complete AV dissociation [28]. Patients may have a history of fainting attacks at the site of blood. Any tendency to bradycardia that might otherwise have been more benign, transient, or possibly unnoticed may be exaggerated in vagotonic patients [19]. In

addition, anxiety or viscous traction, in such individuals, can produce severe bradycardia or atrioventricular heart blocks [3, 29]. A small postural change includes placing legs in the holder, and turning the patient to the left lateral or prone position and CA was reported even after the surgical procedure was over. It is difficult to explain these situations based only on preload changes. Maybe they are due to reflex phenomena similar to those of autonomic dysfunction or hyperreflexia described in patients with a spinal cord section. One should be vigilant during the change of posture of the patient receiving spinal anesthesia [30].

Paradoxically young patients and athletes are frequently classified as low-risk ones, have increased vagal tone, and appear to be at risk of developing severe bradycardia. The highly competitive athlete, in addition, may have "athletic heart syndrome". Its features include sinus bradycardia, sinus dysrhythmias, first-degree and Mobitz type I blockades, and alterations in repolarization. Occasionally, CA has been described during the spinal anesthesia in athletes [31, 32]. Jordi et al. observed the development of first-degree AV block progressing to asystole in patients undergoing spinal anesthesia with the sensory blockade at the T3 dermatome [23]. Retrospective analysis of postoperative holter monitoring indicated persistent first-degree block for six hours after anesthesia. Development of a first-degree block can be a warning sign for the development of asystole. However, the difficulty in diagnosing first-degree block using a cardioscope limits the applicability of this finding [4].

7. **Total spinal following repeat spinal anesthesia:** Total spinal can be there due to a high dose of local anesthetic if due precautions are not taken. If not detected and treated in time, the patient may develop cardiac arrest [33].

8. **Sudden bradycardia & cardiac arrest**: These complications may develop despite vigilance and satisfactory resuscitation, which is yet a mystery. It is observed in young patients undergoing minor surgery. These situations are often attributed as the consequence of mismanagement of the spinal technique and not to an intrinsic risk of the technique itself [32]. Detailed analysis of the hemodynamics in the minute or two leading up to bradycardia or asystole during CNB is a time frame in which intervention is needed to prevent calamities.

Causes of Cardiac arrest following epidural block:

Cardiac arrest can occur during epidural anesthesia [6, 21, 34, 35] due to causes similar to that following spinal anesthesia. In addition, unintentional "total spinal" anesthesia, and local anesthetic systemic toxicity (LAST) are common causes of CA during an epidural block. Absorbed local anesthetic from vascular epidural space can add to bradycardia. Occasional severe toxicity and deaths are reported. While using a mixture of local anesthetics, one should not use maximum doses of two local anesthetics in the belief that their toxicities are independent [36]. Heavy intravenous sedation with drugs such as midazolam can mask early signs of LAST, particularly convulsions. Among all, bupivacaine is considered to be 4–16 times more cardiotoxic than lignocaine. The use of ropivacaine and levobupivacaine may help reduce cardiotoxicity due to stereo-selective binding of sodium and potassium channels resulting in less affinity and strength of inhibitory effect [37]. Jacobson concluded that reduction in preload leading to an increase in vagal activity is responsible for arrest rather than blockade of cardiac accelerator nerves from the study on healthy volunteers receiving epidural [25]. Development of third-degree heart block is reported following thoracic epidural block in a patient having preoperative first-degree heart block [38]. Even though there is a segmental block during epidural, partial sympathetic block can be there in lower segments resulting in preload reduction [39].

A combined spinal-epidural technique (CSEA) may be preferable to a continuous epidural technique as is associated with a lower failure rate, better pain scores, and patient satisfaction. Epidural top-ups of local anesthetic should be given in small incremental doses [40].

Causes of early-onset CA may be vasovagal during needle prick, hypovolemia, compromised cardiovascular status, posture-related changes, and accidental intravascular/intrathecal injection during an epidural block, etc. Late-onset CA may be due to blood loss, myocardial infarction, and delayed spread of local anesthetic after spinal anesthesia, surgical stimulus like traction on mysentry, cementing, posture change, tourniquet release, and use of vasodilators such as nitroglycerine or sodium nitroprusside during total hip replacement, etc.

3. Predisposing factors for cardiac arrest

Although the development of CA during spinal anesthesia is considered as the final step of a spectrum of manifestations that starts with bradycardia, establishing an association among factors related to its development can help identify patients at-risk to develop CA during spinal block [3].

Risk factors for severe bradycardia: Pollard has suggested the risk factors as shown in **Table 2** [3].

According to Carpenter, the level of the block had the weakest correlation with the development of bradycardia [20]. The presence of two or more listed factors in **Table 2** may place these patients at high risk for bradycardia and cardiac arrest under spinal anesthesia [3]. Due to inconsistent reporting, the risk factor associated with the occurrence of bradycardia and cardiac arrest under spinal anesthesia remains uncertain and contradictory [19].

Patients with a background of vagal dominance, and with a history of vasovagal syncope, may be predisposed to severe bradycardia and even cardiac arrest following spinal anesthesia [10]. I.V. supplementary drugs such as fentanyl, dexmeditomidine, droperidol, beta-blockers, and ondansetron [41–45] can be predisposing factors due to alpha- or beta-receptor blocking effect.

Sr. No.	Criteria
1	Age < 50 years
2	Baseline heart rate < 60/minute
3	ASA physical status grade I and II
4	Use of beta-blockers
5	Sensory-level blockade above T6 dermatome
6	Prolonged P-R interval

J. B. Pollard [3].

Table 2.
Risk factors for bradycardia during central neuraxial block.

Sr. No.	Criteria
1	Hypovolemia
2	Preoperative hypertension
3	High sensory nerve block height
4	Age older than 40 years
5	Orthopedic surgery
6	Combined general and spinal anesthesia
7	Chronic alcohol consumption
8	Elevated body mass index
9	Emergency surgery
10	Pregnancy > 20 weeks gestation

Adrian Chin and André van Zundert [40].

Table 3.
Risk factors for hyotension during central neuraxial block.

Risk factors for hypotension: These include hypovolemia, age > 40 to 50 years, emergency surgery, obesity, chronic alcohol consumption, and chronic hypertension, aortocaval compression after 20 weeks of gestation, and alkalinization or excessive doses of local anesthetic (**Table 3**) [7, 22, 46, 47].

CA observed shortly after CNB is due to excessive doses of local anesthetic in the previously hypovolemic patient. Preoperative fasting, dehydration, diuretics and vasodilator drugs for hypertension are common causes. Incidence of CA is more during orthopedic surgeries like hip surgery. Blood loss during surgery, cementing, or postural changes also contribute to CA [16, 48]. The level of sensory blockade in elderly patients is usually higher than that of young adults with the same dose of local anesthetic. According to Biboulet et al. [14], doses as low as 5 mg of bupivacaine, hyper- or isobaric, can cause a sensorial blockade reaching up to T2-T4 [17]. Overdose of local anesthetic using the subarachnoid route is a known cause of CA in elderly patients. It is recommended that the level of the blockade should be limited to T6 and hemodynamic reserves should be evaluated perioperatively to prevent untoward events [48].

When SA is administered by surgeons and non-anesthetist health care providers, the incidence of CA was more [49]. This is due to lack of monitoring, delay in detection, and treatment of complications by non-qualified health care professionals. Lozts et al. postulated that hyperbaric solutions can have delayed cephalad spread even after minutes post-injection and it can take more than 40–60 minutes to fix finally [50]. Obstetric patients have more sympathetic activity so a lower incidence of CA is expected [2, 3]. Adekola et al. observed more cardiac arrests (7.3/10000) in pregnant mothers as compared with non-obstetric patients, however postmortem reports revealed that the causes were not related to spinal anaesthesia [12].

4. Prevention of severe bradycardia, hypotension, and cardiac arrest

Final pathway for the development of severe bradycardia and CA is parasympathetic over activity. Specific strategies to anticipate and prevent vagal predominance

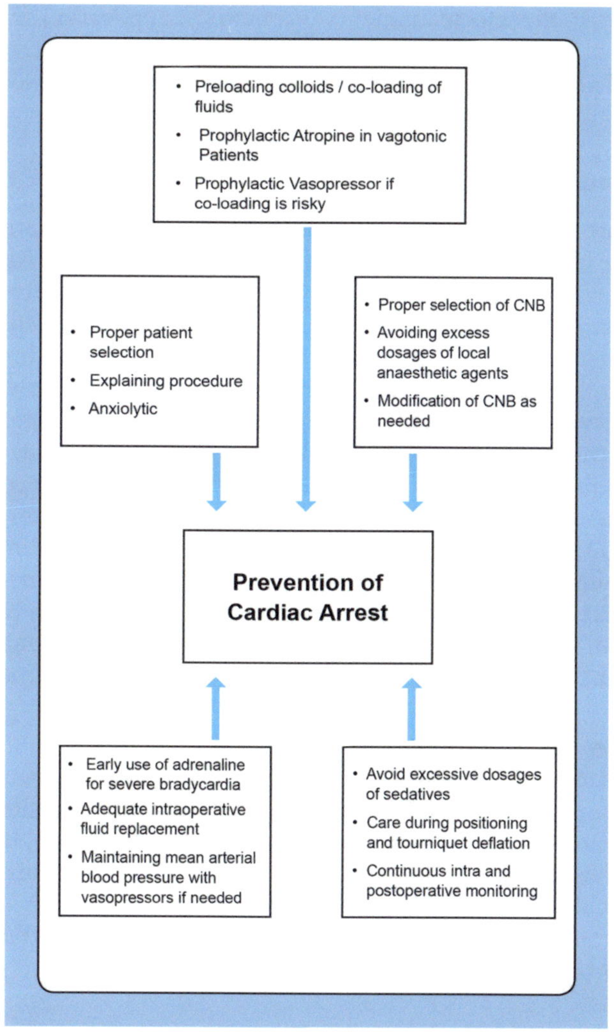

Figure 2.
Prevention of cardiac arrest.

form the mainstay in the management of severe bradycardia and CA under spinal anesthesia (**Figure 2**).

A. Prevention:

a. **Appropriate patient selection:** When two or more risk factors are present (**Table 2**) and when significant intraoperative blood loss or use of vasodilators such as sodium nitroprusside or nitroglycerine is anticipated, one should reconsider the choice of spinal anesthesia [3].

b. **Explaining the procedure to the patient during pre-anesthetic checkup:**

This will help to reduce anxiety and fear, which can trigger severe bradycardia. Anxiolytic like oral hydroxyzine in the apprehensive patients, atropine premedication in the selected patients (vagotonic), application of local anesthetic cream or infiltration before insertion of the needle, administration of CNB in the lateral position, etc., can help to reduce incidence of sudden bradycardia during needle insertion [51].

c. **Prophylactic atropine premedication:**

Routine premedication with atropine is not recommended and does not reduce the incidence of bradycardia and hypotension [52]. Bradycardia of different grades is observed during CNB (mild<60, moderate <50, severe </ min). Clinically significant bradycardia occurs in 10 to 15 percent of spinal anesthetics [53]. The incidence of bradycardia with epidural anesthesia depends on the level and extent of the block. It may be considered in elderly patients having bradycardia and those with the history suggestive of vagotonic symptoms (0.5 mg immediately after spinal anesthesia) [54]. Prophylactic administration of I.V. atropine after spinal did not prevent a decline in blood pressure in parturients even though heart rate was more at 15 and 20th min [55]. I.V. atropine prevented bradycardia when dexmeditomidine sedation was administered but there was increase in the blood pressure so should be used carefully [56]. Epinephrine should be administered in the presence of refractory bradycardia. Early administration of 0.2–0.3 mg adrenaline or drip 0.15 mcg/kg/minute prevents cardiac arrest and subsequent morbidity [3, 40].

d. **Modification in CNB technique:** Hemodynamic consequences can be reduced a) by administering a low dose of local anesthetic with the additive [57], using unilateral spinal anesthesia for lower limb surgery [58] by titrating the required level by using continuous spinal anesthesia [59]. This can reduce the extent of sympathetic block. Care should be executed for local anesthetic toxicity while using a mixture of local anesthetics and epidural dosages when combined spinal epidural anesthesia is administered.

e. **Maintaining adequate preload and prevention of hypotension**: Uncorrected hypovolemia increases the risk of hypotension with the onset of CNB and is an absolute contraindication for spinal anesthesia. Risk factors for hypotension include hypovolemia, age > 40 to 50 years, emergency surgvery, obesity, chronic alcohol consumption, pregnant patient with gestational period of more than 20 weeks, and chronic hypertension (**Table 3**) [40]. In vagotonic patients particularly when blood loss is expected during surgery, preload maintenance is essential [3]. Unfortunately, this is not routinely followed [3, 29]. Preloading with colloids or co-loading with colloids or crystalloids administered within 5–10 minutes is effective [60, 61]. Co-loading should be practiced carefully in patients with preeclampsia.

Change from supine to prone or Trendelenburg/lithotomy to supine posture, tourniquet release, intra-operative blood loss, and use of vasodilators can produce preload changes and need preload correction in anticipation. The position should be resumed if hypotension/bradycardia is observed. 30 centimeter leg elevation increases the venous return and is useful in settings with resource constraints [62].

10–15 degrees left lateral tilt is beneficial in parturient to reduce aortocaval compression reducing preload. Unfortunately, adequacy of preload is difficult to assess clinically. Assessment of inferior vena cava diameter and left ventricular volume by using non-invasive techniques such as ultrasonography (USG) and transthoracic echocardiography can be useful but may not prevent CA [63, 64].

Invasive blood pressure monitoring can help to increase safety in critical patients [65]. Bradycardia may be an early manifestation of reduction in preload and atropine or vasopressor may be needed to treat vagal manifestation and only fluid administration may not be sufficient. Administration of atropine 0.4–0.6 mg is recommended to prevent cardiac arrest.

f. **Vasopressors**: Vasopressors with different modes of action are tried for the prevention and treatment of hypotension in elderly and obstetric patients, particularly when pre- or co-loading is risky as in patients of preeclampsia (**Table 4**).

Ephedrine, phenylephrine, or noradrenaline can be used for prophylaxis. Ephedrine produces tachycardia and is to be avoided in patients where tachycardia is undesirable as in patients with aortic stenosis. It produces tachyphylaxis when used in repeated doses, and hence is administered as intermittent boluses and not as an infusion. Phenylephrine (alpha-agonist) has duration of action of up to 20 minutes. Noradrenaline increases cardiac output due to its alpha-agonist action and additional weak beta-agonist effect. About 8 mg ondansetron blocks Bezold Jarisch reflex activated by serotonin and is used to limit hypotension. Further evidence is awaited for routine use of ondansetron [66–70].

g. **Continuous vigilance throughout the procedure:** Blood loss, altered consciousness, and signs of vagal over activity such as nausea, sweating, bradycardia, change of posture, traction on viscera, and vital parameters are essential throughout the procedure as well as in the postoperative period also. Awareness about delayed CA is necessary [32].

5. Treatment of bradycardia and hypotension

Treatment of bradycardia: Mild bradycardia (<60/min) should be treated in patients with risk factors (3). It is enough to have intra-operative hypotension with bradycardia (<50/min) to rapidly administer atropine plus a vasoconstrictor (e.g., ephedrine). Treatment of moderate and severe bradycardia with hypotension must be quick, intensive, and multimodal. According to Tarkilla et al., atropine is recommended for bradycardia as glycopyrrolate is ineffective [46]. Alexander has suggested that atropine (0.5 mg) or glycopyrrolate (0.2 to o.4 mg) and ephedrine (5 to 10 mg) I.V. can be used for the treatment of bradycardia with hypotension [71]. It does not seem to be wise to administer just one of these drugs and then wait for the result [3, 32]. Pollard recommended a stepwise approach of administering atropine (0.4–0.6 mg), ephedrine (25–50 mg), and epinephrine (0.2–0.3 mg) for the treatment of moderate bradycardia. If there is no improvement after atropine and vasoconstrictors, intravenous epinephrine must be administered without any delay, as recommended by the SOS ALR group in France [74]. Head low position (careful before 30 minutes after spinal) [75] and fluid administration should

	Drug	Receptors	Effects	Dose	Undesirable effects
1	Ephedrine [66]	Alpha- and beta-adrenoreceptors	Maintains arterial pressure by increasing cardiac output and heart rate (beta 1 receptor)	Prophylaxis:10 mg after spinal anesthesia Treatment: rescue dose 5 mg	Weak alpha-activity
2	Mephenteramine [67]	Alpha- and beta-adrenoreceptors	Increases CO and SBP	Treatment of hypotension 5 mg bolus, 2.5 mg/ min infusion	Less significant increase in peripheral resistance
3	Phenylephrine [66, 68]	Alpha-adrenergic agonist causes release of norepinephrine	Increases SVR and MAP *via* arteriolar vasoconstriction resulting in increased CO	Prophylaxis:100 microgram after spinal anesthesia Treatment: rescue dose 50 microgram	Reflex bradycardia
4	Norepinephrine [69]	Potent alpha-agonist and weak beta-agonist	Increase in HR and CO	Prophylaxis: Infusion of 0.07–0.08 mcg/kg/min, Treatment : rescue dose 8 mcg bolus	Bradycardia, weak beta-agonist
5	Theoadrenaline (norepinephrine & theophylline) [70, 71]	Beta 1 adrenoreceptor stimulation, partial agonist at alpha 1 receptor	Increased ionotropic activity Release of nor adrenaline from nerve endings and increased SV, CO	(Ampoule containing cafedrine 200mg/ theoadrenaline 10mg) slow IV 1 ml/min for the treatment of hypotension	Further data awaited
6	Ondansetron [72, 73]	5-HT3 receptors	Inhibits BJR by blocking serotonin binding to 5-HT3 receptors in left ventricle leading to increased BP and HR	4–8mg, 5 min prior to spinal anesthesia	Further data awaited

CS—Cesarean section, CO—cardiac output, SBP—systolic blood pressure, SVR—systemic vascular resistance, MAP—mean arterial pressure, mcg—microgram, BP—blood pressure, HR—heart rate, SV—Stroke volume, IV—intravenous, BJR—Bezold Jarisch reflex. [Number in bracket indicates reference number].

Table 4.
Vasopressors used for prevention and treatment of spinal/epidural anesthesia-induced hypotension.

also be done simultaneously as bradycardia may be the manifestation of reduced preload. The possibility of cephalad spread of hyperbaric local anesthetic and hemodynamic effects must be anticipated. When the level of the sensory block is higher than or at T6, there can be pooling of 20% circulating blood volume in the hepato-splanchnic region and this volume can be mobilized by the use of vasopressors [76]. A transcutaneous pacemaker should be used if bradycardia is not responding [77].

Treatment of hypotension: Incidence of hypotension during spinal is 47% [47]. Systolic blood pressure less than 80% of the baseline value should be treated [68]. Mean arterial pressure should be targeted more than systolic blood pressure. When the same level of dermatomal block is achieved following epidural and spinal anesthesia, the incidence of hypotension is similar, although the onset of hypotension may be slower with epidural anesthesia [3].

20 degrees head low position, co-loading with colloids or crystalloids (around 1000 ml) and vasopressors are used for treatment. Ephedrine is used when there is bradycardia and hypotension [66]. Phenylephrine 100 mcg is used for the treatment of hypotension (100 mcg bolus or 10 mg ampoule in 100 ml saline—100 mcg/ml, i.e., 1 ml/min drip-rate). Phenylephrine can reduce the level of spinal and produce hypertensive crises when administered with atropine [40]. Reflex bradycardia due to hypertension usually limits hypertensive crises. Noradrenaline can also be used instead of phenylephrine with less risk of bradycardia. A combination of caffedrine (covalently linked norephedrine and theophylline) having an inotropic effect and theodrenaline (covalently linked noradrenaline and theophylline) having vasoconstricting effect is used in Germany. The combination has early-onset and long-lasting hypertensive effects [70, 71]. Additional evidence is awaited (**Table 4**).

Treatment of cardiac arrest: Vasodilatation during spinal anesthesia can make resuscitation refractory [3]. Epinephrine is to be administered after CA to maintain coronary perfusion pressure of 15–20 mm of Hg. Rosenberg has recommended 0.01–0.1 mg/kg adrenaline for the treatment of refractory bradycardia but once CA develops one mg of adrenaline must be administered. Spinal anesthesia blocks nerves going to the adrenal glands. Their suppression results in a reduction in circulating levels of noradrenaline and adrenaline during the stress of CA and is an important reason for refractory CA [78]. Adrenaline is not having a vagolytic effect and its use does not preclude the use of other drugs [1]. Veno-arterial ECMO can be used if ROSC is not restored. It may be difficult to find out the cause of cardiac arrest. 12 lead ECG, Troponin test, S. tryptase and 2D Echo would be helpful to diagnose myocardial infarction, anaphylaxis, embolism and hypovolemia. Veno-arterial ECMO may be helpful during this period [79].

After the restoration of circulation, myocardial stunning may need vasopressor support for prolonged period. Refractory cardiac failure may need to leave ventricular assist device [27].

Summary of treatment of bradycardia and cardiac arrest:

1. Mild-to-moderate bradycardia (heart rate – 60/min)—stepwise escalation of therapy.

    a. Atropine 0.4–0.6 mg, IV, b. Ephedrine 25–50 mg, c. Epinephrine 0.2–0.3 mg.

2. Severe bradycardia or cardiac arrest—as shown in the algorithm (**Figure 3**).

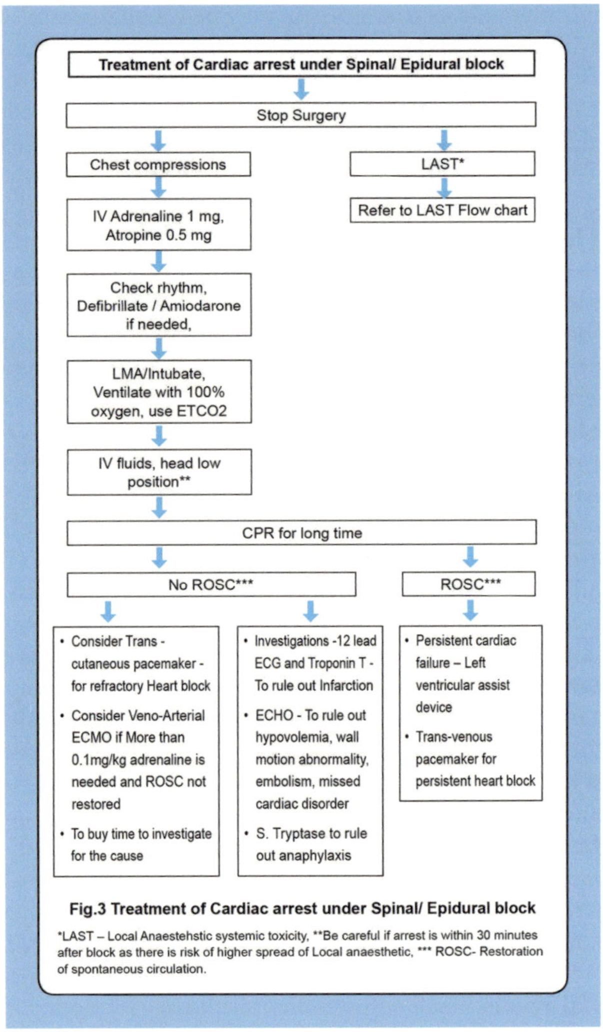

Figure 3.
*Treatment of cardiac arrest under spinal/epidural block. *LAST—Local anesthetic systemic toxicity, **Be careful if arrest is within 30 minutes after block as there is risk of higher spread of local anesthetic. ***ROSC—Restoration of spontaneous circulation.*

Reposition the patient and stop surgical stimulus.

Treatment of local anesthetic systemic toxicity (LAST):

LAST needs a special mention. Seizures should be suppressed immediately to reduce oxygen consumption, and prevent hypoxia and hypercarbia. Administration of a benzodiazepine (midazolam 1 to 2 mg I.V.) is preferred. If ventilation is inadequate, suxamethonium is administered and the airway is secured. The management of ventricular arrhythmias and CA as a result of LAST is different than other CA scenarios and may require prolonged effort [50]. Amiodarone and defibrillation are used for the treatment of ventricular fibrillation. Lignocaine should not be used. Based on animal studies, the bolus dose of epinephrine is to be reduced to ≤1 mcg/kg IV to avoid arrhythmogenic effects. The optimal dose of epinephrine is unknown.

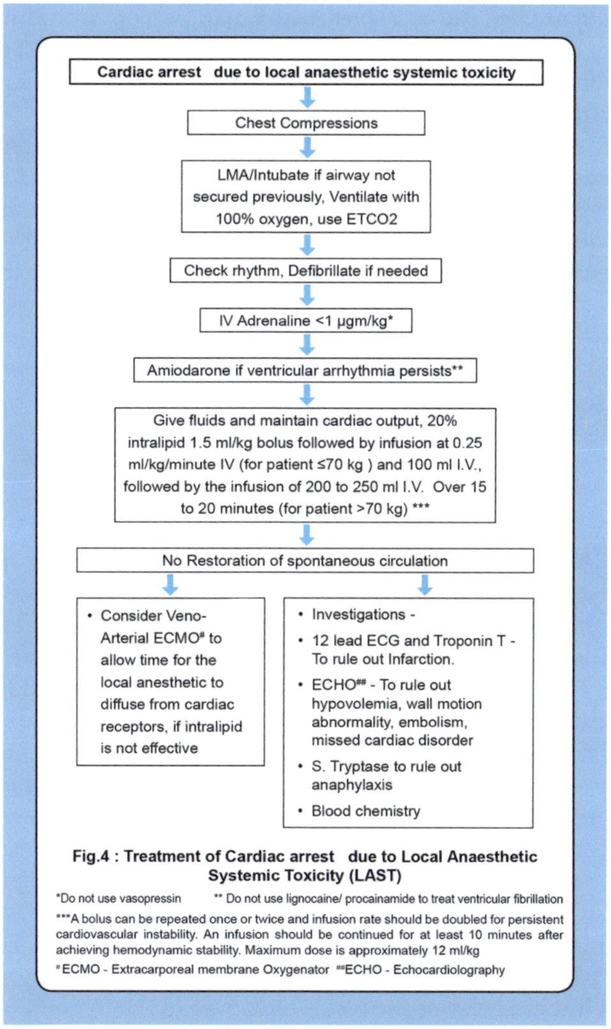

Figure 4.
*Treatment of cardiac arrest due to local anesthetic systemic toxicity (LAST). *Do not use vasopressin. **Do not use lignocaine/procainamide to treat ventricular fibrillation. *** A bolus can be repeated once or twice and infusion rate should be doubled for persistent cardiovascular instability. An infusion should be continued for at least 10 minutes after achieving hemodynamic stability. Maximum dose is approximately 12 ml/kg. #ECMO—Extracarporeal membrane oxygenator, ##ECHO—echocardiolography.*

Vasopressin should not be used as it can lead to pulmonary hemorrhage. Administer 20% lipid emulsion along with advanced cardiac life support or when neurotoxicity is evident. 1.5 mL/kg bolus followed by infusion at 0.25 ml/kg/minute IV (for patient≤70 kg) and 100 ml I.V., followed by the infusion of 200 to 250 ml I.V. over 15 to 20 minutes (for patient >70 kg). A bolus can be repeated once or twice and the infusion rate should be doubled for persistent cardiovascular instability. An infusion should be continued for at least 10 minutes after achieving hemodynamic stability. The maximum dose is approximately 12 ml/kg. Lipid emulsion improves cardiac conduction, contractility, and coronary perfusion by drawing the lipid-soluble local anesthetic out of the cardiac tissue (**Figure 4**).

Propofol should not be used as a substitute for 20 percent intralipid. Cardiopulmonary bypass may be necessary to allow time for the local anesthetic to diffuse from cardiac receptors if advanced cardiac life support and intralipid emulsion are not effective and may be lifesaving [37].

Evolution in the knowledge of the pathophysiology of CNB, better availability of monitoring devices, safer local anesthetic agents and treatment, and now the outcome in the last two decades are better. Institution of timely treatment leads to recovery of patients without any sequelae [1].

Unfortunately, the fact remains that despite timely treatment death may result [9].

CNB is used frequently all over the world and the number of patients developing CA is reported in the current literature. The detailed analysis of these cases will help to prevent catastrophes in the future.

6. When to anticipate cardiac arrest?

Unexpected CA may be observed in ASA grade I patients during spinal anesthesia [1]. Although the common belief is that CA usually occurs within the first 20–30 minutes, [32]; however, this is not true. Cardiac arrest has been reported within 12 to 72 minutes of spinal anesthesia and 180 min after epidural due to the residual sympathetic block [2, 5, 20, 35]. Lesser et al., while using automatic record keeping systems, observed that the mean interval to develop unexpected CA after the administration of spinal anesthesia was 58 minutes [53]. This finding is worrisome since after a short duration of surgical procedures, the situation can arise in the postoperative recovery room or ward when the situation might be worse. Close monitoring should be continued in the postoperative period [21].

Sudden bradycardia and CA may develop in a patient under vigilance with normal vital parameters. It is yet a mystery. Brown et al. reported sudden loss of consciousness and CA during patient chatting with the anesthesiologist [76]. These situations are often attributed as the consequence of mismanagement of the spinal technique and not due to an intrinsic risk of the technique itself [32].

Vigilance will not prevent the episodes of catastrophe but will help to provide timely treatment effectively and uneventful recovery of the patient.

Consequences of cardiac arrest during central neural block:

Despite well-conducted CPR efforts, high mortality rates (26%) were observed in two French reviews by AUROY et al. [15, 16]. Reports during 2001 revealed that 89% of patients had neurological damage or death [30]. The use of atropine with vasopressors resulting in successful resuscitation with minimal or no neurological damage is reported later on in many studies [9, 29, 53]. Caplan pointed out that those patients in whom epinephrine was used after 8 minutes of CA had a worse prognosis [7]. Ayuroy et al. reported that epinephrine was used in less than half of the patients with severe bradycardia and the mortality rate was 25% [48]. If the patient develops CA, prolonged resuscitation efforts may be needed, especially if a high sympathetic blockade is present and also for the treatment of LAST [32, 37].

Evolution in the knowledge of the pathophysiology of CNB, better availability of monitoring devices, safer local anesthetic agents and early treatment, and now the outcome have improved a lot in the last two decades [5, 6, 8]. After restoration of circulation, myocardial stunning may need vasopressor support or left ventricular assist device for refractory cardiac failure [27].

Patient with CA within 20 minutes after spinal has a better prognosis than delayed CA (more than 40 minutes), in which resuscitation is difficult due to blood loss during surgery, postural changes, and surgical procedures like cementing [16]. One should believe and intervene immediately if any detectable abnormalities are seen. Disbelief and insecurity are common patterns in this situation and may influence the outcome [32]. Therefore, the knowledge of the physiologic changes caused by CNB and its complications, proper patient selection, respecting the contraindications of the procedure, adequate monitoring, and constant vigilance are important deciding factors for outcome [8].

Anesthesiologists would face medicolegal problems following such incidents. It is necessary to maintain the proper documentation (preferably electronic medical record systems) of the preoperative status of patients, discussion during informed consent, details of technique, monitoring, perioperative events, consultation, and treatment. Anesthesiologists may be called upon long after the event and proper records will be very helpful to defend. Electronic medical record systems, reporting the adverse events to the national board, and finding out risk factors in a specific group of patients will help to improve patient safety in the future.

7. Discussion

Anesthesiologists are facing problems as well as challenges and have raised queries long ago about unexpected cardiac arrest during CNB which are yet to be answered. Future research is needed in these directions [32].

When CNB is administered, physiological changes are almost always present. It is not clear why do some individuals have these severe complications while the majority of others do not? Efforts to identify the definitive risk population in the preoperative period are needed. Hypovolemia is difficult to diagnose as well as assess clinically during perioperative period and therefore to treat up to the mark. Perioperative treatment of hypovolemia is essential, although it might not be the key factor in preventing hemodynamic instability during CNB [63]. It seems additional knowledge regarding the effect of reduced venous return, vasodilatation, and several reflexes mediated by intrinsic and/or neural mechanisms is needed. Are we missing any links?

We still do not understand what the definitive cause of sudden onset CA is during CNB when vital parameters in immediate pre-arrest period are normal. What happens during the period immediately preceding the cardiac arrest? Is automatic record keeping the answer? Unfortunately, information about this is inadequate and not provided by authors even while reporting an account of their cases recorded by automated anesthesia record keepers [53]. Finding out this information would be difficult without continuous invasive arterial blood pressure monitoring [32]. We need to find out whether this mystery can be solved by using advanced noninvasive hemodynamic monitors such as echocardiography, biomedical impedance, and inferior vena cava dimensions during the perioperative period.

One more dilemma is regarding the dosages of atropine. Whether we should use a higher dose of Atropine (1 mg) to treat bradycardia during CNB as recommended treating other bradyarrhythmias as per AHA 2020 guidelines? Should we use atropine during treatment of cardiac arrest following spinal anesthesia as there is no parasympatholytic action to adrenaline [1]. Atropine is not included in the treatment of asystole as per AHA 2019 guidelines [80].

Are cardiac arrests reported long after spinal/epidural anesthesia has been administered, really due to the anesthetic technique? How to establish the cause effect relationship is a real challenge. CA is reported in postoperative period as late as 72 minutes after epidural anesthesia [5, 20]. What is the adequate timing for sending the patient back to the ward? Guidelines are not uniform and definitive. Is it enough to wait till the recovery of motor and sensory blocks? Sympathetic block outlasts motor block. Is it justified to send the patient inward when he is moving lower limbs or should we wait till the patient voids urine spontaneously? We have to find out user-friendly device to assess sympathetic block.

8. Summary and conclusions

Without any question, central neuraxial blocks are safe and are indispensable techniques in the practice of modern anesthesia. However, safety should not be taken for granted. Although the development of bradycardia is predictable, one should not forget that the possibility of acute evolution to CA is real. The severity of CA increases because ASA grade I young patients may be affected by undergoing elective surgeries unexpectedly.

The definitive etiology of CA following CNB is still not known and seems to be multifactorial. Sympathetic blockade producing a reduction in preload seems to be the founding stone and parasympathetic over activity, the final common pathway of the etiology of CA. Abrupt changes in patient position, intraoperative blood loss, use of vasodilators, release of tourniquet, etc., can trigger the effects resulting from reduced preload contributing to CA, particularly in elderly patients. Patients treated with beta-blockers, the "vagotonic" patients, and patients undergoing hip surgery are more likely to develop CA. Proper selection of patients and type of anesthesia, and adequate monitoring and constant vigilance are essential for early diagnosis, treatment, and successful outcome following CA. CNB technique has to be modified (unilateral spinal, CSE, or continuous spinal) along with invasive monitoring if these blocks are be administered in critical patients having compromised cardiac function. Atropine premedication would be useful in vagotonic patients. Preloading with colloids or co-loading with colloids or crystalloids, vasopressors, head low position may be helpful in preventing and treating hypotension. Early use of adrenaline for treating severe bradycardia, if atropine is not effective reduces the chances of CA and increases the chances of successful revival without subsequent morbidity. A better understanding of the physiologic changes caused by CNB and its complications, availability of safe local anesthetic drugs, and monitoring devices contribute to a successful outcome after CA and complete recovery of the patient. Sympathetic blockade causes significant vasodilatation, which might make CPR difficult, and long-duration CPR may be necessary. Effective and aggressive treatment is necessary to improve the prognosis following CA. ECMO, left ventricular assist device, non-invasive monitors such as abdominal USG (for the size of inferior vena cava), and echocardiography can be useful diagnostic tools if cardiac failure is persistent or CA is refractory. A high index of suspicion and respecting the contraindications of the spinal and epidural block are equally important. Continuous vigilance during and after the procedure till complete recovery after spinal and epidural is essential as unexpected CA can occur at any time during this period.

Electronic medical records and a national registry of cases of CA following central neuraxial block will enable to conduct the research and better understanding of risk factors and etiology of unexpected CA. With the popularity of spinal anesthesia and the reported frequency of these arrests, the potential impact of these interventions on further improving the safety of spinal anesthesia could be substantial.

Author details

Sadhana S. Kulkarni[1*] and Savani S. Futane[2]

1 MGM Medical College Aurangabad, Constituent Unit of MGMIHS, Navi Mumbai, Maharashtra, India

2 Maharashtra Postgraduate Institute of Medical Education and Research, Nashik, Maharashtra, India

*Address all correspondence to: kulkarnisadhana@yahoo.com

IntechOpen

© 2022 The Author(s). Licensee IntechOpen. This chapter is distributed under the terms of the Creative Commons Attribution License (http://creativecommons.org/licenses/by/3.0), which permits unrestricted use, distribution, and reproduction in any medium, provided the original work is properly cited. (cc) BY

References

[1] Limongi JAG, Sant'Anna de Melo Lins R. Cardiopulmonary arrest in spinal anesthesia. Revista Brasileira de Anestesiologia. 2011;**61**(1):110-120

[2] Cook TM, Counsel D, Wildsmith JAW. Major complications of central neuraxial block: Report on the Third National Audit Project of the Royal College of Anaesthetists. British Journal of Anaesthesia. 2009;**102**(2):179-190

[3] Pollard JB. Cardiac arrest during spinal anesthesia: Common mechanisms and strategies for prevention. Anesthesia and Analgesia. 2001;**92**:252-256

[4] Koop SL, Horlocker TT, Warner ME, et al. Cardiac arrest during neuraxial anesthesia: Frequency and predisposing factors associated with survival. Anesthesia and Analgesia. 2005;**100**:855-865

[5] Kumari A, Gupta R, Bajwa SJS, Singh A. Unanticipated cardiac arrest under spinal anesthesia: An unavoidable mystery with review of current literature. Anesthesia, Essays and Researches. 2014;**8**:99-102

[6] Thangavelu R, Bacthavassalame AT, Venkatesh RR, George SK. A case of cardiac arrest during insertion of an epidural needle and before the administration of any epidural medication. Journal of Current Research in Scientific Medicine. 2017;**3**:115-117

[7] Caplan RA, Ward RJ, Posner K, et al. Unexpected cardiac arrest during spinal anesthesia: A closed claim analysis of predisposing factors. Anesthesiology. 1988;**68**:5-11

[8] Alegbeleye BJ. Sudden cardiac arrest under spinal anesthesia in a mission hospital: A case report and review of the literature. Journal of Medical Case Reports. 2018;**12**(1):144-147

[9] Lovstad RZ, Granhus G, Hetland S. Bradycardia and a systolic cardiac arrest during spinal anaesthesia: A report of five cases. Acta Anaesthesiologica Scandinavica. 2000;**44**:48-52

[10] Keenan C, Wang AY, Balonov K, Kryzanski J. Postoperative vasovagal cardiac arrest after spinal anesthesia for lumbar spine surgery. Surgical Neurology International. 2022;**13**:42

[11] Nagrebetsky A, Al-Samkari H, Davis NM, Kuter DJ, Wiener-Kronish JP. Perioperative thrombocytopenia: Evidence, evaluation and emerging therapies. British Journal of Anaesthesia. 2019;**1**:19-31

[12] Adekola OO, Desalu I, Adekunle MO, Asiyanbi GK, Irurhe NK. Complications and outcomes following central neuraxial anesthesia in a sub-Saharan Tertiary Hospital: The legal implication. Egyptian Journal of Anaesthesia. 2015;**31**(2):189-195

[13] Pollard JB. High incidence of cardiac arrest following spinal anesthesia. Anesthesiology. 2002;**96**:515-516

[14] Zuercher M, Ummenhofer W. Cardiac arrest during anesthesia. Current Opinion in Critical Care. 2008;**14**(3):269-274

[15] Auroy Y, Narchi P, Messiah A, et al. Serious complications related to regional anesthesia: Results of a prospective survey in France. Anesthesiology. 1997;**87**(3):479-486

[16] Auroy Y, Benhamou D, Bargues L, et al. Major complications of regional

anesthesia in France. The SOS Regional Anesthesia Hotline Service. Anesthesiology. 2002;**97**:1274-1280

[17] Biboulet P, Aubas P, Dubourdieu J, et al. Fatal and non fatal cardiac arrests related to anesthesia. Canadian Journal of Anaesthesia. 2001;**48**:326-332

[18] Aloweidi A, Alghanem S, Bsisu I, Ababneh O, Alrabayah M, Al-Zaben K, et al. Perioperative cardiac arrest: A 3-year prospective study from a Tertiary Care University Hospital. Drug, Drug Healthcare and Patient Safety. 2022;**14**:1-8

[19] Dyamanna DN, Bs SK, Zacharia BT. Unexpected bradycardia and cardiac arrest under spinal anesthesia: Case reports and review of literature. Middle East Journal of Anaesthesiology. 2013;**22**:121-125

[20] Carpenter RL, Caplan RA, Brown DL, et al. Incidence and risk factors for side effects of spinal anesthesia. Anesthesiology. 1992;**76**:906-916

[21] Liguori GA, Sharrock NE. Asystole and severe bradycardia during epidural anesthesia in orthopedic patients. Anesthesiology. 1997;**86**:250-257

[22] McCrae AF, Wildsmith JAW. Prevention and treatment of hypotension during central neural block. British Journal of Anaesthesia. 1993;**70**:672-680

[23] Jordi EM, Marsch SCU, Strebel S. Third degree heart block and asystole associated with spinal anesthesia. Anesthesiology. 1998;**89**:257-260

[24] Mark AL. The Bezold-Jarish reflex revisited: Clinical implications of inhibitory reflexes originating in the heart. Journal of the American College of Cardiology. 1983;**1**:90-102

[25] Jacobsen J, Sobett S, Brocks V, Fernandes A, Warberg J, Secher NH. Reduced left ventricular diameters at onset of bradycardia during epidural anaesthesia. Acta Anesthesiologica Scandinavica. 1992;**36**:831-836

[26] Ecoffey C, Edouard A, Pruszczynski W, Taly E, Samii K. Effect of epidural anesthesia on catecholamines, renin activity, and vasopressin changes induced by tilt in elderly men. Anesthesiology. 1985;**62**:294-297

[27] Desai N, Chaudhry K, Aji J. Impella left ventricular assist device in cardiac arrest after spinal anaesthesia for caesarean section. BMJ Case Reports. 2015. Available from: https://casereports.bmj.com/content/2015/bcr-2015-211958 [Accessed: June 20, 2022]

[28] Sapire D, Casta A. Vagotonia in infants, children, adolescents and young adults. International Journal of Cardiology. 1985;**9**:211-222

[29] Geffin B, Shapiro L. Sinus bradycardia and asystole during spinal and epidural anesthesia: A report of 13 cases. Journal of Clinical Anesthesia. 1998;**10**:278-285

[30] Lee LA, Posner KL, Domino KB, et al. Injuries associated with regional anesthesia in the 1980s and 1990s: A closed claim analysis. Anesthesiology. 2004;**101**:143-152

[31] Kreutz JM, Mazuzan JE. Sudden asystole in a marathon runner: The athletic heart syndrome and its anesthetic implications. Anesthesiology. 1990;**73**:1266-1268

[32] Barreiro G, Zundert AV, Al-Shaikh B. Unexpected cardiac arrest in spinal anaesthesia. Acta Anaesthesiologica Belgica. 2006;**57**:365-337

[33] Asfaw G, Eshetie A. Case of total spinal anesthesia. International Journal of Surgery Case Reports. 2020;**76**:237-239

[34] Chan KKM, Welch KJ. Cardiac arrest during segmental thoracic epidural anesthesia. Anesthesiology. 1997;**86**:503-550

[35] Pinheiro LC, Carmona BM, Nazareth Chaves Fascio M d, Santos deSouza I, Aquino deAzevedo RA, TimbóBarbosa F. Cardiac arrest after epidural anesthesia for a esthetic plastic surgery: A case report. Parada cardíaca após peridural para cirurgia plástica estética: relato de caso. Revista Brasileira de Anestesiologia. 2017;**67**(5):544-547

[36] Kytta J, Heavner JE, Badgwell JM, Rosenberg PH. Cardiovascular and central nervous system effects of co-administered lidocaine and bupivacaine in piglets. Regional Anesthesia. 1991;**16**:89-94

[37] Lisa Warren MD. Local anesthetic systemic toxicity. Up Todate. 2022. Available from: https://www.uptodate.com/contents/local-anesthetic-systemic-toxicity. [Accessed: May 15, 2022]

[38] Mchugh SM. Development of third-degree heart block due to thoracic epidural anaesthesia. Injury Extra. 2012;**43**(2):18-20

[39] Hopf HB, Weissbach B, Peters J. High thoracic segmental epidural anesthesia diminishes sympathetic outflow to the legs, despite restriction of sensory blockade to the upper thorax. Anesthesiology. 1990;**73**:882-889

[40] Adrian Chin and André van Zundert. Spinal Anaesthesia. 2022. Available from: https://www.nysora.com/techniques/neuraxial-and-perineuraxial-techniques/spinal-anesthesia/2022. [Accessed: May 15, 2022]

[41] Hilgenberg JC, Johantgen WC. Bradycardia after intravenous fentanyl during subarachnoid anaesthesia. Anesthesia and Analgesia. 1980;**59**:162-163

[42] Kim BJ, Kim BI, Byun SH, Kim E, Sung SY, Jung JY. Cardiac arrest in a patient with anterior fascicular block after administration of dexmedetomidine with spinal anesthesia: A case report. Medicine (Baltimore). 2016;**95**:e5278

[43] Fortuana A. Droperidol and spinal anaesthesia. Anesthesia and Analgesia. 1984;**63**:782

[44] Bajwa SJ, Panda A. Alternative medicine and anesthesia: Implications and considerations in daily practice. Ayu. 2012;**33**:475-480

[45] Helmers JH, Briggs L, Abrahamson J, Soni J, Moodley J, Forrler M, et al. A single IV dose of odansetron 8 mg prior to induction of anaesthesia reduces postoperative nausea and vomiting in gynaecological patients. Canadian Journal of Anaesthesia. 1993;**42**:1155-1161

[46] Tarkkila P, Isola J. A regression model for identifying patients at high risk of hypotension, bradycardia and nausea during spinal anesthesia. Acta Anesthesiologica Scandinavica. 1992;**36**:554

[47] Hartmann B, Junger A, Klasen J, et al. The incidence and risk factors for hypotension after spinal anesthesia induction: An analysis with automated data collection. Anesthesia and Analgesia. 2002;**94**:1521

[48] Auroy Y, Benhamou D. Can we explain the high incidence of cardiac arrest during spinal anesthesia for hip surgery? In reply. Anesthesiology. 2003;**99**:755

[49] Charuluxananan S, Thiethong S, Rungreungvanich T, et al. Cardiac arrest after spinal anesthesia in Thailand: A prospective multicenter registry of 40,271 anesthetics. Anesthesia and Analgesia. 2008;**107**:1735-1741

[50] Lotz SMN, Crosgnac M, Katayama M. Anestesia subaracnoidea com bupivacaína a 0.5% hiperbárica : influencia do tempo de permanecia em decubito lateral sobre a dispersao cefálica. Revista Brasileira de Anestesiologia. 1992;**42**:257-264

[51] Mark AL. The Bezold-Jarish reflex revisited: Clinical implications of inhibitory reflexes originating in the heart. Journal of the American College of Cardiology. 1983;**1**:90-102

[52] Hirabayashi Y, Saitoh K, Fukuda H, Mitsuhata H, Shimizu R. Coronary artery spasm after ephedrine in a patient with high spinal anesthesia. Anesthesiology. 1996;**84**:221-224

[53] Lesser JB, Sanborn KV, Valskys R, Kuroda M. Severe bradycardia during spinal and epidural anesthesia recorded by an anesthesia information management system. Anesthesiology. 2003;**99**:859-866

[54] Lakshmi NV. Comparison of atropine with ephedrine in prevention of spinal anesthesia induced hypotension in elderly age group. IJAA. 2019;**6**:1973-1977

[55] Aweke Z, Mola S, Solomon F, Ayalew N, Hailu S, Neme D, et al. Prophylactic efficacy of intravenous atropine with crystalloid co-loading for hemodynamic stability in parturient undergoing cesarean delivery at Dilla University Referral Hospital. A randomized controlled trial. International Journal of Surgery Open. 2021. Available from: https://www.semanticscholar.org/paper/Prophylactic-efficacy-of-intravenous-atropine-with-Aweke- Mola/e03d03d0fbb837a2851644ca054e6ef3060260ef [Accessed: Aug 8, 2022]

[56] Ahn EJ, Park JH, Kim HJ. Anticholinergic premedication to prevent bradycardia in combined spinal anesthesia and dexmedetomidine sedation: A randomized, double-blind, placebo-controlled study. Journal of Clinical Anesthesia. 2016;**35**:13-19

[57] Asehnoune K, Larousse E, Tadié JM, Minville V, Droupy S, Benhamou D. Small-dose bupivacaine-sufentanil prevents cardiac output modifications after spinal anesthesia. Anesthesia and Analgesia. 2005;**101**(5):1512-1515

[58] Casati A, Fanelli G. Restricting spinal block to the operative side: Why not? Regional Anesthesia and Pain Medicine. 2004;**29**(1):4-6

[59] Lux EA. Continuous spinal anesthesia for lower limb surgery: A retrospective analysis of 1212 cases. Local and Regional Anesthesia. 2012;**5**:63-67

[60] Mercier FJ, Diemunsch P, Ducloy-Bouthors A-S, et al. 6% hydroxyethyl starch (130/0.4) vs Ringer's lactate preloading before spinal anaesthesia for caesarean delivery: The randomized, double blind, multicentre CAESAR trial. British Journal of Anaesthesia. 2014;**113**(3):459-467

[61] Ni H-F, Liu H-Y, Zhang J, Peng K, Ji F-H. Crystalloid coload reduced the incidence of hypotension in spinal anesthesia for cesarean delivery, when compared to crystalloid preload: A meta-analysis. BioMed Research International. 2017;**2017**:3462529

[62] Assen S, Tesfaye BJA. Effectiveness of leg elevation to prevent spinal

Anesthesia-induced hypotension during cesarean delivery in the resource-limited area: Open randomized controlled trial. Anesthesiology Research and Practice. 2020;**2020**:5014916

[63] Bhatnagar Donati A, Mercuri G, Iuorio S, Sinkovetz L, Scarcella M, Trabucchi C, et al. Haemodynamic modifications after unilateral subarachnoid anaesthesia evaluated with transthoracic echocardiography. Minerva Anestesiologica. 2005;**71**:75-81

[64] Kundra P, Arunsekar G, Vasudevan A, Vinayagam S, Habeebullah S, Ramesh A, et al. Effect of postural changes on inferior vena cava dimensions and its influence on haemodynamics during caesarean section under spinal anaesthesia. Journal of Obstetrics and Gynaecology. 2015;**35**:667-667

[65] Ituk U, Wong CA. Overview of neuraxial anesthesia. Up To date. 2022. Available from: https://www.uptodate.com/contents/overview-of-neuraxial-anesthesia. [Accessed: May 15, 2022]

[66] Nazir I, Bhat MA, Qazi S, Buchh VN, Gurcoo SA. Comparison between phenylephrine and ephedrine in preventing hypotension during spinal anesthesia for cesarean section. Journal of Anaesthesia and Critical Care. 2012;**2**:92-97

[67] Kansal A, Mohta M, Sethi AK, Tyagi A, Kumar P. Randomised trial of intravenous infusion of ephedrine or mephentermine for management of hypotension during spinal anaesthesia for caesarean section. Anaesthesia. 2005;**60**:28-34

[68] Ferré F, Martin C, Bosch L, Kurrek M, Minville OLV. Control of spinal anesthesia-induced hypotension in adults. Local and Regional Anesthesia. 2020;**13**:39-46

[69] Ngan Kee WD, Lee SWY, Ng FF, Tan PE, Khaw KS. Randomized double-blinded comparison of norepinephrine and phenylephrine for maintenance of blood pressure during spinal anesthesia for cesarean delivery. Anesthesiology. 2015;**122**(4):736-745

[70] Koch T, Wenzel V. Old drugs and new approval procedures: Akrinor remains marketable and an application for reapproval of arginin vasopressin has been made. Der Anaesthesist. 2006;**55**(6):708-710

[71] Marcus HE, Behrend A, Schier R, et al. Anesthesiological management of caesarean sections: Nationwide survey in Germany. Anaesthesist. 2011;**60**(10):916-928

[72] Owczuk R, Wenski W, Twardowski P, et al. Ondansetron attenuates the decrease in blood pressure due to spinal anesthesia in the elderly: A double blind, placebo-controlled study. Minerva Anestesiologica. 2015;**81**(6):598-607

[73] Terkawi AS, Tiouririne M, Mehta SH, Hackworth JM, Tsang S, Durieux ME. Ondansetron does not attenuate hemodynamic changes in patients undergoing elective cesarean delivery using subarachnoid anesthesia: A double-blind, placebo-controlled, randomized trial. Regional Anesthesia and Pain Medicine. 2015;**40**(4):344-348

[74] Alexander M DeLeon, Cynthia A Wong. Spinal anesthesia: Technique. UpTodate. 2022. Available from: https://www.uptodate.com/contents/spinal-anesthesia. [Accessed: May 15, 2022]

[75] Tari SO, Oremu K. Sudden cardiorespiratory arrest following spinal anesthesia. Periodicum Biologorum. 2013;**115**:283-288

[76] Brown DL, Carpenter RL, Moore DC, et al. Cardiac arrest during spinal anesthesia. III. Anesthesiology. 1988;**68**:971-972

[77] John B. Pollard. Cardiac Arrests during Spinal Anesthesia: Review of Persisting Problem; Anaethesia patient safety Newsletter – Circulation. 2001. Available from: file:///H:/cardiac%20arrest%20chapter/2015-2%20references/TCP%20and%20spinal%20brady.html. [Accessed: May 15, 2022]

[78] Rosenberg JM, Wortsman J, Wahr JA, et al. Impaired neuroendocrine response mediates refractoriness to cardiopulmonary resuscitation in spinal anesthesia. Critical Care Medicine. 1998;**26**:533-537

[79] Qin C, Jiang Y, Liu J, Pang H. Venoarterial extracorporeal membrane oxygenation as an effective therapeutic support for refractory cardiac arrest in the setting of spinal anesthesia: A case report and literature review. International Journal of General Medicine. 2021;**14**:73-76

[80] Fred M. Kusumoto, Mark H. Schoenfeld, Coletta Barrett, James R. Edgerton, Kenneth A. Ellenbogen, Michael R. Gold, Nora F. Goldschlager. 2018ACC/AHA/HRS Guideline on the Evaluation and Management of Patients with Bradycardia and Cardiac Conduction Delay; circulation. 2019. Available from: https://www.ahajournals.org/doi/pdf/10.1161/CIR.0000000000000628. [Accessed: May 15, 2022]

Section 6

Acute and Chronic Pain Management

Chapter 9

Outpatient Management of Chronic Pain

Franzes Anne Z. Liongson, Rina Bhalodi, Christopher McCarthy, Sanjay V. Menghani and Ajaz Siddiqui

Abstract

In this chapter, we provide an overview of the most current techniques in the evaluation, diagnosis, and treatment of pain in the outpatient setting. We performed a targeted literature review by searching for the terms such as "chronic pain" and "pain management." Relevant articles were cited, and findings were described in the chapter text. Additionally, we supplemented our review with images from the Spine and Pain Associates' offices at St. Luke's University Health Network (SLUHN) in Bethlehem, PA, as well as medical illustrations by our authors. We begin the review with a description of pain—its definition, components, complexity, and classifications and then provide a stepwise outline of the pharmacologic approach beyond nonsteroidal anti-inflammatory drugs before delving into newer interventional pain management procedures. Subsequently, this chapter is not comprehensive as it does not provide extensive discussion on older, more established procedures such as epidural steroid injections as well as practices falling out of favor such as discograms and neurolysis. Instead, we focus on newer subacute to chronic nonmalignant pain interventions. Finally, we attempt to highlight future directions of the growing field. Overall, we provide an overview of the management of chronic by providing insights into updates to chronic pain management.

Keywords: chronic pain, interventional pain, outpatient medicine, opioids, narcotics

1. Introduction

Pain is a complicated, subjective sensation that results from physical stimuli as well as psychological factors. Pain can vary in location, severity, quality, and consistency. It can occur in response to either physical injury or emotional distress. While there are multiple definitions that have been proposed, the most widely accepted definition of pain, as described by Cohen *et al.* in 2018 is "an unpleasant sensory and emotional experience associated with actual or potential tissue damage or described in terms of such damage" [1].

The pain response is generated by the propagation of nociceptive signals by neurons in the central nervous system (CNS) and peripheral nervous system (PNS) in response to noxious stimuli. Fundamentally, the mechanism of pain comprises detection of noxious stimuli, transduction of noxious stimuli into electrochemical signals, transmission of the electrical signals by neuronal pathways, and modulation through the nervous system to produce the sensation of pain. This process is facilitated by the axons, also known as nerve fibers, which propagate the nociceptive signals to the central nervous system [2].

Pain begins with detection of primary noxious stimuli. Research shows that Transient Receptor Potential (TRP) superfamily of ion channels play a vital role in the detection of pain [3]. Following detection, signals are sent along axons of sensory neurons toward the CNS. The nerve fiber types recognized to play a major role in pain include Aδ and C fibers, two types of primary afferent (sensory) nociceptors. Type Aδ fibers are myelinated nerve fibers with fast conduction speeds that are activated by thermal and mechanical stimuli. They are associated with prickling pain of short duration. Type C fibers are unmyelinated nerve fibers with slow conduction speeds that are activated by thermal, mechanical, and chemical stimuli. They are associated with poorly localized, dull pain. Some C-fibers may also be peptidergic, which means that they express neuropeptides such as substance P (SP), neurokinins, and calcitonin gene-related peptide (CGRP) [4]. There is association between specific TRP channels and specific types of nerve fibers; for example, TRPV1, which is the receptor for capsaicin is associated with sensory neurons having Type C fiber axons [5]. Alternatively, TRPM8, which responds to cold sensation and menthol, is associated with sensory neurons that have Aδ and C fibers [6]. Nerve fibers carry the action potential, an electrochemical signal generated in response to the detected noxious stimuli.

The action potential generated by nociceptors in response to noxious stimuli is transmitted between neurons and culminates with the release of neurotransmitters. Common neurotransmitters and their effects on pain are listed in **Table 1**.

Neurotransmitter	Neurotransmitter Levels in Pain
Prostaglandins (PGE_2, PGI_2)	↑
Leukotriene B_4 (LTB_4),	↑
Nerve Growth Factor (NGF)	↑
Bradykinin (BK)	↑
Adenosine Triphosphate (ATP)	↑
Adenosine	↓, However some evidence suggests prolonged increase in adenosine contributes to chronic pain
Tachykinins (Substance P (SP), Neurokinin A (NKA), and Neurokinin B (NKB))	↑
5-Hydroxytryptamine (5-HT)	Generally ↓ but also ↑ at times
Histamine	↓
Glutamate	↑
Norepinephrine (NE)	↑
Nitric Oxide (NO)	↑ or ↓
Calcitonin Gene-Related Peptide (CGRP)	↑
Gamma-aminobutyric acid (GABA)	↓
Opioid Peptides	↓
Glycine	↓
Cannabinoids	↓

Table 1.
Neurotransmitters and their effects on pain.

Neurotransmitters that act as inflammatory mediators include prostaglandins (PGE_2, PGI_2), leukotriene B_4 (LTB_4), nerve growth factor (NGF), bradykinin (BK), adenosine triphosphate (ATP), adenosine, tachykinins (substance P (SP), neurokinin A (NKA), and neurokinin B (NKB)), 5-hydroxytryptamine (5-HT), histamine, glutamate, norepinephrine (NE), and nitric oxide (NO). Neurotransmitters acting as non-inflammatory mediators include calcitonin gene-related peptide (CGRP), gamma-aminobutyric acid (GABA), opioid peptides, glycine, and cannabinoids [7]. These various neurotransmitters are involved with pain transduction, transmission, and modulation, thus facilitating the mechanism of pain [8, 9].

2. Classification of pain

2.1 Acute versus chronic pain

Pain is classified as either acute or chronic. Acute pain begins suddenly, often due to an injury to the body. It can be caused by, but not limited to, broken bones, burns, sprains, wounds, falls, and medical procedures. Acute pain is not a disease and better classified as a symptom that indicates an inflammatory process that brings attention to tissue damage. Acute pain may affect more than the injured part of the body and can be debilitating due to loss of function, fatigue, or sleep deprivation. Generally, acute pain resolves within 3 months as the body heals. Acute pain can often be treated with the application of ice, analgesics, immobilization, and support bandages.

Acute pain can become chronic pain. Chronic pain is ongoing pain that lasts for more than 6 months and is usually much harder to diagnose and treat than acute pain. Chronic pain occurs when the physical condition causing acute pain remains unresolved in cases such as cancer or arthritis. Chronic pain also occurs when the nervous system is damaged or malfunctions, sending pain signals to the brain without a specific cause. In 2012, the Journal of Pain estimated that the cost of chronic pain was around $600 billion dollars when taking healthcare costs and lowered productivity into account [10]. In 2019, the National Institute for Health Services found that more than 50% of Americans were experiencing chronic pain, and back pain was the lead contributor at 39% [11–13]. Common causes of chronic pain include joint pain due to degenerative damage and overuse, migraines, neuropathic pain, and cancer. More in-depth discussion of chronic pain conditions and treatment options is in the following section of this chapter and summarized in **Table 2**.

2.2 Nociceptive versus neuropathic pain

The two most common types of pain are nociceptive pain and neuropathic pain. Nociceptive pain is caused by tissue damage or injury to the skin, bones, muscles, or joints. Examples include pain from a broken arm, a sprained ankle, a puncture wound, or a fall.

Neuropathic pain (commonly described as "pins and needles") is a numbing or shooting pain that results from damage to the nerves. Common causes of nerve damage resulting in neuropathic pain include uncontrolled diabetes, infections, surgical procedures, radiation treatments, and physical trauma.

Condition	Management
Complex regional pain syndrome (CRPS)	Spontaneous resolution in early or mild cases Physical therapy, psychotherapy, medications (acetaminophen, NSAIDS, and topical anesthetics) Alternative treatments: nortriptyline, gabapentin, pregabalin, amitriptyline, duloxetine, corticosteroids (e.g. prednisolone, methylprednisolone) Severe cases: opioids (e.g. oxycodone, morphine, hydrocodone and fentanyl)
Arthritis	Physical therapy, exercise Symptom management: NSAIDS (ibuprofen, naproxen sodium), Acetaminophen, Counterirritant ointments, Corticosteroids (e.g. prednisone)
Fibromyalgia	Over the counter (OTC) pain relievers (acetaminophen, ibuprofen, naproxen sodium) Antidepressants (Duloxetine (Cymbalta), milnacipran (Savella), Amitriptyline) Anti-seizure drugs, cyclobenzaprine, gabapentin, Pregabalin (Lyrica) Aerobic exercise, muscle strengthening exercises, stress management techniques (meditation, yoga, and massage, sleep hygiene), cognitive behavioral therapy (CBT)
Cancer Pain	Non-opioid medications (e.g. paracetamol, dipyrone, non-steroidal anti-inflammatory drugs, COX-2 inhibitors) Refractory pain: opioids (first: codeine, dextropropoxyphene, dihydrocodeine, tramadol, if pain is still uncontrolled: consider morphine, oxycodone, buprenorphine) Alternative options: Antidepressants, Anti-seizure drugs, Steroids; Other: Physical therapy, Nerve block, Acupuncture, Massage, Relaxation exercises, Meditation, Hypnosis
Chronic Pelvic Pain Syndrome	Physical therapy Hormone medications for pain associated with the menstrual cycle or hormonal changes Antibiotics for pain associated with infections Antidepressant medications (tricyclic antidepressants [TCAs]: amitriptyline, nortriptyline); Neurostimulation; Trigger point injections; Psychotherapy

Table 2.
Chronic pain conditions and treatment options.

3. Chronic pain conditions and their conservative management

3.1 Complex regional pain syndrome

Complex regional pain syndrome (CRPS) is broadly defined as prolonged and excess inflammation and pain following an injury. CRPS has both acute and chronic forms. CRPS is characterized by spontaneous or excessive pain following mild touch or allodynia. Other symptoms include changes in skin temperature, color and swelling. CRPS usually improves over time and severe and prolonged cases are rare but profoundly disabling. Most CRPS is caused by improper function of the peripheral C-fiber nerves. Excess firing of these nerve fibers sends pain messages to the brain and triggers inflammation. Injuries in CRPS typically are subtle and may go unnoticed.

Early or mild cases of CRPS generally resolve on their own. Primary treatments include physical therapy, psychotherapy, and medications. Several classes of medications have been reported as effective for CRPS, but none are FDA approved. Medications include acetaminophen, NSAIDS, and topical anesthetics. Drugs used for other neuropathic pain conditions (discussed in further detail in subsequent sections of this chapter) such as nortriptyline, gabapentin, pregabalin, amitriptyline, and duloxetine have also been shown to be effective. Corticosteroids such as prednisolone and methylprednisolone can be used to treat inflammation, swelling, and edema. Opioids such as oxycodone, morphine, hydrocodone and fentanyl may be required for the most severe cases.

3.2 Arthritis

Arthritis is the swelling and tenderness of one or more joints. The main symptoms of arthritis are joint pain and stiffness, swelling, and decreased range of motion that typically worsens with age. The most common types of arthritis are osteoarthritis and rheumatoid arthritis. While osteoarthritis causes breakdown of cartilage, rheumatoid arthritis is a disease where the immune system attacks the lining of the joints. Treatments vary depending on the type of arthritis and focus on reducing symptoms and improving quality of life. Arthritis is usually diagnosed by physical examination. Analysis of body fluids can identify the type of arthritis. Imaging such as X-rays, CT, and MRI can detect problems within the joint causing symptoms.

Arthritis treatment focuses on relieving pain and improving joint function. The medications used to treat arthritis depend on the type of arthritis. NSAIDS such as ibuprofen and naproxen sodium can relieve pain and inflammation. Acetaminophen has been shown not to be as effective as NSAIDS for arthritis pain. Counterirritant ointments applied over the aching joint may interfere with the transmission of pain from the joint. Corticosteroid medications such as prednisone will reduce inflammation and pain and slow joint damage. Exercise can improve the range of motion, strengthen muscles, and reduce pain.

3.3 Fibromyalgia

Fibromyalgia is characterized by widespread musculoskeletal pain, cognitive difficulties, tenderness, fatigue, numbness or tingling in the arms and legs, heightened sensitivity, sleep disturbances, and emotional and mental distress. Newer guidelines from the American College of Rheumatology require the main factor for diagnosis to be widespread pain throughout the body for at least 3 months. Fibromyalgia affects about 2% of the adult population. Symptoms often begin after a physical trauma or psychological stress. Women are more likely than men to develop fibromyalgia. Fibromyalgia coexists with tension headaches, chronic fatigue syndrome, TMJ, irritable bowel syndrome, postural tachycardia syndrome, depression, and anxiety. The pain, fatigue, and poor sleep quality can interfere with function at home and at work.

The cause of fibromyalgia is unknown; however, many researchers believe that fibromyalgia amplifies painful sensations by affecting the way the brain and spinal cord process signals. This involves the increase in levels of certain chemicals in the brain that signal pain. The brain pain receptors become sensitized and overreact to painful and non-painful signals. Risk factors include sex, genetics, infections, and physical or emotional trauma. Patients with arthritis and lupus are more likely to develop fibromyalgia.

Fibromyalgia is treated with both medications and lifestyle strategies. The main focus of treatment is to reduce pain and improve the quality of life. Common medications to reduce pain include pain relievers, antidepressants, and anti-seizure drugs. Over-the-counter (OTC) pain relievers such as acetaminophen, ibuprofen, or naproxen sodium may be helpful. Opioid medications are not recommended due to significant side effects and addiction and may worsen pain over time. Duloxetine (Cymbalta) and milnacipran (Savella) are FDA approved for treating fibromyalgia and may ease pain and fatigue associated with fibromyalgia. Amitriptyline or the muscle relaxant cyclobenzaprine may be prescribed to promote sleep. The epilepsy drug gabapentin is sometimes used to reduce fibromyalgia symptoms. Pregabalin (Lyrica) is used to treat nerve pain and is FDA approved for treating pain caused by fibromyalgia.

Lifestyle changes include aerobic exercise and muscle strengthening exercises, stress management techniques such as meditation, yoga, and massage, sleep habits to improve the quality of sleep, and cognitive behavioral therapy (CBT) to treat underlying depression.

3.4 Cancer pain

Cancer pain is often caused by cancer compressing on or infiltrating a part of the body, diagnostic procedures, or treatments or from skin, nerve, or other tissue damage caused by hormone imbalance or immune response. Tumors cause pain by crushing or infiltrating tissue, triggering inflammation or infection, or releasing chemicals that stimulate pain. Invasion of the bone by cancer is the most common source of cancer pain. When tumors compress, invade, or inflame parts of the nervous system, they can cause pain. Chronic pain may be continuous or intermittent. Despite pain being adequately controlled by long-acting drugs, breakthrough pain may occasionally occur and is treated with fast-acting analgesics. The presence of cancer pain depends on the location and stage of the cancer. About half of the patients diagnosed with cancer are in pain at a given time and two-thirds of patients with advanced cancer experience debilitating pain. Cancer pain can be either eliminated or adequately controlled in about 80–90% of the cases. Unfortunately, nearly 50% of cancer patients receive suboptimal pain care.

Cancer pain treatment aims to relieve pain with minimal side effects. WHO guidelines recommend prompt administration of drugs when cancer pain occurs. Non-opioid medications such as paracetamol, dipyrone, non-steroidal anti-inflammatory drugs, or COX-2 inhibitors should be administered when pain is not severe. Refractory cancer pain may require more aggressive treatment with mild opioids such as codeine, dextropropoxyphene, dihydrocodeine, or tramadol. Mild opioids are replaced by stronger opioids such as morphine if pain control is still not adequate. More than half of patients with advanced cancer and pain will require strong opioids. Morphine is effective at relieving cancer pain although oxycodone shows superior tolerability and analgesic effect. Side effects of nausea and constipation are rarely severe enough to cause stopping treatment. Sedation and cognitive impairment usually occur with the initial dose and increase with the strength of the opioid. There is some evidence that buprenorphine is another opioid with some evidence of analgesic effect. Other medicines that can also relieve pain, including antidepressants, anti-seizure drugs, and steroids A nerve block procedure can be used to stop pain signals from being sent to the brain. In this procedure, a numbing medicine is injected around or into a nerve. Pain relief may also be enhanced through acupuncture, massage, physical therapy, relaxation exercises, meditation, and hypnosis.

3.5 Chronic pelvic pain syndrome

Chronic pelvic pain occurs in the abdomen, genital area, lower back, or thighs and lasts more than 6 months. The pain may become worse when urinating, having intercourse, walking, or during menstrual periods. Chronic pelvic pain is often caused by irritable bowel syndrome, interstitial cystitis, pelvic floor dysfunction, endometriosis, pelvic injury, and ovarian cysts. Determining the cause of chronic pelvic pain often involves a process of elimination as many different disorders can result in pelvic pain. Pelvic exam can reveal signs of infection, abnormal growths, or tense pelvic floor muscles. Blood and urine tests can check for infections. Ultrasound is useful for detecting masses or cysts in the ovaries, uterus, and fallopian tubes. X-ray, CT scans, and MRI can detect abnormal structure and growths. Laparoscopy allows for a view of pelvic organs to check for abnormal tissues or signs of infection.

There are several treatments depending on the cause of pelvic pain. Hormone medications may relieve pelvic pain that coincides with a particular phase of the menstrual cycle and the hormonal changes that control ovulation and menstruation. Antibiotics can be prescribed for infections that are a source of pelvic pain. Antidepressant medications can be effective for chronic pelvic pain. TCAs such as amitriptyline and nortriptyline have been shown to relieve chronic pelvic pain even in the absence of depression. Physical therapy, neurostimulation, trigger point injections, and psychotherapy can also be an effective part of the treatment plan.

4. Traditional pharmacologic approaches to pain

4.1 Opioids

According to the 2016 CDC Guideline for Prescribing Opioids for Chronic Pain, nonopioids are preferred to opioids for the treatment of chronic pain [14]. If pain cannot be adequately controlled with OTC medications, opioid therapy may be recommended for a limited time. The decision to initiate opioid therapy for the treatment of pain is challenging and should only be made after a thorough assessment has been performed to ascertain the complete nature of the pain, comorbid patient conditions, and pain treatments that have been trialed in the past. Opioids should be prescribed alongside both non-opioid medications and non-pharmacologic treatments and should be closely monitored as prolonged use is not recommended due to risks of addiction, tolerance, and misuse [15].

More than 191 million opioid prescriptions were dispensed to Americans in 2017. Thus, it is important to screen patients for mental illness and substance use disorders that would place them at increased risk for overdose. In an effort to reduce the risk of opioid addiction and misuse, medical societies including the CDC recommend utilizing risk reduction strategies, including written pain agreements prior to starting opioid treatment for chronic pain. These agreements provide opportunities to establish pain goals, discuss the risks and benefits of opioid therapy, and clearly outline the treatment plan that will be utilized to monitor and guide opioid use.

Opioids, sometimes referred to as narcotics, are strong painkillers derived from the opium poppy plant and are used to block pain signals between the brain and the body, providing immediate relief to intense pain by altering the brain's perception of pain. They may be prescribed for low back pain, neuropathic pain, or arthritis pain [14, 16]. Opioids act primarily by binding to the μ-opioid receptor (MOR) on the cell membrane of neurons. Respiratory depression is one of the most dangerous risks associated with opioids and in severe cases can cause apnea. The risk is higher if patients have underlying respiratory conditions such as asthma or sleep apnea. Constipation is also a common side effect associated with chronic opioid use.

Popular examples of opioids include hydrocodone, hydromorphone, methadone, fentanyl, meperidine, morphine, tramadol, and oxycodone. The most common drugs involved in prescription opioid overdose deaths include methadone, oxycodone, and hydrocodone. A recent study showed that 67% of patients who require opioid-based medications were also receiving one or more other prescription drugs. Adverse drug interaction events can be linked to polypharmacy. A recent analysis among chronic back pain patients on long-term opioid analgesics reported that the overall prevalence of drug–drug interactions (DDIs) was 27% [17].

There are numerous drugs that can interact with opioid medications. Several opioids (including codeine, oxycodone, hydrocodone, fentanyl, tramadol, and methadone) are metabolized by the cytochrome P450 (CYP450) system and are associated with DDIs that either reduce opioid efficacy or exacerbate side effects. Morphine, oxymorphone, and hydromorphone are not metabolized by the CYP450 system and are generally involved in fewer DDIs. When prescribing opioids, it is important to remember that they can exacerbate sedation and respiratory when utilized alongside alcohol, anxiolytics, and hypnotics. Opioids can also interact with certain antibiotics, antidepressants, anti-seizure medications, antifungals, and antiretrovirals.

Tramadol is a commonly prescribed opioid that has analgesic properties as well as alternative mechanisms of action. Tramadol is found as a racemic mixture of two enantiomers that have synergistic effects: one enantiomer works as a selective μ agonist and inhibits serotonin reuptake, while the other enantiomer inhibits serotonin and norepinephrine reuptake [18]. Tramadol and its active metabolite (M1) inhibit ascending pain pathways by binding to μ receptors in the central nervous system [18]. Inhibition of reuptake of serotonin and norepinephrine by tramadol and M1 inhibit descending pain pathways to aid in pain relief [18]. It is important to take into consideration that the side effects of tramadol include seizures, NMS, and serotonin syndrome.

Buprenorphine offers a safer alternative for patients who require opioids to manage chronic pain, given the unique pharmacological properties that allow it to provide adequate analgesia with less abuse potential. As a long-acting partial μ receptor agonist and κ receptor antagonist, it leads to analgesia. High dose administration of buprenorphine leads to μ receptor antagonism, achieving the opposite effect. Combination of buprenorphine and naloxone, the pure μ receptor antagonist, is available as Suboxone [18]. The combinatory effects of Suboxone are designed to prevent illicit intravenous use.

4.2 Non-opioid options for pain

There are several well-known and well-utilized non-opioid approaches to pain management beyond non-steroidal anti-inflammatory drugs (NSAIDs) and acetaminophen. Several examples include topical anesthetics, counterirritants, corticosteroids, muscle relaxants, anti-depressants, and anti-seizure medications. **Table 3** provides an overview of pharmacologic approaches and common side effects of each approach.

Topical anesthetics are valuable options in pain management as they achieve relief with a low risk of side effects and drug interactions. There are many formulations available such as creams, ointments, gels, lotions, and patches. Lidocaine 5% patch (Lidoderm) is also FDA approved for the treatment of postherpetic neuralgia. In addition to topical anesthetics, counterirritants (including salicylates, capsaicin, and menthol) can be utilized to provide local and temporary irritation that distracts and interrupts pain signals to the brain. Capsaicin, in the form of Qutenza, is FDA approved for the treatment of pain associated with postherpetic neuralgia.

Drug Class	Examples	Common Side Effects
Anti-seizure Medications	gabapentin, pregabalin	Sedation, dizziness, dry mouth, peripheral edema
Tricyclic Antidepressants (TCAs)	amitriptyline, nortriptyline	Dizziness, dry mouth, blurred vision, nausea, weight gain, constipation
Counterirritants	capsaicin, menthol, salicylates	Local skin irritation
SNRIs	duloxetine, venlafaxine	Diarrhea, nausea, dry mouth, chills
Muscle Relaxants	baclofen, carisoprodol, chlorzoxazone, methocarbamol, tizanidine	Sedation, dizziness, hypotension, nausea, constipation
Steroids	dexamethasone, prednisone	Acne, blurred vision, nausea, insomnia
Opioids	buprenorphine, codeine, fentanyl, hydrocodone, hydromorphone, meperidine, methadone, morphine, oxycodone, oxymorphone, tramadol	Sedation, dry mouth, constipation, nausea
Topical Anesthetics	creams, ointments, gels, lotions, and patches; lidocaine patch	Local skin irritation, bruising

Table 3.
Common pharmacologic approaches to pain management with examples and common side effects.

Steroids are powerful anti-inflammatory medications that can be taken orally or injected. Corticosteroids are used to treat migraines, osteoarthritis, rheumatoid arthritis, and low back pain. Prednisone (Deltasone) and Decadron (Dexamethasone) are examples of corticosteroids.

Muscle relaxants are used to reduce aches and pains associated with muscle strains, sprains, or spasms by relaxing tight muscles and improving the quality of sleep. Muscle relaxants are not typically recommended for treating chronic pain, but they may help with fibromyalgia and low back pain symptoms. Examples of muscle relaxants include baclofen, tizanidine, chlorzoxazone, methocarbamol, and carisoprodol.

Tricyclic antidepressants (TCAs) and serotonin norepinephrine reuptake inhibitors (SNRIs) have been shown to be effective for treating chronic pain through their interactions with norepinephrine. SNRIs are the preferred treatment for neuropathic pain as they are generally better tolerated by patients than TCAs. The most commonly utilized SNRI for chronic pain is duloxetine (Cymbalta), which is FDA approved for treating fibromyalgia as well as diabetic neuropathy. SNRIs have a delayed onset of maximal effect and patients may have to wait weeks before achieving best results. Common side effects include diarrhea, nausea, dry mouth, and dizziness.

TCAs remain inexpensive options for treatment of depression as well as for pain control. The dose utilized for pain control is typically lower than the dose utilized for antidepressant treatment. Commonly utilized TCAs for pain are amitriptyline (Elavil) as well as nortriptyline (Pamelor). Common side effects include dry mouth, dizziness, weight gain, and constipation.

In patients on serotonergic drugs, a rare, but potentially life-threatening condition known as serotonin syndrome can occur when excess serotonin builds up in the body (this can occur if two serotonergic medications are taken concurrently or if an excess of a serotonergic drug is consumed). Symptoms of serotonin syndrome can vary from mild symptoms including diarrhea and nausea to severe symptoms including fever, seizures, and hyperreflexia.

Anti-seizure medications treat chronic neuropathic pain by reducing overactive pain signals from damaged nerves. Examples of anti-seizure medications include pregabalin (Lyrica) and gabapentin (Neurontin). Gabapentin and pregabalin are both FDA approved for postherpetic neuralgia and pregabalin is also FDA approved for diabetic neuropathy and fibromyalgia. Side effects of gabapentin and pregabalin include weight gain, fluid buildup, sleepiness, and drowsiness. Gabapentin and pregabalin cannot be stopped abruptly; they must be withdrawn gradually to minimize withdrawal symptoms such as confusion, delusions, agitation, and sweating.

5. Novel pharmacologic approaches to chronic pain

5.1 Ketamine

Ketamine, a noncompetitive N-methyl-D-aspartate (NMDA) receptor antagonist originally labeled as CI-581, is a phencyclidine derivative that has been in clinical use since its FDA approval in 1970 after which it became recognized for its ability to safely induce short-term anesthesia and analgesia. Its use was limited in clinical practice because of its psychodysleptic, hallucinatory, effects. Recently, ketamine has become the subject of research interest and began to be used in acute, chronic, and cancer pain management [19]. Its potential to be a future pharmacologic treatment option for conditions ranging from major depressive disorder and addiction to asthma and cancer growth is also being studied [20].

Ketamine noncompetitively binds to the ligand-gated NMDA receptors in the central nervous system, particularly in the prefrontal cortex and hippocampus, which results in decreased channel opening frequency and duration. Since activation of the NMDA receptor is believed to play a major role in chronic pain, the effect of ketamine on the NMDA receptor in combination with its effects on non-NMDA pathways involved in pain regulation is believed to be responsible for its analgesic properties [21]. Non-NMDA pathways thought to be associated with the analgesic properties of ketamine include the nicotinic and muscarinic cholinergic receptor antagonism, sodium and potassium channel blockade, high-affinity D2 dopamine receptor and L-type voltage-gated calcium channel activation, GABA-A signaling, and descending modulatory pathway enhancement [22].

The increased use of intravenous ketamine infusions for chronic pain treatment in recent decades motivated the development of consensus guidelines in 2016 by the American Society of Regional Anesthesia and Pain Medicine, the American Academy of Pain Medicine, and the American Society of Anesthesiologists [23, 24]. The results of studies on efficacy of ketamine for chronic neuropathic pain and nociceptive pain are promising although results of the nociceptive pain studies are mixed. A metanalysis of 211 patients from seven studies showed IV ketamine infusions demonstrated analgesia compared to placebo [19, 25]. In this study, the average infusion duration was 5 hours with a median ketamine dose of 0.35 mg/kg, with maximum effect observed between 48 hours and 2 weeks after infusion [25].

Although many pain clinics may administer ketamine intravenously, clinical regimens may encompass either continuous infusion or involve a bolus dose. The most common continuous IV ketamine infusion dose is from 2.0 to 5.0 mcg/kg/min. In some clinics, that continuous infusion dose may be preceded by an IV ketamine bolus of 0.5–1.0 mg/kg [26]. Ketamine infusion time is typically from 30 to 60 minutes in duration for one treatment. In some cases, the infusion duration may be up to 2 hours. The ketamine infusion treatment series generally consists of a total of four to six treatments that are administered two to three times per week, with the number of treatments increased if the patient does not demonstrate adequate response. Adverse effects of ketamine include increased secretions, bronchodilation, hallucinations, visual disturbances, unpleasant dreams, dysphoria, hepatotoxicity, and cystitis. See **Table 4** for a summary of this discussion.

5.2 Cannabis/CBD

Cannabis, also known as hemp, is derived from a genus of flowering plant strains that produce active ingredients such as tetrahydrocannabinol (THC) and cannabidiol (CBD). The mechanism of action of THC comprises activation of cannabinoid receptor type 1 (CB1 receptor) and cannabinoid receptor type 2 (CB2 receptor) [27]. CB1 receptor expression is in the central and peripheral nervous system, while CB2 receptor expression is primarily in the periphery, mostly in cell types involved in immunity, hematopoietic cells, and glia cells [27]. These receptors result in both the analgesic and the psychotropic effects of cannabis [27]. CBD has demonstrated a negative allosteric effect on CB1 receptors and positive modulatory effects on the endocannabinoid system, which results in reduction of psychotropic effects from THC and potentiates the anticonvulsant and analgesic effects when administered concomitantly. Unlike THC, CBD is not psychotropic.

Although plant strains from which cannabis is derived have been grown for at least 12,000 years and there has been evidence of medicine use by Chinese emperors in 2700 BC, cannabis is still considered an investigational drug. Nabilone and dronabinol are synthetic derivatives of THC that are approved by the FDA for treating nausea and vomiting associated with chemotherapy. Clinical trials demonstrate potential for treatment of nausea and vomiting resulting from chemotherapy, appetite stimulation, chronic pain, and muscle spasms [27, 28]. Routes of administration for cannabis and its derivatives include inhalation vias smoking, ingestion, rectal, sublingual, transdermal, ocular, and intravenous [28].

Adverse effects of short-term use of cannabis include impairments in memory, motor coordination, and judgment. At higher doses, cannabis can also result in paranoia and psychosis. Long-term use of use of large quantities of marijuana can lead to addiction, cognitive impairments, chronic bronchitis (if use is via inhalation or smoking), and increased risk of chronic psychotic disorders such as schizophrenia in individuals with a high predisposition [28, 29]. There is also evidence that THC and CBD, the active components of cannabis, act on cytochrome P450 isozymes to influence the metabolism of substances, with THC being an inducer of CYP1A2 and CBD being an inhibitor of CYP3A4 and CYP2D6 [30]. **Table 4** provides a summary of this discussion.

5.3 Infusion therapy

Infusion of IV lidocaine is a modality that can be considered. IV lidocaine is primarily indicated for treatment-resistant peripheral neuropathy [31].

Lidocaine, when used as a local anesthetic, blocks sodium-gated channels, which desensitize peripheral nociceptors. When used as an infusion, IV route, the lower dose blocks the sodium channels of the central nervous system (CNS), mainly affecting the spinal cord and dorsal root ganglia (DRG). Additionally, lidocaine can also affect potassium-gated cannels at the DRG; hyperpolarization cyclic nucleotides channels (HCN); and N-methyl-D-aspartate, (NMDA). The effect on the potassium-gated channels and HCN can contribute to spinal anesthesia. Lidocaine also has anti-inflammatory properties as it decreases cytokines and increases acetylcholine in the CSF, which inhibits spinal pain pathway.

IV lidocaine dosing varies; however, per a recent systematic review, pain clinics have dosed in the following: weight-based of 1–2-mg/kg bolus, a fixed-bolus dose of 50–100 mg, and a 1-mg/kg/hour continuous infusion. Notably, there is also no standard for duration of administration, and serum monitoring is not common practice [32].

Though not an absolute contraindication, careful dosing in patients with cardiac or hepatic failure is essential. The volume of distribution is smaller and the half-life is shorter in the former and the volume of distribution is larger and the half-life is longer in the latter [33]. Other possible complications include headaches, tinnitus, nausea, lightheadedness, paresthesia, hypotension, arrhythmia, respiratory depression, and cardiac arrest [31]. **Table 4** provides a summary of this discussion.

Agent	Dosing	Benefits	Common side effects
Ketamine	continuous IV: 2.0 to 5.0 mcg/kg/min IV bolus: 0.5 to 1.0 mg/kg	chronic neuropathic pain, nociceptive pain	Increased secretions, bronchodilation, hallucinations, visual disturbances, unpleasant dreams, dysphoria, hepatotoxicity, cystitis
Cannabis/ CBD	mild effect: 1.0–2.5 mg moderate effect: 2.5–15 mg maximum: 40 mg/ day	nausea and vomiting resulting from chemotherapy, appetite stimulation, chronic pain, muscle spasms	Impaired memory, impaired motor coordination, impaired judgment, paranoia, psychosis
Lidocaine	continuous IV: 1.0 mg/kg/hour weight-based bolus: 1.0 to 2.0 mg/kg bolus fixed bolus: 50–100 mg	treatment-resistant peripheral neuropathy	Headaches, tinnitus, nausea, lightheadedness, paresthesia, hypotension, arrhythmia, respiratory depression, cardiac arrest
Botulinum toxin (Botox)		headaches, chronic lower back pain	Bruising, pain at the injection site, dysphagia if injections are near the neck and mouth

Table 4.
Novel pharmacologic approaches to pain management with dosages, benefits, and common side effects.

5.4 Additional treatments

5.4.1 Paravertebral injection of botulinum toxin (Botox)

Paravertebral injection of the botulinum toxin (Botox), commonly used in the treatment of headaches, appears to also have a place in the treatment of chronic lower back pain [34]. Botox's mechanism of action involves the reduction of muscle hyperactivity and tension by blocking the presynaptic release of acetylcholine [35].

The most common side effects include bruising and pain at the injection site. Dysphagia can be caused by injections near the neck and mouth. Contraindications include infection near injection site, allergy to medication, Eaton Lambert syndrome, or Myasthenia Gravis. Patients must be 13 years or older and not pregnant or nursing. Botox should be used with caution in patients with neuromuscular conduction disease or taking medications that alter this as well as those with peripheral motor neuron disease [35].

5.4.2 Trigger point injection

Trigger point injections or dry needling is typically used for myofascial pain. They also have a role in alleviating pain from post-mastectomy pain syndrome (PMPS) [36]. These points are identified by palpation, observing for tenderness, referred pain or even twitching of muscle fibers when compressed, commonly referred to as "knots." A needle or an injection containing local anesthetic (avoid bupivacaine as this can be myotoxic) or even saline is inserted at these points directly into the muscle tissue. Care must be taken to avoid any major structures [37].

In order to carry out this procedure, a needle is inserted into the trigger point and "fanning" can be done, which theoretically disrupts connective tissue and causes muscle fiber relaxation and lengthening. Recent studies are currently exploring Radial Extracorporeal Shock Wave Therapy as an alternative to trigger point injections in the treatment of myofascial pain [38].

6. The use of external stimulation devices for chronic pain

6.1 Transcutaneous electric nerve stimulation (TENS)

Transcutaneous electrical nerve stimulation (TENS) is a safe, portable, cost-effective, and noninvasive treatment approach used for pain management in patients who are refractory to pharmacological intervention. Electrical pulses are delivered to adhesive electrode pads positioned on the patient's skin overlying the region where treatment is to be administered [39]. The duration, frequency, and intensity of the electrical pulses delivered by the device can be adjusted by the care provider. The electrode pads are attached to two or more electrode wires connected to the battery-powered TENS device. TENS is believed to relieve pain via decreasing dorsal horn neuron sensitization and increasing gamma-aminobutyric acid (GABA) and glycine levels. **Figure 1** below shows a common setup for outpatient TENS treatment.

Indications for use include musculoskeletal pain, neuropathic pain, osteoarthritis, fibromyalgia, pelvic pain, and lower back pain [40, 41]. The use of TENS is not recommended in patients who have electronic implants such as pacemakers and cardiac

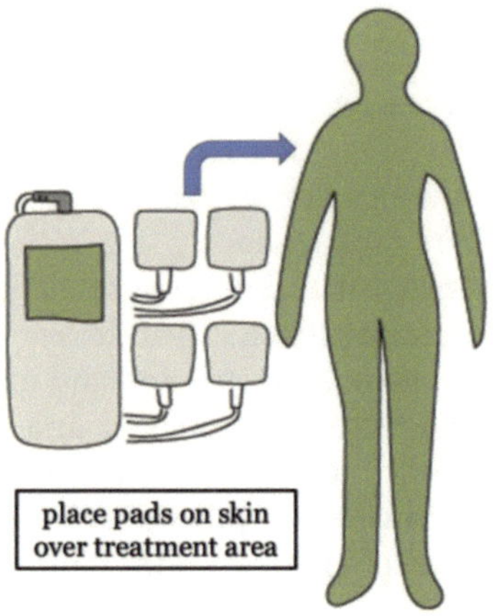

Figure 1.
A schematic of a common setup for TENS treatment.

defibrillators. Caution is also advised before use in individuals who are pregnant, have epilepsy, have active malignancy, have blood clots, have damaged skin, and are immunocompromised [42, 43]. Adverse effects of TENS include skin burns where electrode pads are placed and allergic reaction to electrode pad or its adhesive [39].

6.2 Inferential current stimulation

Interferential current stimulation (ICS) is a convenient, cost-effective, and noninvasive treatment approach used for pain management in patients who are refractory to pharmacologic intervention. In ICS, alternation of two or more sinusoidal currents simultaneously generates interference and maximizes the ability of the current to permeate tissues while maintaining minimal cutaneous nerve stimulation [44]. Intersection and interference of currents in the region to be treated are facilitated by the way the two or more electrodes are placed on the skin for ICS treatment. **Figure 2** shows a schematic of outpatient ICS treatment.

Indications for use include muscle stimulation such as for physiotherapy or rehabilitation, knee osteoarthritis, chronic low back pain, shoulder soft tissue pain, chronic jaw pain, fibromyalgia, incontinence, edema reduction, and myofascial syndrome pain [44–46]. The use of ICS is contraindicated in patients who have implanted electronic devices such as pacemakers, cardiac defibrillators, or hearing aids. Caution is advised before use in patients who are pregnant, have cardiovascular disease, have inflammation or fever, have active malignancy, and have thrombosis. Adverse effects include skin burns, bruises, blisters, or swelling of skin overlying treated region as well as discomfort or muscle soreness in the treated region.

6.3 Pulsed electromagnetic field therapy

Pulsed Electromagnetic Field Therapy (PEMF or PEMT) is a safe, noninvasive treatment approach used for pain management in patients who are refractory to pharmacologic intervention.

The PEMT device consists of a mat comprised of spiral coils and frequency generator that energizes the coils to generate a pulsed electromagnetic field [47, 48]. That electromagnetic field in turn induces electric fields in the patient's conductive

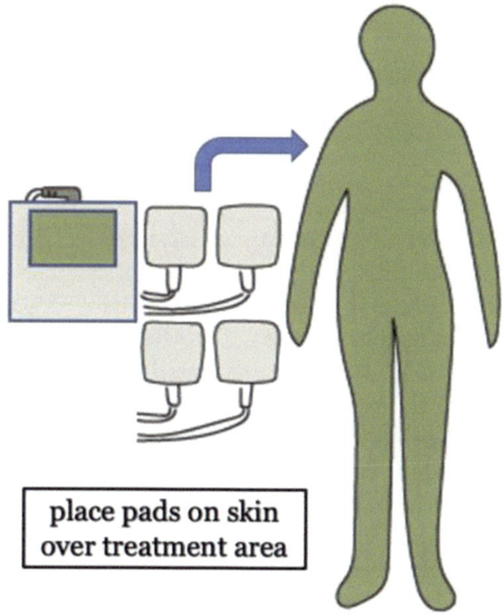

Figure 2.
A schematic of a common setup for ICS treatment.

tissues via inductive coupling. PEMT is believed to cause changes in cellular signaling and modulation of inflammatory cytokines, growth factors, and membrane receptors that produces an analgesic effect [49–51]. **Figure 3** shows a common setup for PEMF/PEMT treatment.

Indications for use include healing of non-union fractures, stress urinary incontinence, cervical fusion, depression, anxiety, brain cancer, fibromyalgia, rheumatoid arthritis, musculoskeletal pain, knee osteoarthritis, chronic pelvic pain, and chronic low back pain [52, 53]. The use of ICS is contraindicated in patients who have implanted devices such as cardiac defibrillators and pacemakers. Caution

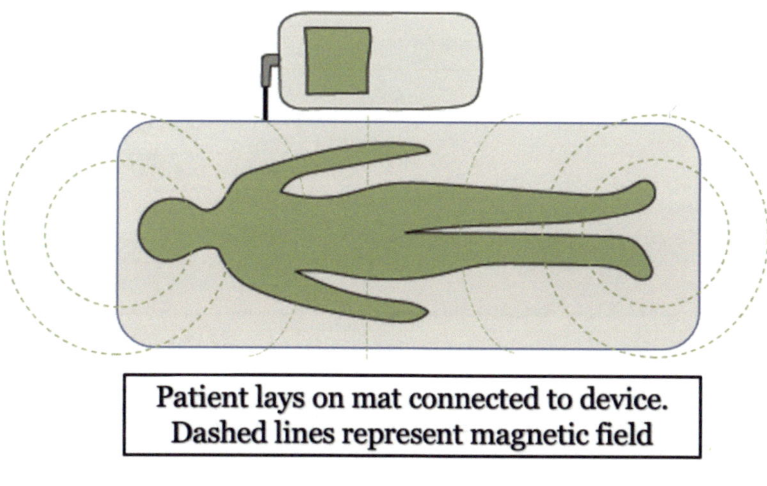

Figure 3.
A schematic of a common setup for PEMF treatment.

is advised before use in patients who are children, are pregnant, have cardiovascular disease, have inflammation or fever, have active malignancy, and have thrombosis. Adverse effects include possible cancer risk from exposure to low-frequency magnetic field.

6.4 Diathermy

Diathermy is a noninvasive treatment approach used for pain management in patients who are refractory to pharmacologic intervention. The technique involves the controlled production of heat within body tissues using high-frequency electromagnetic current generated by diathermies, deep-heating agents such as ultrasound, shortwave, and microwave [54]. The heat generated is believed to increase local circulation, thus promoting toxin removal, facilitating tissue repair, and providing pain relief [55]. **Figure 4** shows a schematic for a common diathermy setup.

Indications for use include rotator cuff disease, bursitis, tendinitis, osteoarthritis, peripheral neuropathy, low back pain, musculoskeletal pain, and fibromyalgia [56, 57]. The use of ICS is contraindicated over wet dressings, reproductive organs, and infected open wounds. It is also contraindicated in patients who are pregnant, have impaired thermal sensation, have implanted devices such as pacemakers, have metal implants, have severe edema, and have bleeding disorders. Caution is advised before use in patients who have cardiac disease, have vascular disease, have active infection or fever, have active malignancy, and have thrombosis. Adverse effects include burns in the treated and adjacent tissues, shock or burn, and excessive heating of metal implants in body such as dental fillings or bone pins.

7. Interventional management of subacute and chronic pain

Interventional pain management, borne of regional anesthesia and neural blockade, has evolved into a multimodal, multidisciplinary approach to treat the incredibly costly and debilitating symptoms of chronic pain. Due to the more

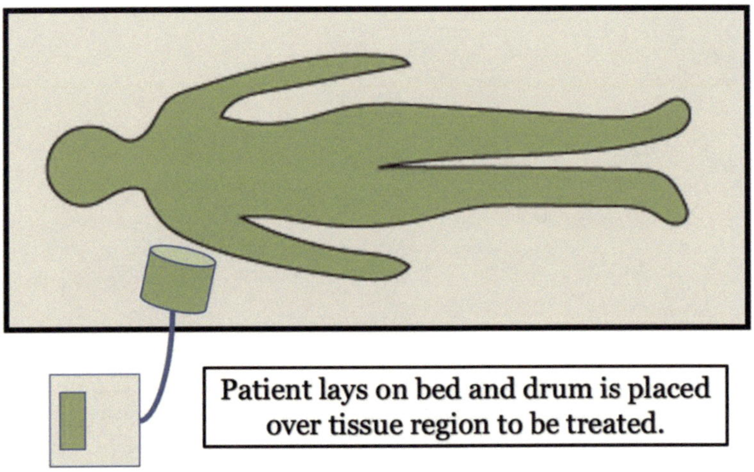

Figure 4.
A schematic of a common setup for induction diathermy treatment via drum method.

invasive nature of interventional procedures, they are not usually first line in the treatment of subacute to chronic pain. Typically, patients are seen in the pain management clinic after failure of pharmacological and/or physical therapy for at least 6 weeks. In 2016, low back and neck pain costs an estimated $134.5 billion dollars and the most common symptom patients present with at interventional pain clinics [58].

Since the 1950s, epidural steroids injections (ESIs) have been used for pain relief of chronic lower back and neck pain, particularly for treatment of radiculopathy. ESI continues to be a mainstay of procedural pain management [59].

Interventional procedure steps may differ and depend on the physician's training and/or patient's body habitus, and the procedures described in this section take that into account in addition to two major pain society guidelines.

7.1 Injectates

7.1.1 Glucocorticoids

Long-acting (depot) glucocorticoids can be used in intra-articular and epidural injections. Two of the most used depot glucocorticoids include methylprednisolone acetate and triamcinolone acetonide. For peripheral intra-articular injections, there is no current standard for dosing of these steroids; however, it is common practice to base the dose on the size of the joint. For methylprednisolone acetate, 10–20, 40–60, and 40–80 mg are used in small, medium, and large joint sizes, respectively. Triamcinolone acetonide dosing is 8–10, 20–30, and 20–40 mg on small, medium, and large joint sizes, respectively.

Contraindications for injectates are septic arthritis due to risk of exacerbation of infection, juxta-articular osteoporosis due to risk of worsening bone density, periarticular fracture as glucocorticoids can inhibit bone healing, and join instability due to risk of weakening adjacent ligaments and capsule [60].

7.1.2 Local anesthetics

The most utilized local anesthetics include lidocaine and bupivacaine, both amides. These anesthetics can be used with or without epinephrine. Epinephrine is added for its vasoconstriction effects that decrease uptake of the local anesthetic into the circulatory system, which affects the cardio-and neuro toxicity and allowing for higher dosages, increases duration of action of the local anesthetic (except for bupivacaine), and decreases bleeding. The addition of epinephrine to local anesthetics is not recommended in procedures on digits of patients with peripheral vascular disease.

In the adult patient, lidocaine without epinephrine dosing should not exceed 4 mg/kg. Lidocaine with epinephrine should not exceed 7 mg/kg. Bupivacaine without epinephrine dosing should not exceed 2 mg/kg meanwhile bupivacaine with epinephrine should not exceed 3 mg/kg. Notably, lidocaine has a higher allowable dose increase with epinephrine when compared to bupivacaine because bupivacaine is more cardiotoxic due to its slower rate of dissociation at diastole, cardiotoxicity being the dose-limiting adverse reaction.

Bupivacaine, typically used at 0.25–0.5% concentration, is longer acting than lidocaine [61]. **Table 5** compares the more commonly used local anesthetics in pain clinics.

Anesthetic Injectate	Concentration (%)	Onset of Action (min)	Duration of Action (min)	Maximum Allowable Dose (mg/kg)	Maximum Total Dose (mg)
Lidocaine	1	2–5	50–120	4	300
Lidocaine (w/epinephrine)	1 (1:200,000)	2–5	60–180	7	500
Bupivacaine	0.25	5–10	240–480	2	175
Bupivacaine (w/epinephrine)	0.25 (1:200,000)	5–10	240–480	3	225

Table 5.
Comparison of commonly used local anesthetics for interventional pain procedures.

7.2 Imaging

Interventional pain clinics rely on either surface landmarks or image guidance such as computed tomography (CT), fluoroscopy, or ultrasound. Historically, surface landmarks were the choice among physicians in performing interventional pain procedures. Imaging is more common now for the accuracy and precision of a procedure as well as improved safety of the patient. Ultrasound guidance, the oldest of the aforementioned imaging modalities, had resurgence across multiple specialties including pain medicine as it is a bedside, point-of-care tool that provides real-time visualization of needle placement and advancement as well as adjacent structures. Ultrasound technology also reduces radiation exposure to both patient and interventionalist [62].

An ultrasound suite requires a smaller footprint when compared to a room that has a C-arm (used for fluoroscopic guidance). Room and equipment setups vary according to physician preference. **Figure 5** below shows an example of a common material setup for ultrasound-guided injection within a room.

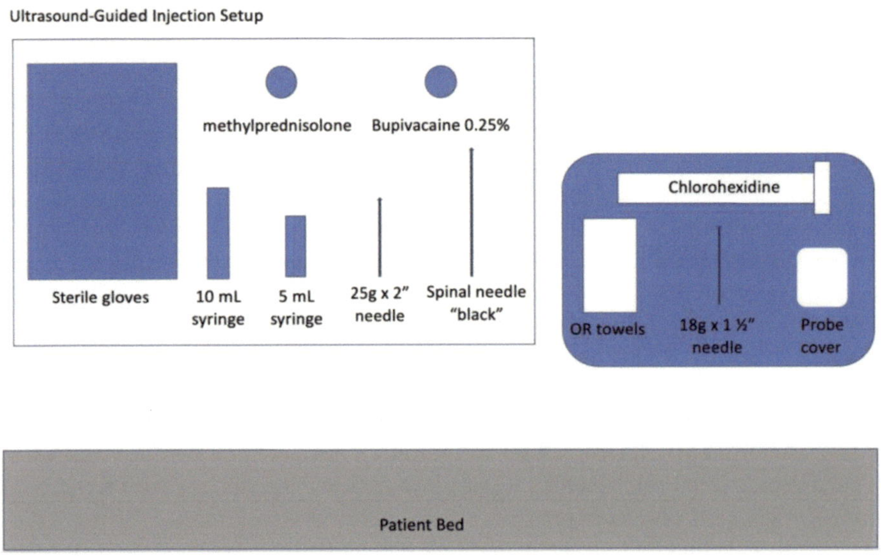

Figure 5.
A schematic of a common setup for ultra-sounded guided procedures (not drawn to scale).

DOI: http://dx.doi.org/10.5772/intechopen.108993

7.3 Joint injections

Most of the procedures listed below can be done with ultrasound or fluoroscopic guidance.

7.3.1 Hip joint injection

The hip joint is the articulation of the acetabulum and the femoral head, also known as the femoroacetabular joint, is essentially a ball-and-socket joint. Notably, 40% of the femoral head is in contact with the acetabulum, lubricated by synovium, at all times—in extension, flexion, rotation, which allow for steady gait, rising from a seated position and general mobilization. This major joint is stabilized by way of ligaments (ischiofemoral, pubofemoral, and iliofemoral) and cartilage, particularly, the labrum. Osteoarthritis of the hip is deterioration of the articular cartilage, and this wear and tear may cause pain that can significantly affect activities of daily living (ADLs) [63]. This procedure can be done via either ultrasound or fluoroscopic guidance.

For performing the procedure under fluoroscopic guidance, anatomical landmarks are first identified by way of fluoroscopy in the AP and oblique views. The patient's hip region is prepped and draped in sterile fashion. The skin and subcutaneous tissues at the needle entry site are infiltrated with a small amount of Lidocaine. The needle is then advanced incrementally under fluoroscopic guidance toward the point where the femoral head meets the femoral neck until os is contacted and the joint space is entered. After negative aspiration, a small amount of contrast solution is injected showing an appropriate arthrogram to ensure that needle termination is not in an adjacent bursa and thereby truly intra-articular. Then, a solution consisting of a local anesthetic mixed with a glucocorticoid is injected slowly. **Figure 6** is an image of a fluoroscopic-guided right hip injection.

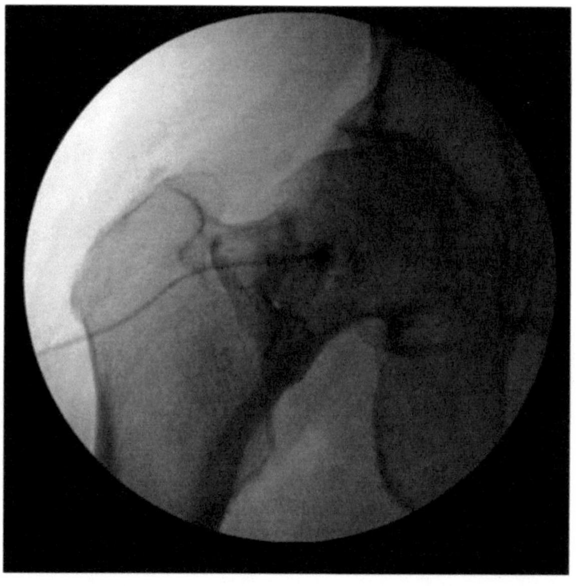

Figure 6.
An example of an image captured during fluoroscopic-guided right hip injection.

For performing the procedure under ultrasound guidance, the patient's hip region is prepped and draped in the usual sterile fashion. A needle is advanced incrementally under ultrasound guidance toward the femoral neck until os is contacted and the joint space is entered. The local anesthetic and glucocorticoid mixture is given after negative aspiration.

Potential risks and complications include infection, small vessel injury, and bleeding. Contraindications include, but are not limited to, acute fracture, bacteremia, septic arthritis, or infection at needle entry site.

7.3.2 Sacroiliac joint injection

Sacroiliac (SI) joint pain is a common cause of mechanical low back pain. It is a pain, when described by patients, radiates to the back, typically below L5, and groin. Typically, degenerative etiology, pregnancy, or trauma can also cause SI joint pain. SI joint injections can be diagnostic as well as therapeutic. The SI joint, as the name suggests, is located between the sacrum and the ilium, bilaterally. Sensory innervation of this joint is not clearly defined; however, it may be lateral branches from dorsal sacral foramen and possibly L5 dorsal rami as well as the superior gluteal nerve [64].

The procedure is typically done with the guidance of fluoroscopy. The patient is prepped in a prone position until the inferior borders of the SI bony plates are parallel on imaging. With intermittent fluoroscopy, needle inserted is inferior until popping sensation is appreciated. Contrast is injected and should outline the SI joint. As with other joint Injections, injectate is local anesthetic and corticosteroid. This can also be done under CT or ultrasound guidance [65]. **Figure 7** shows an image of a right SI joint injection under fluoroscopy.

The risks to this procedure include increased pain at the site of insertion or injection, infection, trauma to nearby anatomy, including nerves. Unsuccessful pain reduction is also possible, when done under fluoroscopic guidance, this appears to be around 10% risk of failure [66].

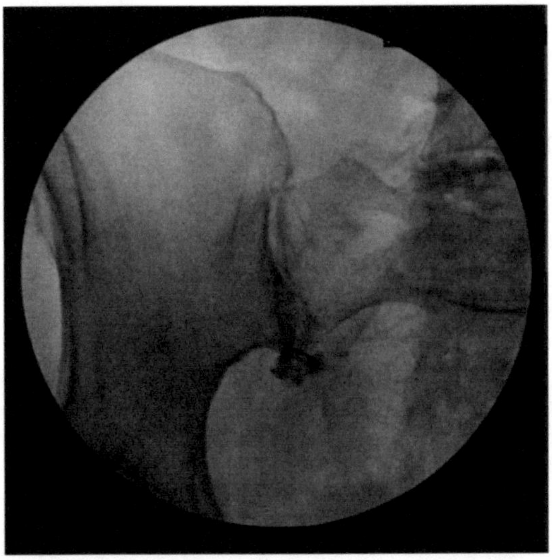

Figure 7.
An example of an image captured during fluoroscopic-guided right SI joint injection performed in the interventional pain clinic.

7.4 Neuronal blockade

Different forms of neural blockade, initially used for surgical anesthesia, have secured their positions in chronic pain management.

7.4.1 Greater occipital nerve

The greater occipital nerve (GON) block can be used as a primary treatment for multiple types of severe headaches or, more commonly, treatment-resistant headaches. A GON block can relieve migraines, cervicogenic headaches, post-dural puncture headaches, and even optic neuralgia. GON block is particularly useful for patients who are not able to tolerate more common pharmacologic regimens, such as those with multiple comorbidities, as well as the elderly and pregnant patient population [67]. The GON stems from the medial branches of dorsal primary rami of the cervical nerve roots C2 – C4, and occasionally C5 and innervates the posterior scalp [68].

To carry out the procedure, the patient is placed in a prone or seated position with slight flexion at neck. Identify the surface landmarks, typically palpated, mastoid process, and occipital protuberance ipsilateral to the headache pain. The GON is about two-thirds of the distance from the mastoid process to the occipital protuberance, about 2 cm lateral and 2 cm inferior from the protuberance. Insert needle from an infero-lateral approach until contact is made with the periosteum and then retract about 1 mm. Aspirate needle at this location to ensure that needle tip is not in the occipital artery and inject with or without a sweeping motion. This can be done with ultrasound guidance and should be noted that GON is typically medial to the occipital artery as shown in **Figure 8**.

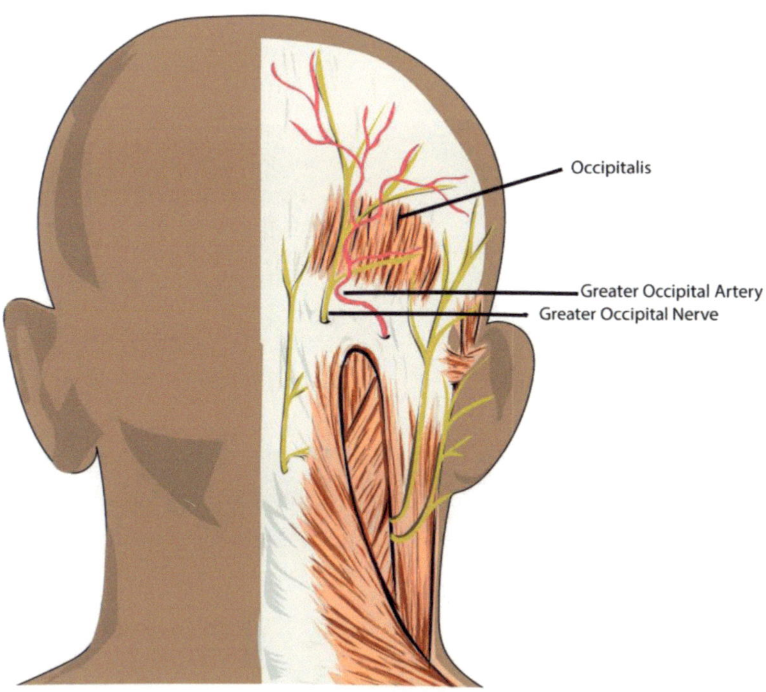

Figure 8.
Anatomic considerations for greater occipital nerve neuronal blockade.

Local anesthetic with or without glucocorticoid is commonly used as the injectate. The use of glucocorticoids can be specifically effective for certain types of headaches such as cluster headaches [69].

As with other nerve blocks, intravascular injection can lead to significant complications. Cushingoid, secondary to excess glucocorticoid, can occur with serial blocks that contain glucocorticoid treatment [70].

7.4.2 Celiac plexus

The blockade of the celiac plexus can be used for intractable abdominal pain, and most commonly pain caused pancreatic cancer [71, 72]. The celiac plexus has three major components, celiac, aortic, and superior mesenteric stemming from the antero-lateral horn of the spinal cord at T5–T12. The celiac plexus innervates the gallbladder, liver, pancreas, and gastrointestinal tract from the stomach to the transverse colon [73].

To carry out this procedure, the patient is positioned in prone and with maximal kyphosis by bolster. Recent evidence suggests that ultrasound-guided celiac plexus blocks are safer and less costly [74]. The surface landmarks are T12 and L1 vertebral bodies. The needle is inserted at the inferior border of the 12th rib, about 6–8 cm from the midline, at a 45-degree posterior to anterior angle, and advanced toward the ventral surface of T12-L1 intervertebral space. Once contact is made with vertebral body, needle is advanced further by 1 cm into the prevertebral fascial plane. This can be confirmed by fluoroscopy [73]. **Figure 9** shows the anatomic considerations for the celiac plexus at vertebral level T12.

If a patient is unable to lie prone, an anterior para-aortic approach can be useful. At the anterior T12 vertebral body, the needle is inserted and advanced toward the abdominal aorta and injected into the antero-crural space. It must be noted that an anterior approach has a higher risk of organ injury [73]. In terms of the injectate used,

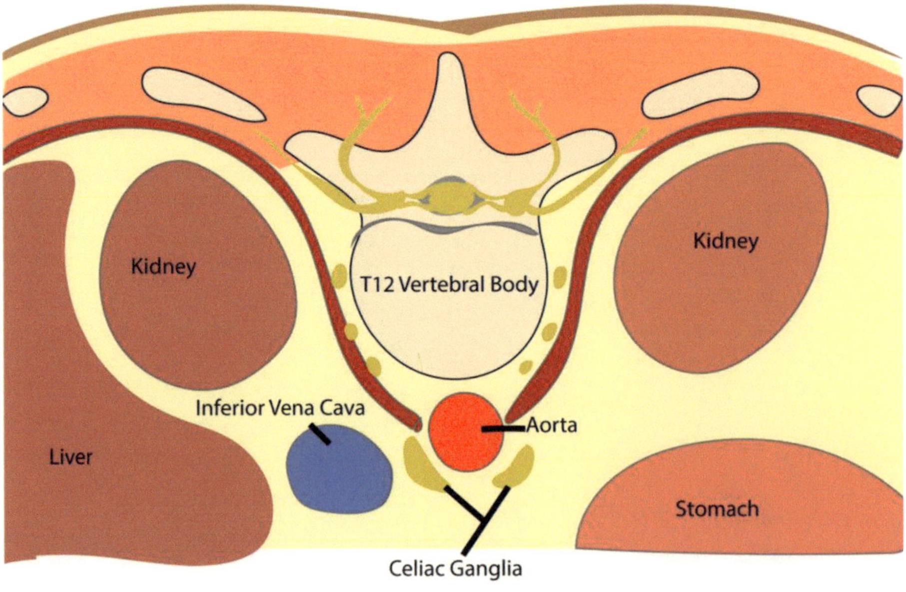

Figure 9.
Anatomic considerations for the celiac plexus.

steroid and local anesthetics are used for benign etiologies of pain and neurolytics are for malignant etiology.

The possible complications from a celiac plexus nerve block or neurolysis include but are not limited to the following: orthostatic hypotension, paresthesia, infection, pneumothorax, paraplegia, and a higher risk of organ damage with the anterior approach [75].

7.4.3 Superior hypogastric plexus

The blockade of the superior hypogastric plexus can be used for chronic pelvic pain caused by multiple etiologies including endometriosis, inflammatory processes, postoperative adhesions, and malignancy [76]. The superior hypogastric plexus is located in the retroperitoneal space, between L5-S1 vertebral bodies.

In the posterior approach, the patient is placed in prone position with emphasized flexion at the lumbar spine by bolster. The surface landmark of L4-L5 intervertebral space is identified, and under fluoroscopic-guidance, the needle is inserted 5–7 cm lateral of the middle of this space, from either side, at a 30-degree oblique and 30-degree caudad angle, toward the anterolateral L5-S1 paraspinous junction. Contrast should spread midline in the AP view and needle tip should be visualized at the anterolateral margin of L5 and spread anterior to the L5 vertebral body. It is important to emphasize the proximity of the superior hypogastric plexus to the iliac vessels [77]. Local anesthetic or neurolytic is commonly used as injectate.

This procedure can cause transient or even permanent retrograde ejaculation as the urogenital system is primarily innervated by the superior hypogastric plexus.

7.4.4 Medial branch block (MBB) injection

Facet joint injection is the injection of a combination of steroid and local anesthetic at the site of the joint, while medial branch block is injected right outside the joint at the medial branch of the dorsal rami. Theoretically, either may have prognostic value for radiofrequency ablation and the latter with more therapeutic value, however, mostly short-term. Common practice at pain management clinics usually requires successful diagnostic medial branch blocks on two separate occasions, which can be followed with radiofrequency ablation [78]. MBBs are indicated for spondylosis, post-laminectomy syndrome, facet arthropathy, and disk degeneration.

To carry out this procedure, the patient is placed in the prone (lumbar) or supine (cervical, anterior approach, other approaches include posterior or posterolateral, dependent on technique of interventionalist) position. Anatomical landmarks are identified with the aid of fluoroscopy in the PA and oblique views [77].

For the Lumbar Spine: The patient's lumbar region is prepped and draped in sterile fashion. The skin and subcutaneous tissues at each needle entry site are infiltrated with a small amount of lidocaine using a needle is incrementally advanced under fluoroscopic guidance in multiple views at each level such that the needle tip is advanced to contact os at the junction of the superior articulating process and the superomedial border of the transverse process at each of the cephalad levels as well as to contact os at the junction of the superior articulating process and the superomedial border of the sacral ala at the S1 level. After negative aspiration is confirmed, a small amount of lidocaine is injected into the cephalad needles and a small amount of 0.25% Bupivacaine is injected at the S1 level.

For the Cervical Spine: The patient's cervical region is prepped and draped in sterile fashion. The skin and subcutaneous tissues at each needle entry site are infiltrated with approximately a total of 3 mL of 1% lidocaine. Needles are advanced under fluoroscopic guidance from the lateral view such that the needle tips are positioned on os at the center of the cuboid masses of the posterior columns of targeted levels. Needle placement should be confirmed via fluoroscopy. At each level, following negative aspiration, a small amount of 0.25% Bupivacaine (or other anesthetic) is injected slowly.

After the procedure, the patient's skin is wiped clean and bandages are placed. **Figure 10** shows an example of an image capture by fluoroscopy for a medial branch block while **Figure 11** is an illustration that shows approximate location of the medial branch in relation to a vertebral body and facet joint.

In terms of anatomic considerations, the C3 deep medial branch, C4, and C6 medial branches are located slightly above the waist of their corresponding articular pillars and C5 medial branch tends to be located right at the waist of the articular pillar. The risks of the procedure include trauma or damage to nearby structures including the spinal cord or adjacent nerves, infection, epidural bleeding, or hematoma.

Other neuronal blocks include stellate ganglion as shown in **Figure 12** for head, neck, and upper arm pain, and genicular nerve for chronic osteoarthritis of the knee as shown in **Figure 13**.

Other procedures include shoulder injections as shown in **Figure 14** and piriformis injection as shown in **Figure 15** for piriformis syndrome, most commonly causing sciatic nerve entrapment and subsequent symptoms. Bursa injections provide relief for bursitis particularly trochanteric, ischial, subacromial, olecranon, and prepatellar.

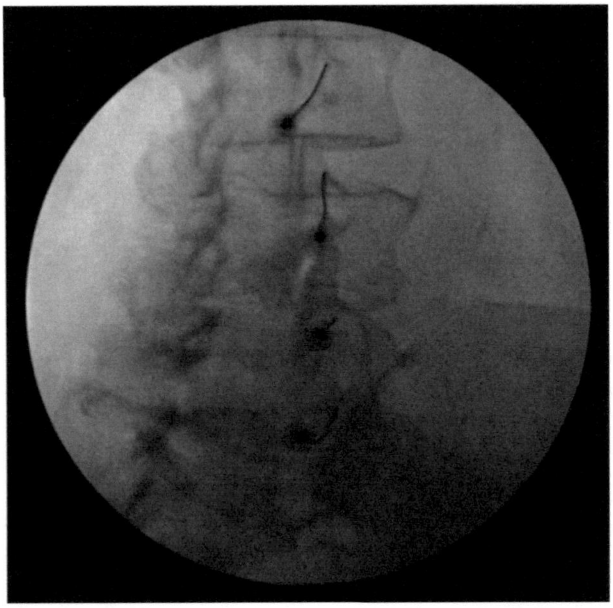

Figure 10.
An example of an image captured during fluoroscopic-guided medial branch block performed in the interventional pain clinic.

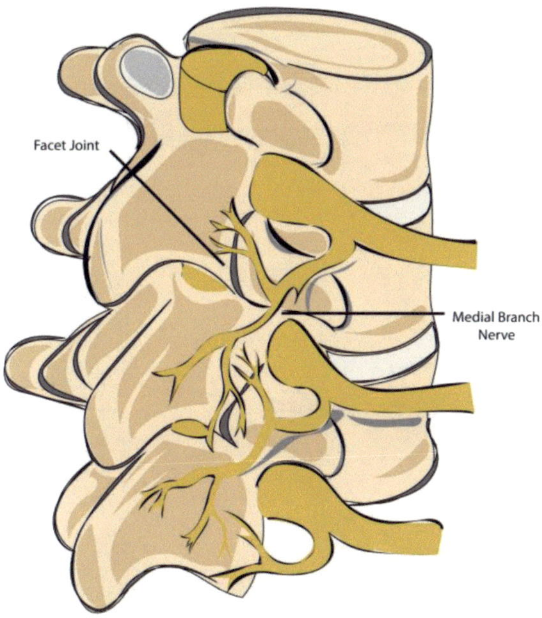

Figure 11.
Anatomical considerations for medial branch blocks.

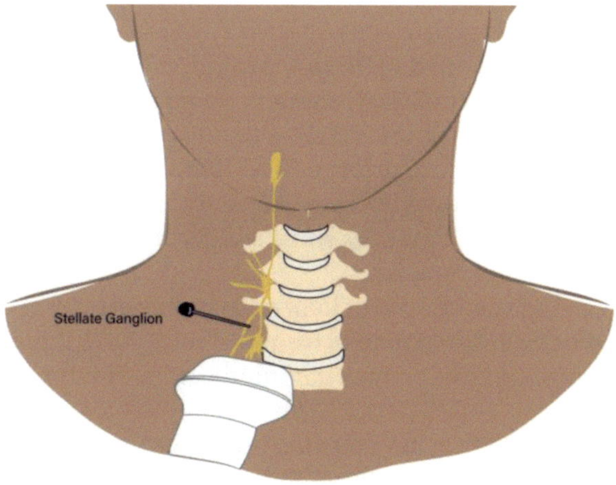

Figure 12.
Anatomical considerations for stellate ganglion blockade.

7.5 Radiofrequency ablation

Literature on radiofrequency ablation (RFA) continues to show mixed results on its cost effectiveness and therapeutic efficacy [79]; despite this, RFA continues to be commonly performed in interventional pain suites, most commonly for facet joint pain as well as SI joint pain.

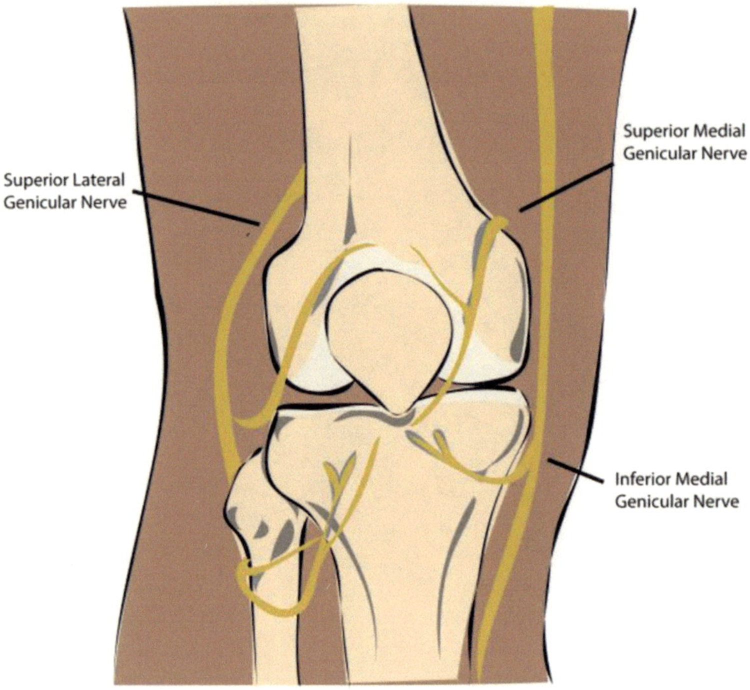

Figure 13.
Anatomical considerations for genicular nerve blockade.

Prior to first time ablation of the MBB for facet joint pain, at least two rounds of successful diagnostic MBBs are usually required. Some hospital systems, such as St. Luke's University Health Network (SLUHN), provide patients with a pain diary after MBB to gauge success of procedure prior to RFA. Repeat ablation may have different prerequisites in different locations. Patients are educated that the goal of RFA is a 50% reduction in pain for about 6–12 months since tempering patient expectations is a mainstay of pain management practice.

RFA is currently being used for facet joint pain by targeting the medial branch of the dorsal ramus (since reimbursement is trending away from intra-articular facet joint injections), discogenic pain (ramus communicans), SI joint pain as well as radicular pain (DRG).

To carry out RFA, the patient is placed in the prone position. Anatomical landmarks are identified by way of palpation with fluoroscopy in the PA and oblique views. The patient's lumbar region is prepped and draped in the usual sterile fashion using chlorohexidine. The skin and subcutaneous tissues are infiltrated with a small amount of 1% Lidocaine at each of the intended needle entry sites. Via fluoroscopy in the AP and oblique views, needle tip is incrementally advanced under fluoroscopic guidance at each level. At each of these levels, the needle tip contacts the os at the superior medial border of the junction of the transverse process of the lumbar levels and to contact the os at the medial aspect of the groove formed by the sacral ala in the superior articular process of S1.

After proper needle placement is confirmed with fluoroscopic guidance at each level, sensory and/or motor stimulation is performed at 2 Hz and 50 Hz, respectively. Small amount of 2% lidocaine is instilled at all levels. After a period of approximately 90 seconds, each level is lesioned at 90 degrees Celsius. Following the initial lesioning,

DOI: http://dx.doi.org/10.5772/intechopen.108993

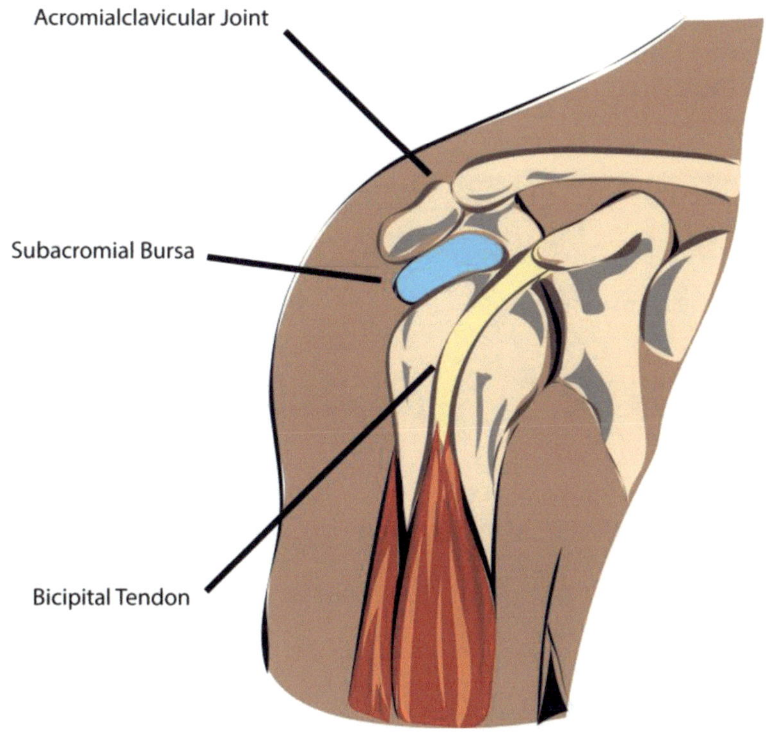

Figure 14.
Anatomical considerations for shoulder injections.

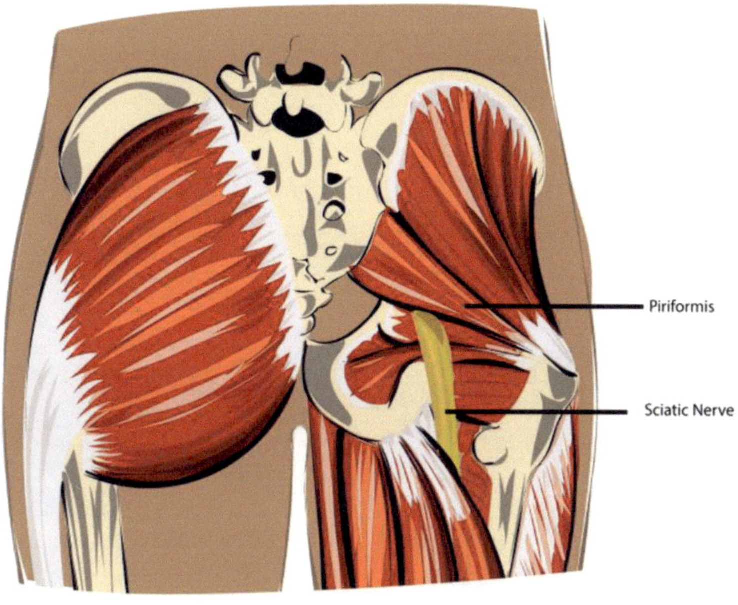

Figure 15.
Anatomical considerations piriformis injection.

each needle tip is repositioned x 2 under fluoroscopic guidance in a clockwise and counterclockwise fashion. Following each reposition, a total of two additional lesions at each side are performed for 90 seconds at 90 degrees Celsius. See **Figure 16** for common settings. After all needles are removed, skin is wiped clean and bandage is placed [77]. **Figure 17** is a schematic of a common room setup for an RFA procedure.

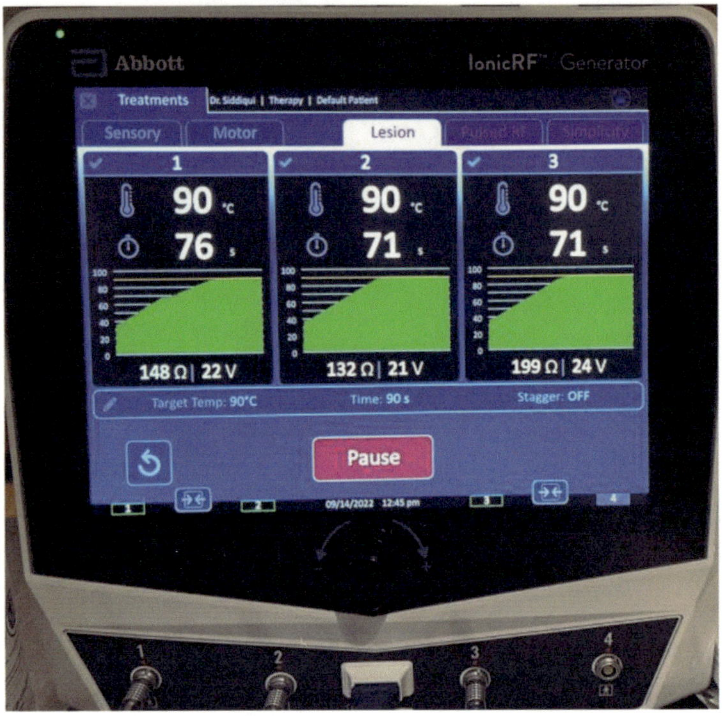

Figure 16.
Initial RFA settings are 90° C for 90 seconds.

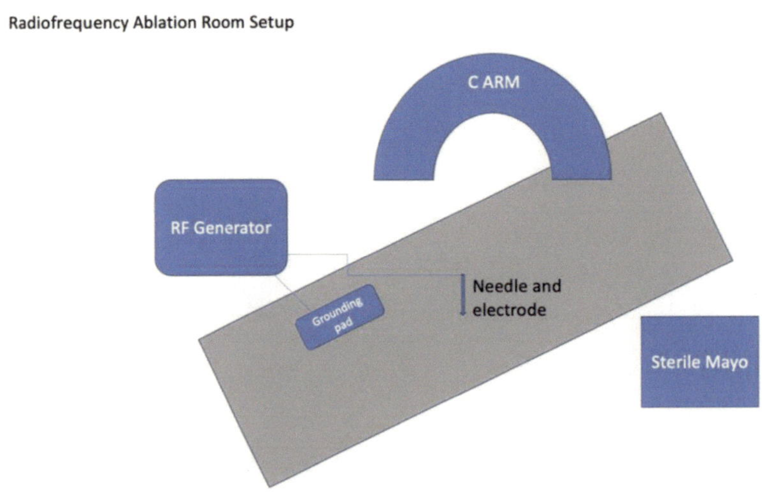

Figure 17.
A schematic of a common setup of an RFA room (not drawn to scale).

Classically, RFA involves thermal energy to cause a lesion and subsequent disruption of a nociceptive pain pathway, by way of Wallerian degeneration. There are currently other iterations including water-cooled radiofrequency ablation (WCRF), cryo-neurolysis, and pulsed radiofrequency ablation [80].

Dizziness and ataxia are possible complications, particularly with cervical RFA. There is also the possibility of infection, cutaneous numbness, dysesthesia, postprocedural pain, and trauma to adjacent structures.

The above discusses conventional continuous radiofrequency ablation. There is also pulsed radiofrequency ablation (PRF) that delivers sort bursts of current and water-cooled radiofrequency ablation (WCRF), a method that uses a continuous flow of water to regulate the flow of current and prevents the needle from overheating.

7.6 Spinal cord stimulation

Spinal cord stimulators (SCS) are indicated for persistent pain status post spinal surgery also known as failed back surgery syndrome (FBSS), and it is moderately effective for radicular pain. It can also be used for Complex Regional pain syndrome (CRPS), painful diabetic neuropathy, and even postherpetic neuralgia and axial low-back pain. Notably, in Europe, SCS is used in refractory angina and peripheral vascular disease [81]. Psychiatric evaluation clearance is common place practice prior to a SCS trial. SCS is typically done in two stages, including a trial device and if effective (50% reduction in pain [82]) final device placement, both done under fluoroscopy.

A SCS trial includes the following steps: The patient is placed in the prone position with legs, abdomen, and arms padded, neck should be noted in neutral position with minimal discomfort. Patient is prepped in sterile fashion. Anatomical landmarks are identified by way of palpation and fluoroscopy in the AP view and the skin overlying the initial intended insertion site is infiltrated with a small amount of 1% Lidocaine. A Touhy needle is incrementally advanced using a loss-of-resistance technique with the aid of fluoroscopy in both the AP and lateral views into the appropriate epidural space. An 8-contact lead is subsequently passed through the Touhy needle and advanced into the epidural space under the aid of fluoroscopy to where the tip of the lead was is at the targeted endplate. The lead is confirmed posterior by way of fluoroscopy in the lateral view and in the AP view [77].

The patient's pain is adequately captured with initial stimulation and the introducer needles are removed with tips in place. The electrodes are secured with adhesive strips. Impedance is checked and multiple electric combinations were utilized to provide coverage of the patients' area of pain. **Figure 18** shows an example of a fluoroscopic image of a trial spinal cord stimulator placed in the thoracic spine.

Of note, prophylactic and postsurgical broad-spectrum antibiotics are used at SLUHN for the placement of the trial device.

If the SCS trial is successful, the final device is placed where an incision is made for tunneling the cables leads and a second incision is made to place the pulse generator above the iliac crest after which the lead cables are connected by tunneling to the pulse generator.

General lead placement locations are navigated by the location of pain [83]. **Table 6** below shows suggested lead placement based on symptomatic location of pain.

One of the most common complications of SCS is lead migration or damage causing decreased efficacy of treatment [84]. A more rare but potentially catastrophic

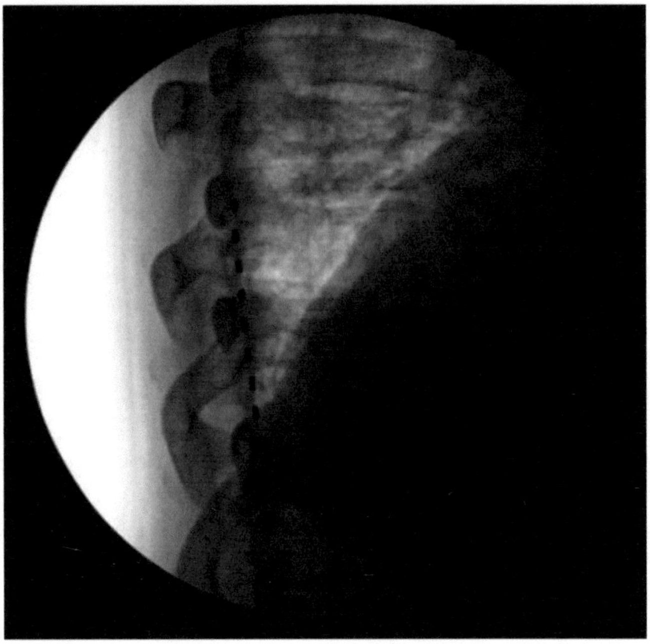

Figure 18.
An example of an image captured during fluoroscopic-guided thoracic epidural spinal cord stimulator leads trial.

Location of Pain	Lead Placement
Neck	C3 and Up
Shoulder	Above C5
Hand	C5-C6
Anterior Thigh	T7, T8, T11–12
Posterior Thigh	T11-L1
Foot	L1
Low Back	T9-T10

Table 6.
Location of pain and associated lead placement for spinal cord stimulation.

complication is a spinal epidural hematoma, which can occur days to weeks after completion of procedure. Spinal epidural hematoma is a medical emergency and should be considered if patient experiences new onset severe back pain and/or neurological impairment [85]. Other complications include spinal cord trauma and tolerance to treatment, particularly in long-term use [86].

The progressing advancement of SCS has allowed for broadening of indications and will likely continue to do so. Placement of the device after a successful trial is usually completed by a Neurosurgeon or Orthopedic Spine surgeon who specializes in this placement, which can lead to a bottleneck in demand for the device placement. **Table** 7 provides a summary of this discussion.

Intervention	Indications	Complications
Spinal Cord Stimulator	Refractory to conservative management • Failed Back Surgery Syndrome (FBSS, post-laminectomy), usually about 12 months after surgery • Complex Regional Pain Syndrome • Painful diabetic neuropathy • Postherpetic neuralgia • Axial low-back pain In Europe • Refractory Angina • Peripheral Vascular Disease	Decreased Efficacy • Lead migration • Instrument damage • Tolerance to treatment Rare but catastrophic • Spinal epidural hematoma • Spinal cord trauma

Table 7.
Common indications and complications of Spinal Cord Stimulators indications.

8. Discussion

The primary goal of the outpatient pain clinic is to help patients improve their quality of life by reducing pain, decreasing dependence on narcotic pain medications, and supporting increased activity levels, thereby allowing a return to a sense of function. Pain may be complex, vague, and wildly subjective, but it can be targeted with a systematic approach that is consistently applied for every patient that presents to the clinic. A thorough history and physical should precede a decision on treatment approach.

The initial evaluation begins with a history of present illness (HPI) and a review of medical history. There are several "red flags" that may significantly alter the treatment plan and warrant further workup; therefore, a thorough history is essential to determine the appropriate treatment approach. When evaluating pain, it is important to take note of location, radiation of pain, duration, quality, severity, exacerbating factors, alleviating factors, history of trauma to the area, as well as the impact this pain has on activities of daily living (ADL). It is also important to note what treatments have already been trialed, including pain medications, external stimulation devices, and surgeries. Pain procedures and alternatives methods are helpful for patients who are not appropriate for more invasive surgical treatment, or for those whom surgery has failed, such as spinal cord stimulators for Failed Back Surgery Syndrome.

The physical exam begins the moment the patient steps foot into the office. General inspection includes overall gait, posture, range of motion, effort, even work of breathing. A neurological exam includes deep tendon reflexes, dermatome and myotome distributions, as well as strength (which can be indicative of neurological and/or musculoskeletal impairment), and tenderness on palpation. Provocation tests are helpful in discerning between symptoms that correlate with more than one etiology and a cluster of positive provocative tests increases accuracy of a diagnosis. For example, if a patient presents with neck pain, a Spurling's test is sensitive but not specific for acute radiculopathy if pain radiates into ipsilateral arm and Lhermitte is specific but not sensitive for cervical spinal cord compression.

Typically, interventional procedures are considered only after a patient has not improved or has experienced only limited improvement on more conservative measures such as medications and/or physical therapy for about 6 weeks. Those whose pain impedes on their ability to participate in physical therapy may also benefit from interventional procedures. Different prerequisites depend on the proposed treatment, and they are illustrated in the charts below (**Figures 14–18**). It can be argued that some procedures, especially less invasive procedures such as ultrasound-guided large joint injections, may be appropriate before this timeframe if the goal is to prevent dependence on narcotics, polypharmacy, or the multitude adverse effects pain medications can have.

Since back pain is the most commonly presenting chief complaint in an outpatient pain clinic, it is important to differentiate between organic and nonorganic back pain etiologies. Nonorganic back pain is more suspected if three or more of the following symptoms are positive: pain with axial compression or passive rotation, negative straight-leg raise with patient distraction, regional disturbance that does not follow dermatomal distributions, overreactions to physical examination, and non-anatomic specific tenderness. This does not mean this patient is not feeling pain; however, it may mean that certain procedures are not indicated. Avoidance of more invasive procedures would be prudent if organic back pain is ruled out. Patient with nonorganic back pain may benefit from optimization of medical and mental health, perhaps further workup, or appropriate referrals in addition to other treatments such as aforementioned external stimulation devices for distraction therapy, trigger point injections and/or SNRIs for conditions such as fibromyalgia, or even cannabis/CBD.

When a patient's back pain is suspicious for organic causes, it is helpful to keep broad stroke interventional mainstays in mind. Classically, radicular symptoms, spinal stenosis, and discogenic pain improve with ESI, facet joint dysfunction responds well to MBB, and SI joint dysfunction with SI joint injections. Newer interventions include RFA after a certain number of successful MBBs as well as the ablation of SI joint nerve, SCS for FBSS, and even radicular pain may be appropriate. Pain Management Physicians may wait at least 12 months after surgery prior to considering a trial of SCS for FBSS as it may take this long to recover from spinal surgery. External stimulation devices can be used in patients who cannot or will not undergo more invasive procedures. The chart seen in **Figure 19** is a general guide on how an interventionalist can organize the initial presenting symptoms with a potential treatment.

Research regarding number of ESIs prior to indications of surgical intervention is limited. For some interventional pain medicine physicians, surgery may be considered if subsequent ESIs continue to provide waning or minimal levels of relief either by percent of relief or temporal measures. There are multiple reasons why a patient may never be an appropriate candidate for surgery independent of ESI count.

Navigating the course of action, prerequisites and expectations of different treatments can be daunting for both patient and referring physician. The diagrams below illustrate example steps of some of the major interventional pain procedures, from the moment a patient walks into the clinic until day of procedure. The steps to a diagnostic MBB can be seen in **Figure 20** while the prerequisites for radiofrequency ablation of the Medial Branch can be seen in **Figure 21** as well as its continued use for treatment. **Figure 22** shows the process prior to an epidural steroid injection and in **Figure 23** the steps prior to SI joint injection. These may differ in different practices and can change as literature and policies are updated. It should be noted that the initial treatment is sometimes also known as diagnostic since a failure in that treatment may warrant further workup for source of pain.

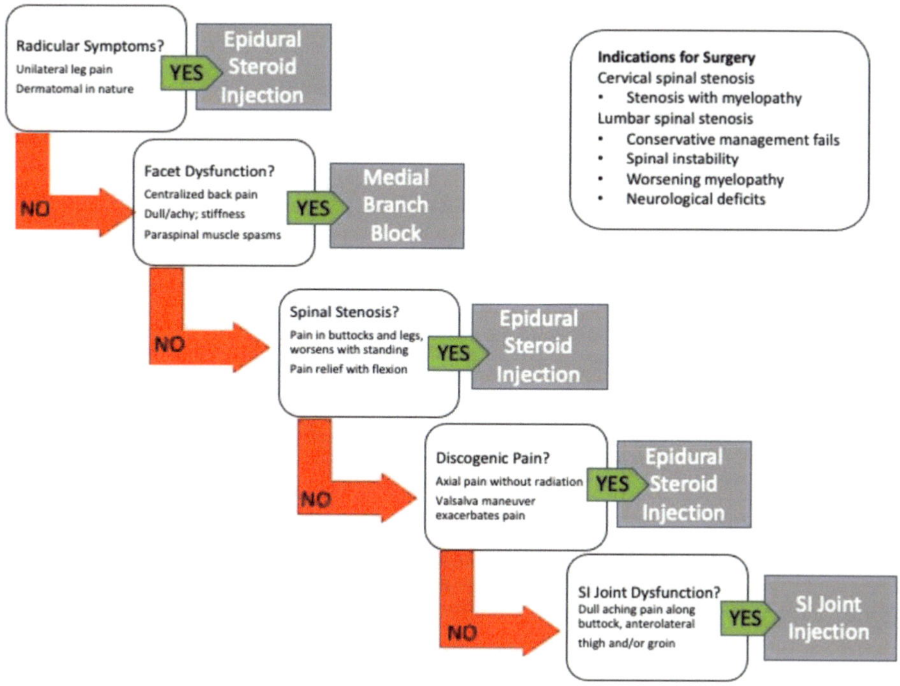

Figure 19.
An example of a common pathway for epidural steroid injection and SI joint injection.

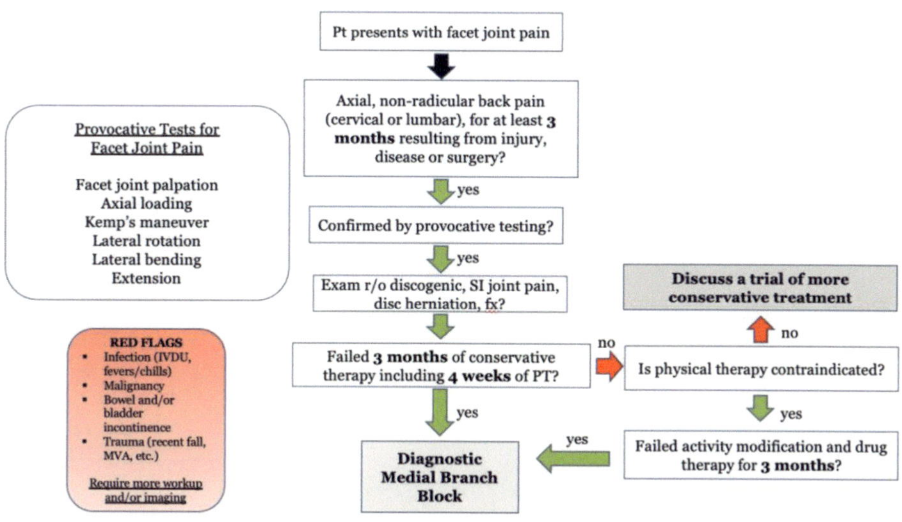

Figure 20.
An example of a common pathway including requirements prior to a diagnostic MBB.

The benefits pain management contributes to medicine are vast and the potential contributions are boundless. This chapter pays tribute to the foundations of this specialty while highlighting newer innovations and expanding on already-established

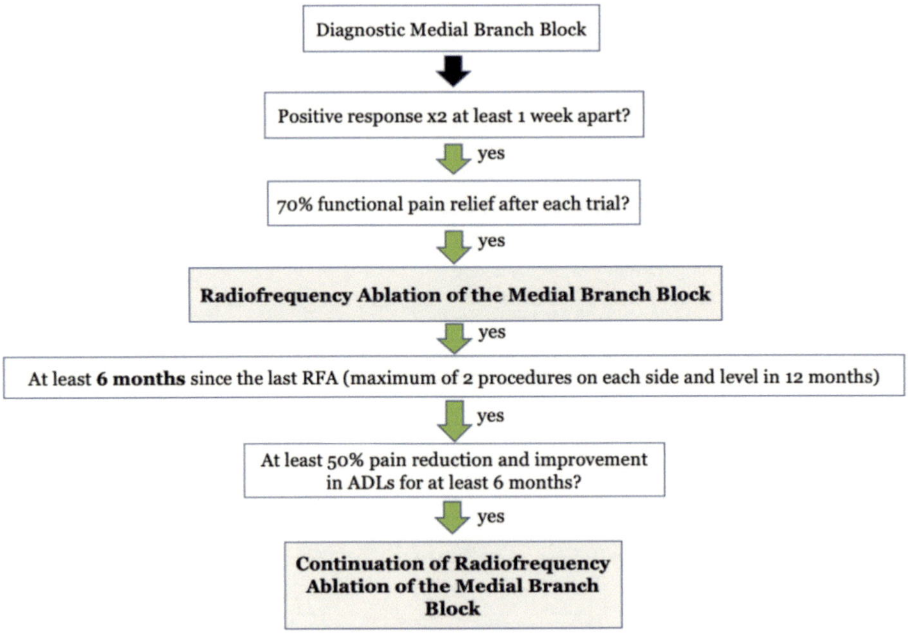

Figure 21.
An example of a common pathway including requirements prior to initial RFA of the MBB and continuation treatment.

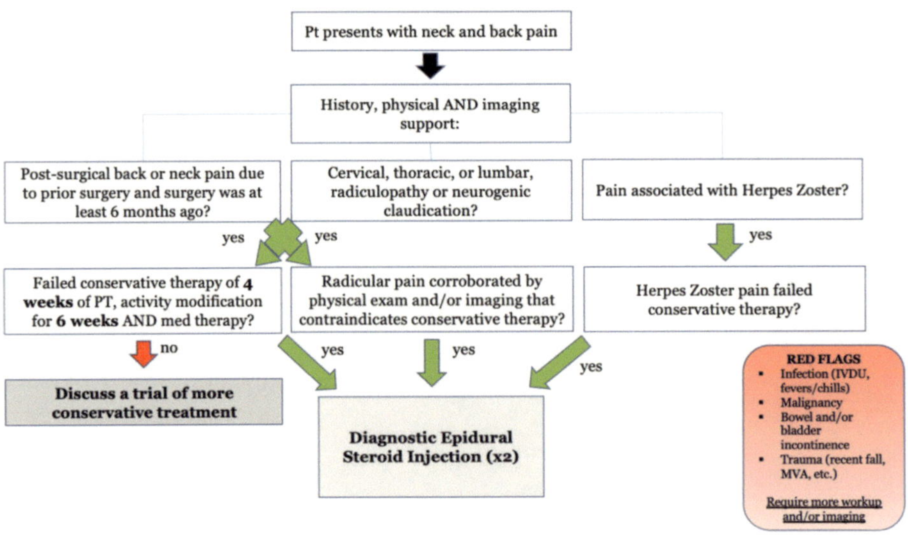

Figure 22.
An example of a common pathway including requirements prior to diagnostic ESI.

modalities that may be safer, faster, and more accessible such as ultrasound-guided procedures or advancement of current technology.

In 2019, COVID-19, a disease caused by the virus SARS-Cov-2, quickly spread resulting in a global pandemic and subsequent lockdown. The organic effects of this disease as well as the mental health consequences may have an interesting effect on the patient population presenting to outpatient pain clinics. The importance of a

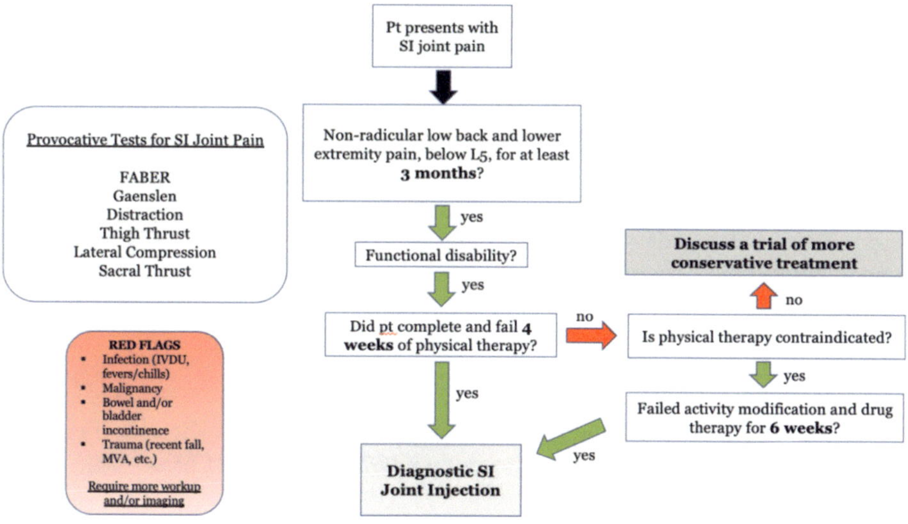

Figure 23.
An example of a common pathway including requirements prior to diagnostic SI joint injection.

targeted evaluation as well as continued advancement of safer more efficacious treatments, invasive and noninvasive, will likely be more important than ever.

This chapter review is not comprehensive as there is a less detailed focus on already-established procedures such as epidural steroid injections and the multitude of peripheral nerve blocks, which are arguably the pillars of interventional pain management. Instead, this chapter focuses on the innovations that are becoming more common in clinical practice. Since pain management is a robust and advancing field, this chapter may not include newer procedures or lesser studied ones.

There are multiple procedures that have grown out of favor from common practice including discograms as they are painful, facet joint injections as medial branch block, and subsequent ablation provides longer relief for this type of back pain, neurolysis due to its increased risks when compared to neural blockade and ablation, and even intrathecal pumps, which are a good treatment option but require long-term maintenance and troubleshooting.

In contrast, there are forms of therapy such as prolotherapy, which is essentially the repeated injection of irritant or platelet-rich plasma (PRP) injections, which is the injection of autologous platelets into affected joint space to trigger connective tissue growth and/or repair and subsequent theoretical pain relief that are awaiting larger, more in-depth studies prior to acceptance into common practice.

Pain medicine's core specialties include Anesthesiology, Psychiatry, Physical Medicine and Rehabilitation, and Neurology. The diversity of the specialty allows for a multifaceted projection of innovation such as aforementioned prolotherapy and PRP injection as well as the augmentation of the perception of pain and visualizing biomarkers of pain, which expands the scope and impact of outpatient pain management.

9. Conclusions

This chapter briefly describes the mechanism and pathways contributing to the perception of pain before discussing the current pharmacologic and non-pharmacologic agents that modulate these pathways as well as interventional pain approaches that are becoming more commonly used. In the outpatient pain management clinic, the focus is on subacute to chronic, non-cancer pain—its etiologies, evaluation, and subsequent management including the wide array of noninvasive treatments such as ketamine, external stimulation devices, and CBD, as well as more invasive modalities of treatment. We review the mainstay of interventional pain procedures and highlight its innovations such as radiofrequency ablation and spinal cord stimulators. As more research is conducted and technology advances, it is imperative to update medical health professionals on how to better help patients improve their quality of life and regain their function.

Acknowledgements

Sanjay V. Menghani's training is supported by an F30 Ruth L. Kirschstein individual predoctoral NRSA fellowship from the NIGMS (5F30GM139246-02).

Conflict of interest

The authors declare that the work for this book chapter was conducted in the absence of any commercial or financial relationships that could be considered a conflict of interest.

Author details

Franzes Anne Z. Liongson[1*], Rina Bhalodi[1], Christopher McCarthy[1], Sanjay V. Menghani[2,3] and Ajaz Siddiqui[4]

1 St. Luke's University Hospital Network (SLUHN), Bethlehem, USA

2 University of Arizona College of Medicine – Tucson, Tucson, USA

3 Medical Scientist Training MD-PhD Program, University of Arizona College of Medicine – Tucson, Tucson, USA

4 Spine and Pain Associates, St. Luke's University Hospital Network (SLUHN), Bethlehem, USA

*Address all correspondence to: franzes.liongson@sluhn.org

IntechOpen

© 2022 The Author(s). Licensee IntechOpen. This chapter is distributed under the terms of the Creative Commons Attribution License (http://creativecommons.org/licenses/by/3.0), which permits unrestricted use, distribution, and reproduction in any medium, provided the original work is properly cited.

References

[1] Cohen M, Quintner J, van Rysewyk S. Reconsidering the international association for the study of pain definition of pain. Pain Reports. 2018;**3**(2):e634

[2] Basbaum AI, Bautista DM, Scherrer G, Julius D. Cellular and molecular mechanisms of pain. Cell. 2009;**139**(2):267-284

[3] Stucky CL, Dubin AE, Jeske NA, Malin SA, McKemy DD, Story GM. Roles of transient receptor potential channels in pain. Brain Research Reviews. 2009;**60**(1):2-23

[4] Dubin AE, Patapoutian A. Nociceptors: The sensors of the pain pathway. The Journal of Clinical Investigation. 2010;**120**(11):3760-3772

[5] Tominaga M, Caterina MJ, Malmberg AB, Rosen TA, Gilbert H, Skinner K, et al. The cloned capsaicin receptor integrates multiple pain-producing stimuli. Neuron. 1998;**21**(3):531-543

[6] Lawson SN, Waddell PJ. Soma neurofilament immunoreactivity is related to cell size and fibre conduction velocity in rat primary sensory neurons. The Journal of Physiology. 1991;**435**:41-63

[7] Yam MF, Loh YC, Tan CS, Khadijah Adam S, Abdul Manan N, Basir R. General pathways of pain sensation and the major neurotransmitters involved in pain regulation. International Journal of Molecular Sciences. 2018;**19**(8):2164

[8] Pak DJ, Yong RJ, Kaye AD, Urman RD. Chronification of pain: Mechanisms, current understanding, and clinical implications. Current Pain and Headache Reports. 2018;**22**(2):9

[9] Kuner R, Kuner T. Cellular circuits in the brain and their modulation in acute and chronic pain. Physiological Reviews. 2021;**101**(1):213-258

[10] Gaskin DJ, Richard P. The economic costs of pain in the United States. The Journal of Pain. 2012;**13**(8):715-724

[11] Manchikanti L, Singh V, Falco FJ, Benyamin RM, Hirsch JA. Epidemiology of low back pain in adults. Neuromodulation. 2014;**17**(Suppl 2):3-10

[12] Almomani F, Alghwiri AA, Alghadir AH, Al-Momani A, Iqbal A. Prevalence of upper limb pain and disability and its correlates with demographic and personal factors. Journal of Pain Research. 2019;**12**:2691-2700

[13] Lucas J, Connor E, Bose J. Back, lower limb, and upper limb pain among U.S. adults, 2019. NCHS Data Brief. 2021;(415):1-8

[14] Dowell D, Haegerich TM, Chou R. CDC guideline for prescribing opioids for chronic pain - United States, 2016. MMWR - Recommendations and Reports. 2016;**65**(1):1-49

[15] Rosenblum A, Marsch LA, Joseph H, Portenoy RK. Opioids and the treatment of chronic pain: Controversies, current status, and future directions. Experimental and Clinical Psychopharmacology. 2008;**16**(5):405-416

[16] Katz N, Benoit C. Opioids for neuropathic pain. Current Pain and Headache Reports. 2005;**9**(3):153-160

[17] Pergolizzi JV Jr, Labhsetwar SA, Puenpatom RA, Joo S, Ben-Joseph RH,

Summers KH. Prevalence of exposure to potential CYP450 pharmacokinetic drug-drug interactions among patients with chronic low back pain taking opioids. Pain Practice. 2011;**11**(3):230-239

[18] Edinoff AN, Kaplan LA, Khan S, Petersen M, Sauce E, Causey CD, et al. Full opioid agonists and tramadol: Pharmacological and clinical considerations. Anesthesiology and Pain Medicine. 2021;**11**(4):e119156

[19] Culp C, Kim HK, Abdi S. Ketamine use for cancer and chronic pain management. Frontiers in Pharmacology. 2020;**11**:599721

[20] Nowacka A, Borczyk M. Ketamine applications beyond anesthesia - A literature review. European Journal of Pharmacology. 2019;**860**:172547

[21] Niesters M, Martini C, Dahan A. Ketamine for chronic pain: Risks and benefits. British Journal of Clinical Pharmacology. 2014;**77**(2):357-367

[22] Yang Y, Maher DP, Cohen SP. Emerging concepts on the use of ketamine for chronic pain. Expert Review of Clinical Pharmacology. 2020;**13**(2):135-146

[23] Cohen SP, Bhatia A, Buvanendran A, Schwenk ES, Wasan AD, Hurley RW, et al. Consensus guidelines on the use of intravenous ketamine infusions for chronic pain from The American Society of Regional Anesthesia and Pain Medicine, The American Academy of Pain Medicine, and The American Society of Anesthesiologists. Regional Anesthesia and Pain Medicine. 2018;**43**(5):521-546

[24] Orhurhu V, Orhurhu MS, Bhatia A, Cohen SP. Ketamine infusions for chronic pain: A systematic review and meta-analysis of randomized controlled trials. Anesthesia and Analgesia. 2019;**129**(1):241-254

[25] Bell RF, Kalso EA. Ketamine for pain management. Pain Reports. 2018;**3**(5):e674

[26] Clark JD. Ketamine for chronic pain: Old drug new trick? Anesthesiology. 2020;**133**(1):13-15

[27] Romero-Sandoval EA, Fincham JE, Kolano AL, Sharpe BN, Alvarado-Vázquez PA. Cannabis for chronic pain: Challenges and considerations. Pharmacotherapy: The Journal of Human Pharmacology and Drug Therapy. 2018;**38**(6):651-662

[28] Aviram J, Samuelly-Leichtag G. Efficacy of Cannabis-based medicines for pain management: A systematic review and meta-analysis of randomized controlled trials. Pain Physician. 2017;**20**(6):E755-Ee96

[29] Volkow ND, Baler RD, Compton WM, Weiss SRB. Adverse health effects of marijuana use. New England Journal of Medicine. 2014;**370**(23):2219-2227

[30] Chayasirisobhon S. Mechanisms of action and pharmacokinetics of Cannabis. The Permanente Journal. 2021;**25**(1):1-3

[31] Kim YC, Castañeda AM, Lee CS, Jin HS, Park KS, Moon JY. Efficacy and safety of lidocaine infusion treatment for neuropathic pain: A randomized, double-blind, and placebo-controlled study. Regional Anesthesia and Pain Medicine. 2018;**43**(4):415-424

[32] Masic D, Liang E, Long C, Sterk EJ, Barbas B, Rech MA. Intravenous lidocaine for acute pain: A Systematic Review. Pharmacotherapy. 2018;**38**(12):1250-1259

[33] Thomson PD, Melmon KL, Richardson JA, Cohn K, Steinbrunn W, Cudihee R, et al. Lidocaine pharmacokinetics in advanced heart failure, liver disease, and renal failure in humans. Annals of Internal Medicine. 1973;**78**(4):499-508

[34] Jazayeri SM, Ashraf A, Fini HM, Karimian H, Nasab MV. Efficacy of Botulinum Toxin Type A for Treating Chronic Low Back Pain. 2011;**1**(2):77-80

[35] Sim WS. Application of botulinum toxin in pain management. The Korean Journal of Pain. 2011;**24**(1):1-6

[36] Khoury AL, Keane H, Varghese F, Hosseini A, Mukhtar R, Eder SE, et al. Trigger point injection for post-mastectomy pain: A simple intervention with high rate of long-term relief. npj Breast Cancer. 2021;**7**(1):123

[37] Borg-Stein J, Iaccarino MA. Myofascial pain syndrome treatments. Physical Medicine and Rehabilitation Clinics of North America. 2014;**25**(2):357-374

[38] Suputtitada A, Chen CPC, Ngamrungsiri N, Schmitz C. Effects of repeated injection of 1% lidocaine vs. radial extracorporeal shock wave therapy for treating myofascial trigger points: A randomized controlled trial. Medicina. 2022;**58**(4):479

[39] Johnson MI, Paley CA, Howe TE, Sluka KA. Transcutaneous electrical nerve stimulation for acute pain. Cochrane Database of Systematic Reviews. 2015;**2015**(6):Cd006142

[40] Bjordal JM, Johnson MI, Ljunggreen AE. Transcutaneous electrical nerve stimulation (TENS) can reduce postoperative analgesic consumption. A meta-analysis with assessment of optimal treatment parameters for postoperative pain. European Journal of Pain. 2003;**7**(2):181-188

[41] Mulvey MR, Bagnall AM, Johnson MI, Marchant PR. Transcutaneous electrical nerve stimulation (TENS) for phantom pain and stump pain following amputation in adults. Cochrane Database of Systematic Reviews 2010(5):Cd007264.

[42] Wu LC, Weng PW, Chen CH, Huang YY, Tsuang YH, Chiang CJ. Literature review and meta-analysis of transcutaneous electrical nerve stimulation in treating chronic back pain. Regional Anesthesia and Pain Medicine. 2018;**43**(4):425-433

[43] Huang J, Yang C, Zhao K, Zhao Z, Chen Y, Wang T, et al. Transcutaneous electrical nerve stimulation in rodent models of neuropathic pain: A meta-analysis. Frontiers in Neuroscience. 2022;**16**:831413

[44] Dias LV, Cordeiro MA, Schmidt de Sales R, Dos Santos M, Korelo RIG, Vojciechowski AS, et al. Immediate analgesic effect of transcutaneous electrical nerve stimulation (TENS) and interferential current (IFC) on chronic low back pain: Randomised placebo-controlled trial. Journal of Bodywork and Movement Therapies. 2021;**27**:181-190

[45] Fuentes JP, Armijo Olivo S, Magee DJ, Gross DP. Effectiveness of interferential current therapy in the management of musculoskeletal pain: A systematic review and meta-analysis. Physical Therapy. 2010;**90**(9):1219-1238

[46] Moore JS, Gibson PR, Burgell RE. Neuromodulation via interferential electrical stimulation as a novel therapy in gastrointestinal motility disorders. Journal of Neurogastroenterology and Motility. 2018;**24**(1):19-29

[47] Yang X, He H, Ye W, Perry TA, He C. Effects of pulsed electromagnetic field therapy on pain, stiffness, physical function, and quality of life in patients

with osteoarthritis: A systematic review and meta-analysis of randomized placebo-controlled trials. Physical Therapy. 2020;**100**(7):1118-1131

[48] Ross C, Overholt T, Xu R, Badlani G, Evans RJ, Matthews CA, et al. Pulsed electromagnetic field (PEMF) as an adjunct therapy for pain management in interstitial cystitis/bladder pain syndrome. International Urogynecology Journal. 2022;**33**(3):487-491

[49] Tepper OM, Callaghan MJ, Chang EI, Galiano RD, Bhatt KA, Baharestani S, et al. Electromagnetic fields increase in vitro and in vivo angiogenesis through endothelial release of FGF-2. The FASEB Journal. 2004;**18**(11):1231-1233

[50] Schnoke M, Midura RJ. Pulsed electromagnetic fields rapidly modulate intracellular signaling events in osteoblastic cells: Comparison to parathyroid hormone and insulin. Journal of Orthopaedic Research. 2007;**25**(7):933-940

[51] Capone F, Dileone M, Profice P, Pilato F, Musumeci G, Minicuci G, et al. Does exposure to extremely low frequency magnetic fields produce functional changes in human brain? Journal of Neural Transmission. 2009;**116**(3):257-265

[52] Martiny K, Lunde M, Bech P. Transcranial low voltage pulsed electromagnetic fields in patients with treatment-resistant depression. Biological Psychiatry. 2010;**68**(2):163-169

[53] Hug K, Röösli M. Therapeutic effects of whole-body devices applying pulsed electromagnetic fields (PEMF): A systematic literature review. Bioelectromagnetics. 2012;**33**(2):95-105

[54] Page MJ, Green S, Mrocki MA, Surace SJ, Deitch J, McBain B, et al. Electrotherapy modalities for rotator cuff disease. Cochrane Database of Systematic Reviews. 2016;**2016**(6):Cd012225

[55] Rabini A, Piazzini DB, Tancredi G, Foti C, Milano G, Ronconi G, et al. Deep heating therapy via microwave diathermy relieves pain and improves physical function in patients with knee osteoarthritis: A double-blind randomized clinical trial. European Journal of Physical and Rehabilitation Medicine. 2012;**48**(4):549-559

[56] Ferreira RM, Torres RT, Duarte JA, Gonçalves RS. Non-pharmacological and non-surgical interventions for knee osteoarthritis: A systematic review and meta-analysis. Acta Reumatológica Portuguesa. 2019;**44**(3):173-217

[57] Fu T, Lineaweaver WC, Zhang F, Zhang J. Role of shortwave and microwave diathermy in peripheral neuropathy. The Journal of International Medical Research. 2019;**47**(8):3569-3579

[58] Dieleman JL, Cao J, Chapin A, Chen C, Li Z, Liu A, et al. US health care spending by payer and health condition, 1996-2016. Journal of the American Medical Association. 2020;**323**(9):863-884

[59] Manchikanti L, Knezevic NN, Boswell MV, Kaye AD, Hirsch JA. Epidural injections for lumbar radiculopathy and spinal stenosis: A comparative systematic review and meta-analysis. Pain Physician. 2016;**19**(3):E365-E410

[60] Pountos I, Georgouli T, Blokhuis TJ, Pape HC, Giannoudis PV. Pharmacological agents and impairment of fracture healing: What is the evidence? Injury. 2008;**39**(4):384-394

[61] Tetzlaff JE. The pharmacology of local anesthetics. Anesthesiology Clinics of North America. 2000;**18**(2):217-233 v

[62] Neal JM, Brull R, Chan VW, Grant SA, Horn JL, Liu SS, et al. The ASRA evidence-based medicine assessment of ultrasound-guided regional anesthesia and pain medicine: Executive summary. Regional Anesthesia and Pain Medicine. 2010;**35**(2 Suppl):S1-S9

[63] Glenister R, Anatomy SS. Bony Pelvis and Lower Limb, Hip. In: StatPearls. Treasure Island (FL): StatPearls Publishing LLC; 2022

[64] Cox RC, Fortin JD. The anatomy of the lateral branches of the sacral dorsal rami: Implications for radiofrequency ablation. Pain Physician. 2014;**17**(5):459-464

[65] Harmon D, O'Sullivan M. Ultrasound-guided sacroiliac joint injection technique. Pain Physician. 2008;**11**(4):543-547

[66] Polly DW Jr. The sacroiliac joint. Neurosurgery Clinics of North America. 2017;**28**(3):301-312

[67] Xavier J, Pinho S, Silva J, Nunes CS, Cabido H, Fortuna R, et al. Postdural puncture headache in the obstetric population: A new approach? Regional Anesthesia & Pain Medicine. 2020;**45**(5):373

[68] Fernandes L, Randall M. Idrovo LPeripheral nerve blocks for headache disordersPractical Neurology. 2021;**21**:30-35

[69] Brandt RB, Doesborg PGG, Meilof R, de Coo IF, Bartels E, Ferrari MD, et al. Repeated greater occipital nerve injections with corticosteroids in medically intractable chronic cluster headache: A retrospective study. Neurological Sciences. Feb 2022;**43**(2):1267-1272

[70] Lavin PJ, Workman R. Cushing syndrome induced by serial occipital nerve blocks containing corticosteroids. Headache. 2001;**41**(9):902-904

[71] Rana MV, Candido KD, Raja O, Knezevic NN. Celiac plexus block in the management of chronic abdominal pain. Current Pain and Headache Reports. 2014;**18**(2):394

[72] Rosland JH, Geitung JT. CT guided neurolytic blockade of the coeliac plexus in patients with advanced and intractably painful pancreatic cancer. Scandinavian Journal of Pain. 2018;**18**(2):247-251

[73] Kambadakone A, Thabet A, Gervais DA, Mueller PR, Arellano RS. CT-guided celiac plexus neurolysis: A review of anatomy, indications, technique, and tips for successful treatment. Radiographics. 2011;**31**(6):1599-1621

[74] Minaga K, Takenaka M, Kamata K, Yoshikawa T, Nakai A, Omoto S, et al. Alleviating pancreatic cancer-associated pain using endoscopic ultrasound-guided neurolysis. Cancers. 2018;**10**(2):1-17

[75] Yousefshahi F, Tahmasebi M. Long-lasting orthostatic hypotension and constipation after celiac plexus block; A case report. Anesth Pain Medicine. 2018;**8**(1):e63221

[76] Hou S, Novy D, Felice F, Koyyalagunta D. Efficacy of superior hypogastric plexus neurolysis for the treatment of cancer-related pelvic pain. Pain Medicine. 2019;**21**(6):1255-1262

[77] Stogicza AR. Interventional Pain: A Step-by-step Guide for the FIPP Exam. 1st ed 1 online resource (XVIII, 205 p. 148 illus., 80 illus. in color.) p

[78] Cohen SP, Doshi TL, Constantinescu OC, Zhao Z, Kurihara C, Larkin TM, et al. Effectiveness of lumbar facet joint blocks and predictive value before radiofrequency denervation: The facet treatment study (FACTS), a randomized, controlled clinical trial. Anesthesiology. 2018;**129**(3):517-535

[79] Maas ET, Juch JNS, Ostelo R, Groeneweg JG, Kallewaard JW, Koes BW, et al. Cost-effectiveness of radiofrequency denervation for patients with chronic low back pain: The MINT randomized clinical trials. Value in Health. 2020;**23**(5):585-594

[80] Lee CH, Chung CK, Kim CH. The efficacy of conventional radiofrequency denervation in patients with chronic low back pain originating from the facet joints: A meta-analysis of randomized controlled trials. The Spine Journal. 2017;**17**(11):1770-1780

[81] Caylor J, Reddy R, Yin S, Cui C, Huang M, Huang C, et al. Spinal cord stimulation in chronic pain: Evidence and theory for mechanisms of action. Bioelectronic Medicine. 2019;**5**(1):12

[82] Deer TR, Mekhail N, Provenzano D, Pope J, Krames E, Leong M, et al. The appropriate use of neurostimulation of the spinal cord and peripheral nervous system for the treatment of chronic pain and ischemic diseases: The neuromodulation appropriateness consensus committee. Neuromodulation. 2014;**17**(6):515-550 discussion 50

[83] Barolat G, Massaro F, He J, Zeme S, Ketcik B. Mapping of sensory responses to epidural stimulation of the intraspinal neural structures in man. Journal of Neurosurgery. 1993;**78**(2):233-239

[84] Kumar K, Buchser E, Linderoth B, Meglio M, Van Buyten JP. Avoiding complications from spinal cord stimulation: Practical recommendations from an international panel of experts. Neuromodulation. 2007;**10**(1):24-33

[85] Franzini A, Ferroli P, Marras C, Broggi G. Huge epidural hematoma after surgery for spinal cord stimulation. Acta Neurochirurgica. 2005;**147**(5):565-567 discussion 7

[86] Hayek SM, Veizi E, Hanes M. Treatment-limiting complications of percutaneous spinal cord stimulator implants: A review of eight years of experience from an academic center database. Neuromodulation. 2015;**18**(7):603-608 discussion 8-9

Chapter 10

Acute Post-Operative Pain Management

Samina Khatib, Syed S.N. Razvi, Mudassir M. Shaikh and Mohammad Moizuddin Khan

Abstract

Despite major advances in the field of anesthesia and medicine, postoperative pain continues to be undermanaged in a significant proportion of patients. The consequences of undermanaged pain are deleterious for both patients and the healthcare system. This review aims to give the readers a practical and updated approach to acute postoperative pain management. This chapter deals with the definition of pain, the physiology and pathophysiology of pain, and various approaches to the management of acute pain. A review of the literature was done to understand the methods of pain management with a major focus on the literature of the last decade (2010–2022). A literature search was done on PubMed and Google Scholar using keywords "acute postoperative pain" and "pain physiology." The research papers on the basics of pain physiology, the prevalence of acute post-operative pain and methods of acute postoperative pain management were reviewed. A brief practical approach for acute postoperative pain using pharmacological and non-pharmacological approaches and a brief discussion have been done on the approach for special group of patients. The management of acute postoperative pain can be done using various pharmacological and non-pharmacological methods. The approach for each patient has to be tailored depending on the individual patient's needs.

Keywords: acute postoperative pain, nociception, opioids, opioids, pain management, anesthesia

1. Introduction

Anesthesia as a specialty has primarily originated from the human endeavor to control pain. In the evolution of medicine and surgery, complex surgeries have been made possible due to the pain relief given by the science of anesthesia. As modern anesthesiology evolved, the role of anesthesiologists is not confined only to operating and recovery rooms but extends to surgical wards also. Pain management in the postoperative period is one of the most essential components of postsurgical care.

1.1 What is pain?

The International Association for Study of Pain defines pain as "an unpleasant sensory and emotional experience associated with or resembling that associated with actual or potential tissue damage" [1]. Pain is a multidimensional experience with the following components: objective, subjective, physiological, emotional, and psychological [1]. Differences in pain experience are influenced by the biological response, psychological state, personality traits, and social traits [2]. A large systemic review of literature pooled from 165 studies showed that in the first 24 hours after major surgery (abdominal, thoracic, orthopedic, and gynecological), the mean incidence of moderate to severe pain was 30% and 11%, respectively [3]. The incidence of these pain levels varied by analgesic technique, with lower incidence with patient-controlled analgesia and epidural analgesia. A questionnaire survey of Asian countries by Vijayan et al. showed that only 30% of patients in India receive adequate pain management [4]. These and a large number of other surveys and studies show an unacceptable level of acute postoperative pain [5–11].

1.2 Pain can also be classified as physiological pain or pathological pain

Physiological pain is a "normal" sensation and includes a range of transient sensations we experience in response to stimuli that are of sufficient intensity to threaten to damage the tissue or produce small localized areas of injury, but which neither provoke an extensive inflammatory response nor damage the nervous system. Pathological pain is a sensation that arises as a consequence of either the inflammatory response that accompanies tissue injury or as a result of damage to the nervous system [12]. Pathological pain involves the disruption of the normal selectivity or specialization of the somatosensory system [12].

1.3 Physiological pain

The term "nociception" is a process by which information about tissue damage is conveyed to the central nervous system. Nociceptors are specialized, free, unmyelinated nerve endings that convey a variety of stimuli into nerve endings that the brain interprets as pain. Many patients can experience pain in the absence of a noxious stimulus.

The process of pain transmission is illustrated in the **Figure 1** and involves four steps [12]:

1. Transduction: The conversion of energy from a noxious thermal, mechanical, or chemical stimulus into electrical energy by nociception.

2. Transmission: It is the process of transfer of these signals from the periphery to the spinal cord and brain.

3. Perception: The appreciation of these signals in higher structures as pain.

4. Modulation: It is the descending inhibitory/facilitator input from the brain that influences the nociceptive transmission at the level of the spinal cord.

1.4 Pain pathways and neurobiology of nociception

The etiology of acute postoperative pain is multifactorial. Surgical tissue injury releases histamine and inflammatory mediators (bradykinin, prostaglandins, serotonin, and nerve growth factor), which in turn activate peripheral nociceptors. These

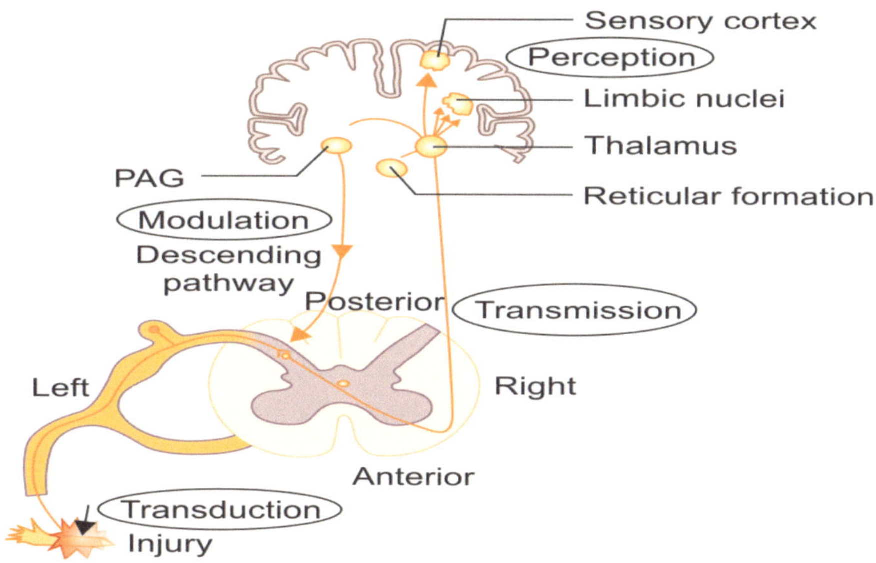

Figure 1.
Pain pathway [13].

nociceptors transmit the nociceptive information to the central nervous system by transduction and transmission [12].

Noxious stimuli are transduced by peripheral nociceptors and transmitted by A-delta and C nerve fibers to the dorsal horn of the spinal cord, where integration of peripheral nociceptive and descending modulatory input (i.e., serotonin, norepinephrine, GABA, enkephalin) occurs. After complex modulation, this information is passed on through the spinothalamic tract and spinoreticular tracts to higher centers where the pain is perceived. Some inputs pass to ventral and ventrolateral horns to initiate segmental spinal reflexes, which are associated with increased skeletal muscle tone, inhibition of phrenic nerve function, or decreased gastointestinal motility. The constant release of inflammatory mediators in the periphery sensitizes functional nociceptors and activates dormant ones (enlisted in **Table 1**). Further, it leads to a decreased threshold for activation and an increased rate of discharges. The surgical injury besides causing sensitization of primary and central pathways also leads to feelings of fear, anxiety, and frustration [2]. Intense noxious input from the periphery may lead to central sensitization and hyperexcitability causing a persistent post-injury change in central nervous system in addition to functional changes in the dorsal horn (spinal sensitization). This may lead to acute pain progression to chronic pain [12].The International Association for the Study of Pain defines chronic pain as persistent or recurrent pain lasting longer than 3 months [12].

The systemic response to surgery may contribute to perioperative morbidity and mortality. There are several systemic responses to surgery, including sympathetic nervous system activation, the neuroendocrine stress response, and inflammatory immunologic changes. Commonly observed pathophysiologic changes [14, 15] include:

1. Neurohumoral alteration (peripheral sensitization) occurring at the site and in regions immediately adjacent to the injury

2. Alternations in synaptic function and nociceptive processing within the spinal cord and limbic cortex

1. Bradykinin
2. Histamine
3. Substance P
4. Leukotriene
5. Prostaglandins
6. Arachidonic acid metabolites
7. Prostaglandin E2
8. Nerve Growth factor
9. Interleukin-1
10. Interleukin-4
11. Interleukin-6
12. Interleukin-8
13. interleukin-10
14. Tumor necrosis factor

Table 1.
List of cytokines/inflammatory mediators that contribute to acute effects of postoperative pain.

3. Sympatho-adrenal activation resulting in an elevation of heart rate and blood pressure and diminution in regional blood flow

4. Neuroendocrine response leads to hyperglycemia and a negative nitrogen balance and alternation in synaptic function.

The neurohumoral responses (peripheral sensitization) and central sensitization have already been explained in the physiology of pain.

Following extensive tissue injury (following surgery), nociceptive impulses stimulate sympathetic cells in the hypothalamus and preganglionic neurons in the anterior lateral horn. Surgical trauma results in increased plasma concentrations of epinephrine and norepinephrine. The magnitude and duration of catecholamine release are directly related to patient factors such as the type of surgery, inherent sympathetic response, patient age, and genetic polymorphisms. Pathophysiological changes associated with increased sympathetic tone and altered regional perfusion are illustrated in **Figure 2** [15].

1. Increased incidence of postsurgical hypertension that ranges from 5 to 50%

2. Increased peripheral vascular resistance associated with increased contractility and myocardial oxygen consumption. This can precipitate myocardial ischemic episodes

3. Due to the redistribution of blood to high-priority organs, microcirculation to injured tissue, viscera, and adjacent musculature may be reduced. This may lead to impaired wound healing, enhanced sensitization of nociceptors, muscle spasm, visceral/somatic ischemia, and acidosis

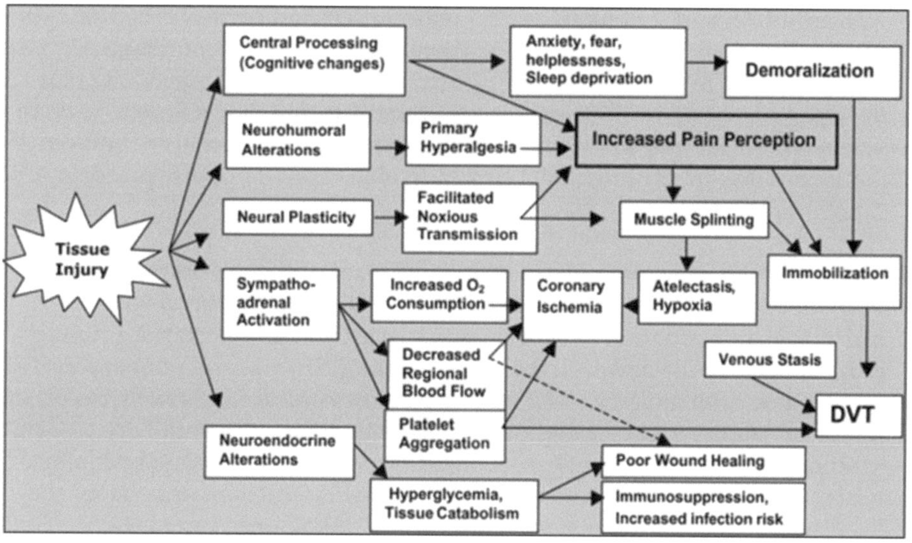

Figure 2.
Pathophysiology of postoperative pain [15].

4. Renal hypo-perfusion may occur, leading to activation of renin angiotensin aldosterone axis. Angiotensin released may further accentuate the redistribution by causing vasoconstriction and further hypoperfusion to injured tissue, skin, and visceral organs

5. Catecholamines, angiotensin, and other surgical-stress-related factors may release platelet fibrinogen activation and accelerate coagulation. In a patient with atherosclerosis, this may further reduce blood flow in critically stenosed vessels.

1.5 Neuroendocrine responses

Following tissue injury (the nociceptive impulses reach via the spinal cord and midbrain reticular formation), the neurogenic stimuli affect the hypothalamus, secretory target organs, or both and cause a neuroendocrine response [15, 16]. This is also called the stress response to injury and is characterized by increased secretion of catabolic hormones such as cortisol, glucagon, growth hormone, and catecholamines and a decreased release of anabolic hormones such as insulin and testosterone. This results in substrate mobilization, followed by hyperglycemia and a negative nitrogen balance. Associated changes include gluconeogenesis, glycogenolysis, proteolysis, and breakdown of lipid stores. These changes have short-term benefits of enhanced energy production; however, if this response is amplified or prolonged, catabolic aspects of stress response ensue, which can have a negative impact on the postsurgical outcome. The effects may be the following:

1. Protein loss leads to muscle wasting and fatigue.

2. Impaired immunity secondary to diminished immunoglobulin synthesis and impaired phagocytosis. The activated cells (secondary to nociception) in the preoptic region secrete pro-opiomelanocortin, which in turn facilities the release of ACTH, β-endorphin, and other anterior pituitary hormones. The trauma-related

release of IL-6 and IL-1 β can also increase ACTH and cortisol secretion. The relation between plasma IL-6 and cortisol levels is linear in postsurgical patients. The prolonged nitrogen balance and sustained secretion of glucocorticoids result in impaired wound healing, decreased immunity, and diminution in protein synthesis, which may inhibit cell division, production of collagen, and acute convalescence; in already debilitated individuals, this can cause postoperative infections.

3. The levels of β endorphin increase threefold, and this can lead to immunosuppression, complement release, decreased peripheral vascular resistance, and initiation of shock. Also, plasma levels of posterior pituitary-derived octapeptide and arginine vasopressin (AVP) rise and remain elevated for up to 5 days after surgery. AVP may cause postsurgical fluid retention, plasma hyperosmolarity, and oliguria. Pain transmission from the periphery to CNS produces complex neuroendocrine stress response involving hypothalamic, pituitary, adrenocortical, and sympathoadrenal interactions apart from the localized release of inflammatory mediators (leukotriene, cytokines, prostaglandins, TNF).

4. Endocrine response: There occurs increased secretion of ACTH, cortisol, glucagon, aldosterone, renin, and angiotensin-II, leading to increased levels of blood glucose, free fatty acids, ketone bodies, and lactate as part of the stress response. There occurs sodium and water retention. A hypermetabolic, catabolic state follows leading to negative nitrogen balance and protein catabolism leading to delayed convalescence and wound healing.

5. Coagulation: The stress response leads to a hypercoagulable state due to decreased levels of anticoagulants and increased levels of procoagulants, inhibition of fibrinolysis, increased platelet reactivity and increased plasma viscosity. This leads to hypercoagulable events such as deep vein thrombosis, vascular graft failure, and myocardial ischemia [17].

6. Immunological: There occurs immunosuppression due to stress response. Hyperglycemia contributes to depression of immune function and poor wound healing.

7. Cardiovascular: The activation of the sympathetic nervous system leads to increased myocardial oxygen consumption, coronary vasoconstriction, and decreased coronary vasodilatation leading to tachycardia, raised blood pressure, and contributing to myocardial ischemia, and infarction.

8. Gastrointestinal: The sympathetic overactivity may decrease gastrointestinal motility and contribute to the development of paralytic ileus.

9. Respiratory: The postoperative respiratory function is markedly decreased especially after upper abdominal and thoracic surgery. There is a spinal reflex-mediated inhibition of phrenic nerve activity leading to decreased postoperative pulmonary function. Patients with postoperative pain have shallow breathing and inadequate cough and are therefore susceptible to the development of postoperative pulmonary complications.

2. Preemptive analgesia and enhanced recovery after surgery

Surgery produces a biphasic insult on the human body. First of all, during surgery, there is trauma to the tissue followed by an inflammatory process at the site, which is also responsible for noxious input. Both these processes sensitize the pain pathways. They occur at a peripheral level where there is a reduction in the threshold of nociceptive afferents at a central level with increased excitation of spinal neurons involved in pain transmission. This concept has implications in acute postoperative pain management and has led to the concept of preemptive analgesia [18]. This concept states that the analgesic intervention preceding surgical injury is more effective in relieving acute postoperative pain than the same treatment following surgery. It works by preventing central sensitization in central nervous system to intense noxious stimuli, thus preventing pain hypersensitivity and hyperexcitability [18].

Enhanced recovery after surgery (ERAS) protocols are multimodal perioperative care plans intended to accelerate the recovery process after surgical procedures by maintaining preoperative organ function and reducing the intense stress response following surgery [19]. Initiated by Professor Henrik Kehlet in the 1990s, ERAS, enhanced recovery programs (ERPs) or "fast-track" programs have become an important focus of perioperative management. These programs are designed to curtail the physiological and psychological responses to major surgery leading to a reduction in postoperative complications and hospital stays, improvements in cardiopulmonary function, earlier restoration of bowel activity, and earlier recommencement of normal activities. The ERAS protocols help to improve the quality of perioperative care with aim of alleviating the loss of functional capacity and speeding up the recovery process [20].

For ERAS programs, optimal pain management plays a key role. The complex nature of nociception and mixed mechanisms of generating surgical pain is responsible for the failure of unimodal analgesia to adequately address postoperative pain, hence the need for multimodal analgesia. Multimodal analgesia includes using multiple strategies and analgesics acting at various points of the pain pathway to manage postoperative pain. These strategies include patient education; local anesthetics-based infiltration, peripheral nerve blocks, neuraxial analgesia, and a combination of analgesic drugs that act via different mechanisms on different receptors within the pain transmission pathway to provide synergistic effects, superior analgesia, and physiological benefits [11]. The multimodal, evidence-based, and procedure-specific analgesic regimens should be the standard of care to achieve optimal analgesia with minimal side effects and facilitate the achievement of important ERAS milestones such as early mobilization and oral feeding [20]. Thoracic epidural analgesia (T6–T11) remains the gold standard for postoperative pain control in patients undergoing open abdominal surgery. Initiation of neural blockade before surgery and its maintenance throughout the surgery decreases the need for anesthetic agents, opioids, and muscle relaxants [20]. Epidural analgesia provides better postoperative static as well as dynamic analgesia for the first 72 hours to accelerate the recovery of gastrointestinal functions, decrease insulin resistance, and impact positively cardiovascular and respiratory functions. Intra-thecal analgesia is a valuable analgesic technique to improve early postoperative analgesia and facilitate surgical recovery [20]. Opioid side effects are dose-dependent and can cause a delayed recovery. Opioid-sparing analgesic strategies such as regional anesthetic techniques should be implemented in a context of a multimodal analgesic regimen.

Continuous wound infusion of local anesthetics leads to improved postoperative analgesia and reduces opioid consumption; however, the effect on the recovery of bowel function is unclear. The use of intravenous lidocaine infusion, abdominal truncal blocks, intra-peritoneal anesthetic, and multimodal approach using NSAID, COX2 inhibitors, and paracetamol decreases opioid consumption by 30% and dose-dependent side effects [20].

In ERAS, the attenuation and treatment of postoperative ileus are also important [20]. The prolonged ileus can be prevented by the use of opioid-sparing strategies, thoracic epidural analgesia, intravenous lidocaine, NSAIDs/COX-2inhibitors, ketamine, etc. The use of opioid antagonists such as alvimopan and metitrexone, the use of laxatives, and gum-chewing are useful strategies to reduce side effects related to opioids [20].

3. Assessment of pain

This step is vital for effective pain management. Pain assessment should be done during rest as well as during movement. The assessment should be done before and after every treatment to evaluate the effectiveness of the treatment. In conditions where the pain is intense or in the intensive care units, and surgical wards, pain assessment, treatment, and re-evaluation should be done frequently or at regular intervals. Documentation of pain and response to treatment and adverse effects on a vital sign sheet is very much essential for proper treatment. It facilitates proper communication between staff and also facilitates auditing and quality control. Special attention should be paid to patients who cannot communicate their pain, e.g., those who are cognitively impaired, pediatric patients, unconscious patients, etc.

3.1 Self-assessment tools

Patient self-report is the most useful tool and the gold standard, and one should always listen to the patients and believe what they say. Several patient self-assessment tools are available:

1. Facial expression (Faces scale): A pictogram of six faces with different facial expressions from a happy smiling face to a teary-eyed face is used to assess pain. This scale is useful where there is a communication problem such as pediatric patients, the elderly, or those patients who do not understand the local language.

2. Verbal Rating Scale (VRS): Patients are asked to rate their pain on a five-point scale as none, moderate, severe, and very severe.

3. Numerical rating scale (NRS): It consists of a 0–10 scale where 0 correlates to no pain and 10 to the worst possible pain.

4. Visual analog scale (VAS) consists of a graduated straight 100 mm line marked at one end with the term “no pain and the other end “worst possible pain.”

The VRS and NRS are used most frequently while VAS is used mainly as a research tool.

Postoperative pain control is often not isolated to the surgical site but includes other locations such as sore throat following intubation and also injection sites [21]. One approach is preparing a body map and marking the sites with pain and individual

Sub-scale	Description	Score
Facial expression	Relaxed	1
	Partially tightened	2
	Fully tightened	3
	Grimacing	4
Upper limbs	No movement	1
	Partially bent	2
	Fully bent with finger flexion	3
	Permanently retracted	4
Compliance with ventilation	Tolerating movement	1
	Coughing but tolerating ventilation for most of the time	2
	Fighting ventilator	3
	Unable to control ventilation	4

Figure 3.
Behaviorial pain scale [24].

pain scores, but this is a tedious and impractical approach for the postoperative period. The multidimensional tools are under validation such as the Clinically Aligned Pain Assessment (CAPA) tool that measures five dimensions of pain including comfort, change in pain, pain control, functioning, and sleep [22]. It may improve assessment of pain in the postoperative period and leads to increased communication between patient and healthcare professionals and increases patient satisfaction levels [22].

For patients who are unable to self-report, e.g., dementia or patients who are unable to verbalize due to different reasons, standardized objective assessment tools have been designed and validated. One is the "Pain assessment in Advanced Dementia" (PAINAD) scale, the electronic pain assessment tool (e-PAT), Abbey pain scale, Dolopus-2, ADD Protocol, Observation Pain Behavioral tool, are some of the recommended tools for individuals with severe cognitive impairment [23]. Also Critical Care Pain Observation Tool and Behavioral Pain Scale are useful for pain assessment in patients who are unable to verbalize in critical care [23]. The surrogate measures such as opiate consumption may also be useful. The cardio-respiratory parameters are unreliable for pain assessment. The trends in pain assessment scores are more helpful than isolated pain scales [23]. An example of an assessment tool in non-verbal patients is illustrated in **Figure 3** [24]. This is the behavioral pain scale for assessing pain in critically ill patients on a ventilator [24]. A score of 0 indicates no pain, mild pain is indicated by a score of 0–3, moderate pain by a score of 3–6, and severe pain by a score of 6–8.

4. Goals of postoperative pain management

Effective pain management not only decreases patient suffering but also reduces morbidity. It also facilitates early recovery and discharge from the hospital and reduces treatment costs. The goals of proper pain management are to improve the quality of life, facilitate postoperative recovery, reduce morbidity and improve functional outcomes, reduce hospital stay, prevent chronic pain, and promote patient satisfaction [21].

4.1 Principles for acute perioperative pain management

Optimal perioperative pain management should done by charting out a pain management plan based on individual patient's needs. For this, one needs to evaluate every patient preoperatively to assess the medical history, presence of coexisting diseases, psychological conditions, history of chronic pain, substance abuse, and other concomitant medications [21]. A multimodal pain management plan, which includes pharmacological and non-pharmacological techniques, needs to be formulated based on the patient history. The patients and their families as well as the healthcare personnel need to be informed and educated regarding the pain management plan and its goals. In the postoperative period, tracking and documentation of pain are of utmost importance using an appropriate pain assessment tool. The medication and treatment technique should be altered based on the patient's response and the presence of any adverse events. Education of healthcare workers about proper storage, disposal, and record-keeping of opioids and tapering the doses after hospital discharge are important steps. Pain specialists may be consulted for patients with special needs and those with uncontrolled pain.

5. Treatment of acute postoperative pain

Several options are available for treating postoperative pain including systemic (opioid and non-opioid) analgesics, regional analgesic techniques, and non-pharmacological methods. By taking into account each patient's preferences and making an individualized assessment of the risk and benefits of each treatment modality, the clinician can optimize the postoperative analgesic regimen for each patient.

6. Opioid medications

The action of opioids is mediated through three types of opioid receptors, namely MOR (mu), DOR (delta), and KOR (kappa), with varying levels of affinity to each type of opioid receptor and also varying interactions with these receptors (agonists, partial agonists, antagonists). They exert analgesic effects, influence mood, and behavior, and affect respiratory, cardiovascular, gastrointestinal, neuroendocrine, and immune systems [25]. The analgesic efficacy of opioids is limited by the development of tolerance or due to side effects such as nausea, vomiting, pruritis, sedation, or respiratory depression. Opioids may be administered by subcutaneous, transcutaneous, transmucosal, or intramuscular routes, but the most important routes commonly employed are intravenous and oral. Opioids may also be delivered at specific anatomic sites such as intrathecal or epidural space. Long-acting opioids should be avoided in the immediate postoperative period except in patients who are already taking them before surgery [26]. When treating opioid-naïve adults, clinicians should avoid basal infusions with intravenous PCA, as it does not provide additional analgesia and is associated with nausea, vomiting, and respiratory depression [26].

7. Side effects of opioid medications

The side effects of opioids are depicted in **Table 2**. The commonly used opioids and their routes of administration, side effects, and management are described briefly

Common	Occasional	Rare
Gastrointestinal		
Nausea	Delayed gastric emptying	Biliary colic
Vomiting		
Constipation		
Neurological		
Sedation	Hallucination	Delirium
Drowsiness	Mood disturbance	Seizure
Cognitive dysfunction	Anxiety	Addiction
	Myoclonus	
Respiratory		
Cough reflex inhibition	Dry mouth	Respiratory depression
	Bronchospasm	Non cardiac pulmonary edema
Others		
Miosis	Pruritus	Hyperalgesia
	Muscle rigidity	Allodynia
		Tolerance
		Physical dependence

Table 2.
Side effects of opioids [27].

in **Table 3**. The incidence of life-threatening adverse events, such as respiratory depression, is rare and occurs within 24 hours. A systematic review of observational studies reported the incidence of postoperative opioid-induced respiratory depression as five in 1000 [27]. Also, those with preexisting cardiac disease, pulmonary disease, and obstructive sleep apnea are at increased risk of opioid-induced respiratory depression [27]. Other common side effects of opioid administration are sedation, dizziness, nausea, vomiting, constipation, physical dependence, and tolerance. Physical dependence and addiction are important concerns that can act as a barrier to pain management. Less common side effects are delayed gastric emptying, hyperalgesia, immunologic and hormonal dysfunction, muscle rigidity, and myoclonus. The most common side effects of opioids are constipation and nausea, which are difficult to manage. Mostly tolerance does not develop in them, especially to constipation. This may lead to discontinuation or under-dosing and inadequate analgesia.

8. Non-opioid medications

These have been enlisted and described briefly in **Table 4** and are discussed as follows.

a. **Acetaminophen (Paracetamol):** It is used most often in conjunction with other medications as a part of multimodal analgesia protocol [16]. When used as a part of multimodal analgesia, it leads to faster recovery, higher levels of

Opioid	Route of administration with sample dosing	Side effects (Adverse reactions)	Cautions/ contraindications
Morphine	• IV 2–5 mg prn every 1–2 hours • IM/SC 5-10 mg every 4 hours or prn every 2 hours • Epidural: 2–4 mg (preservative free) • Spinal: 0.1–0.3 mg (preservative free)	• Hypotension • Bronchospasm • Pruritus • Nausea/vomiting • Confusion, agitation	Side effects also with neuraxial administration
Codeine Available alone or in combination with acetaminophen	PO 30–60 mg every 4 hours maximum 240 mg/day	• Nausea and vomiting • Drowsiness • Confusion, agitation • Constipation	To be avoided in renal and hepatic dysfunction
Fentanyl	• IV bolus: 0.001–0.005 mg/kg (can be titrated up to 0.05 mg/kg) • Epidural: 0.025–0.1 mg (diluted in local anesthetics or saline) • Spinal: 0.005–0.2 mg	• Respiratory depression • Epidural/spinal administration: pruritus and delayed respiratory depression	Muscle rigidity with high doses, Smaller doses needed in elderly
Tramadol	• PO 50–100 mg every 4 hours • IV/IM slowly 50–100 mg every 4 hours • Do not exceed 400 mg /day	Nausea, dizziness, dry mouth	• 30% of effect reversible with naloxone • Should not be used with drugs that increase serotonin
Tapentadol	PO 50–100 mg every 4–6 hours (short acting preparations) or every 12 hours (long-acting preparations)		• Should not be used along with drugs that increase serotonin • To be avoided in renal dysfunction
Hydrocodone	• P.O 5–10 mg every 6 hours (short-acting) • P.O 20 mg once daily(long-acting) • Intravenous/subcutaneous		• QTc interval prolongation in higher doses • (>160 mg/day) • Caution in renal dysfunction
Oxycodone Available alone or in combination acetaminophen	• P.O 5 mg every 4 hours (short-acting) • P.O 10 mg every 12 hours (long –acting)		Caution in renal dysfunction
Oxymorphone	• P.O 5 mg every 4 hours (short-acting) • P.O 5 mg every 12 hours (long –acting)		• To be taken on empty stomach for increasing bioavailability • Cautious use in renal dysfunction
Hydromorphone	• P.O 5 mg every 4 hours (short-acting) • P.O 8 mg every 24 hours (long –acting) • IV/SC: 0.5–1 mg every 4 hours		Caution in renal dysfunction

Table 3.
Commonly used opioids for acute pain: Routes of administration, side effects, and contraindications [28, 29].

Drug	Routes of Administration and Sample Adult dosage	Side effects/Adverse reactions	Cautions/ contraindications
Paracetamol/ Acetaminophen. Centrally acting Non-opioid analgesic	PO 0.5–1 gm./4 hours i.v, maximum dose 4gm./ 24 hours	Potential for hepatotoxicity when exceeding recommended dose	Neonates. History of G6-PD deficiency
Nefopam: Non-opioid, non-steroid, centrally acting	IV slow 20 mg every 4–6 hours not exceeding 120 mg/day	Nausea, vomiting, tachycardia, pain at the injection site, rare-hallucinations, convulsions, pruritis, etc.	In patients receiving medications which increase serotonin (MAOIs, SNRIs, SSRIs, TCAs, Pethedine and tramadol)
Diclofenac (NSAID)	PO-25–50 mg/8 hours, Deep I.M 75 mg/day, 25–50 mg IV infusion in 15–60 minutes, 6 mg/hour, maximum of 150 mg/day	Inhibits platelet function, causes gastric ulcers or upper GI bleeding, bronchospasm, tinnitus, water retention, acute renal failure in patients with pre-existing renal impairment	Contraindicated in aspirin allergy, asthma, severe renal impairment, gastric ulcers
Ketorolac (NSAID)	Normal adult dosage 30 mg IV once daily or 30 mg iv every 6 hours (not exceeding 120	Same as Diclofenac	Similar to other NSAIDs, Concurrent anticoagulants, antiplatelet or any other condition. Not to be used intraoperative in cases with expected massive bleeding
Naproxen (NSAID)	Po 250 m–500 mg	Same as Diclofenac	Same as other NSAIDs
Parecoxib (NSAID-selective COX-2 inhibitor)	IV/IM initial dose of 40 mg followed by 20–40 mg every 12 hours (not exceeding 80 mg /day)	Water retention. Acute renal failure in patients with pre-existing renal impairment or dehydration	Same as other NSAIDs. Allergies to sulphonamide or aspirin, heart failure, coronary artery disease cerebrovascular disease. Previous CABG or coronary stent pregnant or lactating women. Uncontrolled hypertension
Etrocoxib (NSAID selective COX-2 inhibitor)	PO 60–120 mg/day, 120 mg for acute pain - not to be continued for more than 8 days	Water retention. Acute renal failure or previous renal impairment	Same as parecoxib
Gabapentinoids	Gabapentin:300–1200 mg preoperatively an hour before surgery. Pre-gablin 75–300 mg	Dizziness, Visual disturbances, Ataxia	Caution in elderly patients and in those with co-morbidities.
Ketamine NMDA antagonist	0.3–0.5 mg /kg/hour bolus. 0.1–0.2 mg/kg/hour infusion	Hyper salivation, nausea and vomiting, and psychotomimetic effects - vivid dreams, blurred vision, hallucinations, nightmares and delirium. Prevents CPSP	Not to be used as part of ERAS regime. Caution in liver disease, coronary – artery disease, psychiatric conditions

Table 4.
Non-opioid group of drugs for postoperative pain management [28].

satisfaction, fewer opioid adverse effects, and a decrease in the length of hospital stay. A statistically significant decreased mean consumption in mean cumulative 24-hour morphine consumption is observed with paracetamol compared with placebo after major surgery. When given prophylactically, it is associated with lesser postoperative nausea and vomittimg, and this is postulated to be due to superior pain control.

b. **Nefopam**: It is a non-opioid, centrally acting analgesic drug [30]. It acts through centrally mediated nociceptive activation of triple monoamine descending inhibitory pathways. Its anti-hyperalgesic properties are due to its modulatory effect on glutaminergic transmission. Because of this property, it can be used for neuropathic pain besides treatment of acute nociceptive pain. When used as a part of a multimodal regime, it has opioid-sparing effects. It has no adverse effects on respiratory and hemostatic functions and has no antipyretic properties. It can cause sweating, nausea, vomiting, malaise, hallucinations, convulsions, pruritis, erythema, urticaria, etc. [30] Cautious use is needed in patients receiving medications that increase the serotonin levels [30].

c. **Non-steroidal Anti-inflammatory Drugs (NSAIDs):** The primary mechanism of action of NSAIDs is the inhibition of cyclooxygenase (COX) and inhibition of the synthesis of prostaglandins, which are the primary mediators of peripheral sensitization and hyperalgesia. They can also exert their effect through inhibition of spinal COX [11]. There are two isoforms of COX, i.e., COX 1 and COX 2. Recently, COX 3 variant has been described, which may have a role in the central action of NSAID'S. There are two types of NSAIDs: non-selective inhibitors and selective COX-2 inhibitors. Selective COX-2 inhibitors provide anti-inflammatory relief without compromising gastric mucosa integrity. The commonly used non-selective NSAIDs are diclofenac, naproxen, ketorolac, ibuprofen, sulindac, etc. The commonly used selective COX-2 inhibitors are celecoxib, etoricoxib, parecoxib, etc.

Used as sole agents, NSAIDs generally provide effective analgesia for mild to moderate pain. NSAIDs are also traditionally considered useful adjuvants to opioids for the treatment of moderate to severe pain. NSAIDs may be given orally or parenterally and are particularly useful as a component of a multimodal analgesia regimen.

a. **Gabapentinoids:** Gabapentin and pregabalin are antiepileptic drugs, also used in the treatment of neuropathic pain. These drugs cause depressed neuronal excitability due to the interaction with the $\alpha 2\delta$ calcium channel subunit. Also, there is enhanced descending inhibition and diminished descending serotonergic facilitation and modulation of the affective component of pain [25]. While prior studies [31] showed that there was a reduction in postoperative narcotic requirements with the benefits of decrease in the risk of postoperative nausea and vomiting. Recent meta-analysis however, showed no clinically significant improvement in pain relief with gabapentinoids [27]. However, there was a greater risk of dizziness and visual disturbance. A large range of the doses have been reported, ranging from 300 to 1200 mg for gabapentin and from 75 to 300 mg for pregabalin, given either preoperatively or postoperatively [31].

b. **Ketamine:** Ketamine is generally used as an intraoperative anesthetic agent. But, in subanaesthestic doses, it is a useful analgesic.The NMDA antagonistic properties of ketamine are responsible for attenuating central sensitization and opioid tolerance. The subanaesthetic dose of ketamine reduces the rescue analgesia requirement and pain intensity. In addition, perioperative ketamine reduces 24-hour patient-controlled analgesia (PCA) morphine consumption and postoperative nausea and vomiting and has minimal adverse effects. The side effects of ketamine are: hypersalivation, nausea, and vomiting, psychotomimetic effects such as vivid dreams, blurred vision, hallucinations, nightmares, and delirium. These act as deterrent to its routine use as an analgesic. Ketamine also reduces the likelihood of transition to chronic postsurgical pain. Although ketamine can be used effectively as part of a multimodal pain management regime currently, it is not recommended as a routine part of most ERAS postoperative pain strategies [2].

Patient-controlled analgesia (PCA): It is based on the idea that whenever the patient has pain, the patient can self-administer the analgesic drug, without having to request and wait for the healthcare staff [32]. PCA is useful in the acute pain setting where there is inadequate pain control from the initial opioid administration in the emergency department, and continued opioid dosing has been proven to improve patient outcomes [32]. Postoperative patients, especially those with indwelling nerve or epidural catheters, are ideal candidates for PCA. The ability of postsurgical patients to titrate and administer their pain medication allows for superior pain control compared to scheduled nurse dosing. Patients in labor pain are also well-established candidates for epidural PCA [32]. The pain associated with contractions, when exacerbated by induction agents such as oxytocin, can be adequately reduced and controlled by the patient [32]. A PCA device can be programmed for several variables such as demand dose (bolus), lockout interval, and background infusion. Compared to traditional analgesic regimens, PCA provides superior postoperative analgesia and improves patient satisfaction. Local anesthetics and opioids are commonly used medications for PCA. For intravenous PCA, opioids can be used as the sole analgesic. For epidural PCA, they are used or in combination with local anesthetics.

Opioids commonly used for PCA are: The pure Mu opioid receptor agonists (morphine, fentanyl, hydromorphone, meperidine, sufentanil, alfentanil, and remifentanil), Mu opioid receptor agonist-antagonists (butorphanol, nalbuphine, and pentazocine), and partial Mu opioid receptor agonists (buprenorphine, dezocine) [32]. Despite the availability of several analgesics, morphine is still considered the gold standard for PCA. The local anesthetics used for epidural analgesia and indwelling nerve catheter PCA are: bupivacaine, levobupivacaine, and ropivacaine [32]. Other medications added to intravenous PCA in order to reduce side effects and improve pain control include: ketamine, naloxone, clonidine, magnesium, ketorolac, lidocaine, and droperidol [32].

The opioid dosing is depicted in **Table 5**. However, the medication dose, which is given in PCA, must be tailored according to individual patients' analgesic needs. The patients should be oriented, alert, and demonstrate the ability to administer the demand dose for pain. The basal or continuous infusion is started if the patients are using frequent demand doses or if the pain is severe. The suggested basal dose is 30–50% of the average hourly dose [29]. For opioid-tolerant patients, one should consider the patient's current opioid regimen, clinical condition (cause and its severity), side effects from opioids, baseline sedation, and need for opioid rotation. First,

Opioid	Demand(PCA) dose	Lock-out interval (minutes)	1-hour dose limit	Continuous dose	Nurse bolus prn	Nurse bolus interval (hours)
Morphine	1 mg (0.5–2.5 mg)	10–30 minutes	4 mg	30–50% of hourly dose	2–4 mg	2
Hydromorphone	0.2 mg (0.1–0.5)	10–30	0.8 mg		0.5–1 mg	2
Fentanyl	10mcg (5–25)	10–30	40mcg		25mcg	2

Table 5.
Intravenous patient-controlled analgesia for opioid-naïve patients [29].

the total opioid dose used in the previous 24 hours is estimated, and then an equianalgesic opioid conversion table is used for calculating the IV dose of opioid intended for use in PCA. The hourly dose is the new IV dose from this step divided by 24 hours to obtain the basal/hourly dose. The PCA demand dose is 10–20% of this new opioid dose as PRN every hour [29].

9. Neuraxial analgesia

The analgesia provided by epidural is site-specific and superior to that with systemic opioids. The use of this technique may even reduce morbidity and mortality [10].

1. **Single-dose neuraxial opioids:** Administration of a single dose of opioid may be efficacious as a sole analgesic or as an adjuvant, when administered intrathecally or epidurally. The hydrophilic opioids: morphine and hydromorphone tend to remain in CSF and produce delayed analgesia with a longer duration of effect. However, they cause more frequent side effects because of the cephalic or supraspinal spread. Neuraxial administration of lipophilic opioids such as fentanyl and sufentanil provides quick onset of analgesia. Their rapid clearance from CSF leads to less incidence of side effects such as respiratory depression.

2. **Continuous epidural analgesia:** Analgesia delivered through an indwelling epidural catheter is a safe and effective method for management of acute postoperative pain. Analgesia through the epidural route can provide analgesia superior than the systemic opioids. Intraoperative use of epidural with general anesthesia results in less pain and faster recovery than general anesthesia followed by systemic opioids [15, 18].

9.1 Analgesic drug for epidural

1. **Local anesthetics:** Epidural infusion of local anesthetics alone may be used for postoperative analgesia, but provides better analgesia when given in combination with opioids.

2. **Opioids:** Opioids used alone for postoperative epidural infusion do not cause motor block or hypotension from the sympathetic blockade [18]. Analgesic site of action for continuous hydrophilic opioids is primarily spinal. It is useful when the epidural insertion is not congruent with the surgical site. Continuous epidural

infusion of morphine may provide superior analgesia with fewer side effects compared to intermittent doses.

Local anesthetic and opioid combinations: The epidural infusion of LA-opioid combination is advantageous than the infusion of LA or opioid alone. This combination provides superior postoperative analgesia, limits time for regression of sensory blockade, and decreases the dose of local anesthetic. Continuous epidural analgesia of LA-opioid combination provides superior analgesia than the intravenous patient-controlled analgesia with opioids [14].

Patient-controlled epidural analgesia (PCEA): Like intravenous PCA, PCEA allows individualization of postoperative analgesia requirements and may have several advantages over continuous epidural infusion, including lower drug use and better patient satisfaction. PCEA may also provide analgesia superior to than intravenous PCA [15]. PCEA is a relatively safe and effective technique for postoperative analgesia.

The drug doses for continuous epidural infusion and PCEA drug doses are given in **Table 6**.

Adjuvant drugs: A variety of adjuvants may be added to epidural infusion to enhance analgesia while minimizing side effects. Clonidine acts centrally as an agonist on alpha-2a adrenergic receptors [33]. Clonidine also mediates its effects through the spinal dorsal horn alpha-2 receptors via the primary afferents, interneurons, and through the descending noradrenergic pathways. Clonidine enhances the analgesic activity of opioids and local anesthetics and prolongs the duration of blocks [33, 34]. Two proposed mechanisms for the analgesic effects produced by clonidine include the reduction of glutamate and excitatory neuropeptide release from central afferent terminals, as well as the hyperpolarization of dorsal horn neurons [33]. Epidural dose of clonidine is 5–20 micrograms/hour. Its side effects are hypotension and bradycardia [1].

Location of epidural catheter: The insertion of an epidural catheter congruent to incision dermatome results in optimal postoperative analgesia with lesser side effects (lower extremity block, urinary retention) and a decrease in morbidity [10, 18]. There is a summary of neuraxial opioids, their adverse effects, and management of same in **Table 7**.

	Epidural Analgesia	Dose for continuous infusion (lumbar/thoracic)	Patient controlled analgesia (lumbar/thoracic)	Continuous peripheral nerve analgesia
Ropivacaine OR	0.2% (2 mg/ml)	6–12 ml/hour	Background 4–6 ml/hour	0.2%
Bupivacaine OR	0.1–0.2% (1–2 mg/ml)		Bolus dose 2 ml (2–4 ml) Minimum lockout interval – 10 minute	0.1 to 0.125%)
Levobupivacaine	0.1 to 0.2% (1–2 mg/ml)		Recommended max. Hourly dose (bolus + background) = 12 ml	0.1 to 0.2%
			Type of block	
			Interscalene /Infraclavicular	5–9 ml/hr.
			Axillary	5–10 ml/hr.
			Femoral	7–10 ml/hr.
			Popliteal	3–7 ml/hr.

Table 6.
Local anesthetics dose for postoperative patient controlled anaesthesia [28].

Adverse reactions	Risk factors	Evaluation	Treatment
Respiratory depression/ Sedation	• Opioid naïve Extremes of age, Obesity, Preexisting respiratory disease • Obstructive sleep apnoea • Concurrent use of sedatives	Respiratory route < 10 min. Sedation score > 2	Supplemental oxygen, open airway. Naloxone IV 0.4–0.2 mg every 2–3 minutes (till awake or normal respiration) Followed by infusion in patients on long acting opioids –dose- 2-5 mcg/kg/hour titrate as per response
Hallucination/ delirium/ cognitive failure	High dose, depression, drug abuse, elderly, preexisting cognitive impairment Impaired liver/ renal function	Rule out other causes and side effects of other drugs	• Decrease dosage • Opioid rotation • -Major or minor tranquilisers • Haloperidol 2–5 mg IM every 4–8 hours
Rigidity/ myoclonus/ seizures	• High dose • Preexisting epilepsy • Neurotoxity from M3G norpethidine or tramadol		• Opioid rotation to opioids with inactive metabolites • Lorazepam PO 0.5–1 mg BID • Clonazepam PO 0.5-1 mg • Baclofen 10mgBID-TID
Nausea/ vomiting	Female, history of nausea/ vomiting	Rule out other causes	• Pre-emptive anti-emetics, • Opioid rotation • Anti-emetics
Pruritus			• Diphenhaydramine 25 mg i.v OR • Nalbuphine 1-5 mg i.v OR • Naloxone 0.25–2 mcg/kg/ hour
Urinary retention	Common with neuraxial opioid	Evaluate for full bladder and urinary voiding every 1–2 hours postoperatively	Cold pack, catheterization, Naloxone 0.001–0.002 mg/kg IV titrate according to clinical response
Constipation			• Stool softeners, stimulants like • Bisacodyl 1–2 tablets HS • Lactulose 30 ml HS • Milk of magnesia 30 ml HS TID

Table 7.
Adverse reactions from neuraxial opioids and treatment.

10. Regional analgesia

The use of peripheral nerve blocks (PNBs) as a single injection or as continuous infusion can provide site-specific analgesia superior to the systemic opioids and may even result in improvement in various outcomes [14]. The PNBs may have several advantages over systemic opioids (i.e., good analgesia and lesser opioid-related side effects) and neuraxial techniques (i.e., less risk of spinal hematoma, better hemodynamic instability). All this can lead to faster recovery, reduced stay in the hospital, decreased incidence of nausea and vomiting, early rehabilitation, and greater patient satisfaction [34]. Absolute contraindications to the use of peripheral nerve blocks include allergy to local anesthetics, inability to cooperate due to dementia or similar conditions, or patient refusal. PNBs should not be given if there is an active infection at the injection site, or if there are preexisting neural deficits in area of distribution of the block, and in patients with coagulopathies or on antithrombotic drugs [35].

11. Upper extremity blocks

The regional blocks can be given using a nerve stimulator or ultrasound visualization for locating the nerves. The nerve stimulator causes muscle contractions when the corresponding nerve is stimulated. Commonly used local anesthetics include bupivacaine and ropivacaine. Once the local anesthetic is placed, the patient can expect pain relief and limb heaviness for the duration of the local anesthetic action and adjuncts used [36].

- **Interscalene block**: The interscalene block covers most of the brachial plexus; however, the ulnar (C8-T1) nerve is spared [36]. It is useful for patients undergoing surgery of the shoulder, upper arm, and elbow. It is not an effective block for hand surgery as the inferior trunk is spared. This block is contraindicated in patients who have respiratory disorders because of higher possibility of ipsilateral phrenic nerve block resulting in diaphragmatic hemiparesis. This can lead to a 25% reduction in pulmonary function. Furthermore, the recurrent laryngeal nerve may be blocked, which could result in incomplete airway obstruction if there is already an existing vocal cord palsy.

- **Supraclavicular block:** The indications for supraclavicular block are: the surgeries of the distal two-thirds of the upper extremity, and surgeries from the mid-humerus to the fingertips [37]. Sparing of distal branches, especially the ulnar nerve, can occur. Besides the general contraindications applicable to PNBs, caution is advised for patients with severe pulmonary disease as local anesthesia spread can cause diaphragmatic paresis or pneumothorax [37].

- **Infraclavicular block**: It is indicated for postoperative pain control for upper extremity surgeries such as the elbow, forearm, wrist, and hand, and when positioning is restricted due to limited abduction at the shoulder [38].The shoulder area may be spared since the superficial cervical plexus C1–C4 innervates it. The skin of the axilla and proximal medial arm requires an additional intercostobrachial nerve block to provide full anesthesia. There may also be an incomplete radial nerve sensory block [38]. The infraclavicular block has the advantages that pneumothorax can be avoided and that it is suitable for catheter usage. The disadvantage is that the brachial plexus is located deeper and the angle of approach is more acute making it challenging unless the anesthesiologist is experienced in performing it [38]. The procedure is also challenging in patients with obesity for the same reasons.

- **Axillary block**: provides surgical anesthesia for elbow, forearm, and hand procedures, cutaneous anesthesia for superficial procedures of the inner part of the arm.The block anesthetizes the nerves of the brachial plexus at the level of the individual nerves [39]. The axillary approach is the safest of the four approaches, as it does not cause the blockade of the phrenic nerve. Also, it does not have the potential to cause pneumothorax, making it an ideal option for day -case surgery [39]. However, the general risks of accidental intravascular and intraneural injection still exist.

- **Intercostobrachial block:** The intercostobrachial nerve arises from the second thoracic nerve root. It is not a component of the brachial plexus and therefore, cannot be given by any brachial plexus approach [40]. For this block, the patient is positioned supine with the arm abducted to expose the axillary fossa. The intercostobrachial nerve is located in the subcutaneous tissue of the medial portion of upper arm. For this block, the needle is advanced subcutaneously, across the medial aspect of the arm while injecting 5–10 cc of local anesthetic [40].

- **Radial nerve block**: The radial nerve comes out between the brachioradialis tendon and the radius, just proximal to the styloid process [41]. The needle is inserted subcutaneously, just proximal to the styloid process of the radius, aiming medially, and 3–5 cc of local anesthetic is injected. A radial nerve block will provide anesthesia and/or analgesia to the dorsal radial side of the hand. This includes anesthesia dorsally to the thumb, index and middle fingers, and the lateral aspect of the ring finger [41]. It is used as a sole or adjunctive therapy for interventions of the hands and fingers, for the management of acute pain in the radial nerve's distribution, for the diagnosis and treatment of radial tunnel syndrome, and for the diagnostic prognostication procedure in injury to the radial nerve [41].

- **Median nerve block:** The median nerve is located between the tendons of the flexor palmaris longus and the flexor carpi radialis [42]. The needle should be inserted between the two tendons until it passes through the fascia, and it is to be moved further until it touches the bone. The needle direction should then be changed in a way that the local anesthetic is injected in lateral and medial directions. A median nerve block is a simple, safe, and effective procedure. It provides analgesia to the palmar aspect of the thumb, index finger, middle finger, the radial portion of the palm, and ring finger [42].

- **Ulnar nerve block**: The ulnar nerve runs between the ulnar artery and flexor carpi ulnaris tendon, which is just superficial to the ulnar nerve [43]. The block is administered by placing the needle under this tendon close to its attachment, just above the styloid process of the ulna, and by moving further for 5 mm to 10 mm. A total of 3–5 cc of local anesthetic is injected at this location. It is used for surgical procedures in the distribution of the ulnar nerve either as a sole block or combined with ulnar or radial nerve blocks for a complete hand block. It can act as a rescue for inadequate brachial plexus blocks. An ulnar nerve block is used as an alternative to sedation for painful procedures such as fracture reduction and to provide pain relief in burns [43].

12. Lower extremity blocks

- **Lumbar plexus block:** The lumbar plexus (LP) is formed within the body of the psoas major muscle by the four spinal nerves of L1–L4. In 60% of people, the lumbar plexus receives a contribution from the nerve root of T12 as well [44].

The LPB is used to provide analgesia following injuries or surgeries of the hip or thigh (e.g., acetabular fractures, femoral neck or mid-shaft fractures, hip replacement, hip arthroscopy, knee replacement). It has also been used for chronic pain conditions such as herpes zoster. It is important to note that the LPB is unlikely by itself to produce complete anesthesia for hip replacement surgery due to the innervation of the posteromedial hip capsule deriving from branches of the sacral plexus and sciatic nerve [44].

- **Femoral nerve block:** The femoral nerve is one of the largest branches of the lumbar plexus. The femoral nerve arises from the ventral rami of the L2, L3, and L4 spinal nerves and is located in the femoral triangle inferior to the inguinal ligament. The femoral nerve is the most lateral of the structures within the triangle, which also contains the femoral artery and femoral vein at its medial end [45]. The femoral nerve block is useful for anterior thigh and knee procedures [45].

- **Fascia iliaca compartment block:** This block is considered an anterior approach to the lumbar plexus where local anesthetic (LA) is injected proximally beneath the fascia iliaca. In this, there occurs blockade of the femoral nerve (FN), obturator nerve (ON), and lateral cutaneous nerve of the thigh (LCNT) simultaneously [46]. Unlike the FN block, the needle is not placed adjacent to the FN, thus reducing the risk of neuropraxia. Indications for FICB include perioperative analgesia for fractured neck of femur, hip and knee surgery, above knee amputation, and application of plaster cast to femoral fracture in pediatric patients. Complications include block failure, hematoma, neuropraxia, local anesthetic systemic toxicity (LAST), quadriceps weakness, perforation of peritoneal cavity contents, and bladder puncture [46].

- **Obturator nerve block:** An ONB is performed commonly to prevent thigh adductor jerk during transurethral resection of bladder tumor, to provide analgesia for knee surgery, to treat hip pain, and to improve persistent hip adductor spasticity [47].The proximal approach comprises a single injection of local anesthetic into the interfascial plane between the pectineus and obturator externus muscles. The proximal approach may be superior for reducing the dose of local anesthetic and providing successful blockade of the obturator nerve, including the hip articular branch, when compared with the distal approach.

- **Sciatic nerve block:** The sciatic nerve originates from the sacral plexus (L4-S3) and provides most of the motor and sensory innervation to the leg: [48] The sciatic nerve is an important major nerve of the lower extremity, supplying the vast majority of the motor and sensory function to the lower limb. It is the motor nerve for the posterior thigh and all muscles below the knee. Sensory function is provided to the posterior thigh, posterior knee joint, and everything below the knee, except a narrow band on the medial lower leg, supplied by the saphenous nerve. The long course of the sciatic nerve, from the sciatic notch in the gluteal region to the popliteal fossa, allows for multiple possible sites for an anesthetic blockade.

- **Popliteal nerve block:** The popliteal nerve block is a block of the sciatic nerve in the popliteal fossa with the patient lying in a prone position. The block is useful for surgeries of the lower leg, particularly the foot and ankle. It anesthetizes the same dermatomes as both the anterior and lateral approaches to the sciatic nerve [48].

- **Saphenous nerve block**: The saphenous nerve block is indicated for procedures related to the lower leg or foot along its neural distribution [49]. It is most commonly used in conjunction with a popliteal sciatic nerve block to provide complete anesthesia of the lower leg for various surgical and nonsurgical procedures.

- **Pericapsular nerve group block**: The pericapsular nerve group (PENG) block is an interfascial plane block used for blocking the articular branches supplied by femoral, obturator, and accessory obturator nerves. PENG block is useful in anterior and lateral hip arthroplasties and hip fractures. It is performed with the patient in a supine position by depositing 15–20 ml of local anesthetic in the plane between the psoas tendon and the pubic ramus under direct ultrasound visualization [50]. The main advantage of PENG block is that it provides better analgesia of the hip without causing any motor block. As there6is no muscle weakness so the patient can participate in physical therapy early [50].

- **Femoral nerve block, fascia iliaca compartment block or lumbar plexus block** has been used to manage postoperative analgesia in hip surgeries. These blocks cause the weakness of quadriceps muscles, and hence, the patients are predisposed to falling. These blocks also result in incomplete analgesia to the hip as there is a sparing of few articular branches to the hip [44, 45].

- **iPACK block**: IPACK block is an acronym for infiltration of local anesthetic into the interspace between the popliteal artery and the posterior capsule of the knee and was first introduced in 2012 [51].The iPACK block is used for postoperative analgesia in total knee arthroplasties and cruciate ligament repair. Posterior knee sensory supply is through the articular branches of the tibial nerve with contributions from the obturator nerve. In the iPACK block, 15–20 ml of local anesthetic is injected under ultrasound guidance in the tissue plane popliteal artery and posterior aspect of the capsule of the knee joint. The main advantage of the iPACK block is that it is a motor-sparing block and does not result in foot drop or loss of sensorimotor function of the leg and foot [51].

13. Truncal blocks

Several non-epidural/truncal regional analgesia techniques can be used for management of postoperative thoracic and abdominal pain. Truncal blocks include the blocks of chest wall and anterior abdominal wall. The chest wall blocks are thoracic paravertebral, intercostal blocks, pectoral blocks, serratus anterior plane block, suprascapular, interpleural analgesia, and cryoanalgesia. The blocks of anterior abdominal wall are transverses abdominis plane block (TAP), rectus sheath block, quadrates lumborum blocks, erector spinae blocks, ilioinguinal, iliohypogastric nerve [52]. The ultrasound-guided regional blocks have revolutionized the management of perioperative pain. The unique feature of this is that no nerve or plexus needs to be identified. The local anesthetic is injected into a particular muscle plane, which spreads and reaches the intended nerves. The current research is leading us to an era where ultrasound will become a basic necessity for practice of regional anesthesia [52].

13.1 Chest wall blocks

- **Thoracic paravertebral blocks**: have been used for thoracic, breast, upper abdominal surgery and treatment of rib fracture pain. The paravertebral space lies on either side of the vertebral column. The thoracic paravertebral space (TPVS) is continuous with the intercostal space laterally, epidural space medially, and contralateral paravertebral space via the prevertebral and epidural space [53].The classical technique involves contacting the tranverse process of the vertebra, walking the needle above it, and gradually advancing it till there is a loss of resistance. A pressure measurement technique can also be used. Pressure in the erector spinae muscle is higher in inspiratory phase than expiration. Once the superior costotranseverse ligament is traversed and TPVS is entered, the pressure inversion occurs and expiratory pressure is higher [53]. Other approaches are medial approach and paravertebral-peridural block technique [53]. The local anesthetics can be administered as a single injection or as a continuous infusion through a catheter. This block may provide analgesia equal or superior to that of thoracic epidural and is a valuable alternative to thoracic epidural [18, 19].

- **Intercostal blocks:** These are used for pain management in the chest wall for conditions such as incisional pain, thoracotomy, herpes zoster, rib fracture, breast surgery, and upper abdominal surgery [54]. The block is given by walking off the needle along the inferior border of the rib and advancing 1–3 mm anteriorly where a give way or "pop" is felt as it advances through the fascia of internal intercostal muscle, and then 3–5 ml of local anesthetic is injected after negative aspiration [54]. Ultrsound-guided block decreases the possibility of pneumothorax, allows administration of LA before the division of lateral branch, which is necessary to achieve anesthesia of the entire dermatome [54]. The block is simple, but one needs to be careful to avoid pneumothorax and intravascular injections of LA [54]. If multiple blocks are to be given, the concentration should be reduced and total dose of LA should be calculated to avoid toxicity.

- **Serratus anterior plane block:** It is indicated in pain management of thoracoscopy, thoracotomy, and breast surgery and in rib fractures (effective in lateral rib fractures and ineffective in anterior and posterior rib fractures) [55]. Superficial serratus anterior plane block is given under ultrasound guidance by injecting LA anterior to the serratus anterior muscle and for the deep SAPB, the local anesthetic is injected anteriorly to the rib and deep to the serratus anterior muscle [55].The SAPB targets the lateral cutaneous branches of the thoracic intercostal nerves, which run inferior to each rib at mid-axillary line, they run through the intercostal muscles and serratus anterior muscle, innervating the musculature of lateral thorax [55].

- **Pectoralis nerve block**: The pectoral nerve blocks: PEC 1 block and PEC2 block, are novel techniques to block the pectoral nerves, intercostal nerves 3–6, intercostobrachial nerves, and the long thoracic nerves. These blocks are useful for surgeries such as insertion of breast expanders, submuscular prostheses, ports, pacemakers, implantable cardiac defibrillators, anterior thoracotomies, sentinel node biopsy, and axillary dissection [56].The PEC1 block is given under ultrasound guidance in the fascial plane between pectoralis major and minor muscle, while PEC2 is an extension of PEC1 with second injection being given in the plane between pectoralis minor and serratus anterior muscles often at the level of third rib [56].

13.2 Blocks of anterior abdominal wall

- **Transversus abdominis plane block** is an approach for blocking the abdominal wall neural afferents to provide postoperative analgesia to the parietal peritoneum, skin and muscles of the anterior abdominal wall. The transversus abdominis plane compartment can be sited with landmarks or ultrasound guidance or identified intraoperatively by surgeons. The landmark technique can be used exclusively for posterior approach and involves identification of lumbar triangle of Petit and the plane between the internal oblique and transversus abdominis muscles with tactile pops [57]. However, these may be difficult to locate in obese patients and absent or variable in other patients. Ultrasound-guided posterior approach involves placing the probe in mid-axillary line superior to the iliac crest (over the triangle of Petit) and identifying the target fascial plane. Another TAP block for upper abdominal surgery is by oblique subcostal approach. Another four-point, single-shot approach technique is recently described that combines the posterior and oblique subcostal techniques [58]. There can be needle-related complications such as breach of the peritoneum and injury to viscera and those related to LA toxicity [58].

- **Rectus Sheath Block:** It is an anterior abdominal block that reduces postoperative pain associated with midline incisions around the umbilicus and laparoscopic surgery. Ultrasound-guided rectus sheath block will block the ventral rami of 7th–12th thoracolumbar nerve by injecting the LA into the space between the rectus muscle and posterior sheath [59]. Potential complications are related to LA toxicity and needle injury, namely injury to epigastric vessels and wound infections. These are rare with ultrasound-guided blocks [59]. A study showed that rectus sheath block provided analgesia equivalent to epidural analgesia in colorectal surgery with advantage of lesser incidence of hypotension [60].

- **Qudratus Lumboram block**: It is also called as interfascial plane block as the block is given by injecting LA into the thoracolumbar fascia, which is the extension of abdominal wall fascia posteriorly and embodies the back muscles: quadratus lumboram, psoas major, and erector spinae [61].The block provides analgesia for abdominal and pelvis surgeries: gynecologic, obstetric, and urologic surgeries. It is also useful in hip, femur, and lumbar vertebral surgeries. There are no reports of LA-related toxicity with this block and also no infectious complications. Variants of block have been described relative to the site of deposition of LA around quadratus lumboram: lateral, anterior, posterior, and intramuascular [61].

- **Erector Spinae block**: It is a newer regional technique and can be used for analgesia related to anterior, posterior, and lateral thoracic and abdominal areas. The ESP block is performed between the T5–T7 paraspinal levels and can be performed at lower levels as well. The block is given under ultrasound guidance with needle being advanced through trapezius muscle, rhomboid major muscle, and erector spinae muscle toward the transverse process and LA deposited below the erector spinae nuscle [62].

- **Ilioinguinal and iliohypogatric nerve blocks:** These blocks are used for postoperative analgesia in lower abdominal surgeries and cesarean section. The block involves the blocking of ilioinguinal and iliohypogastric nerves in the plane between the transversus abdomini and internal oblique muscles [63]. In the conventional blind method, this plane is reached by the "click" felt during needle insertion at this point. With this blind method, there are possibilities of missing the plane between the transversus abdominis and internal oblique. Also there are chances of complications such as bowel perforation, injury to blood vessels, urinary retention, and femoral nerve blockade [63]. Ultrasound-guided procedure avoids these complications and helps in accurate drug placement after identifying the nerves and thus lesser dose of LA [63].

14. Adjuncts to regional nerve blocks

The duration of action of local anesthetics in PNB varies but may last up to 24 hours. Patients who have had a single-shot PNB may complain of slightly greater postoperative discomfort between 16 and 24 h compared with those who have had only systemic analgesics [64]. Rebound pain may occur after single-shot PNBs, resulting in sleep disturbances, difficulties employing enhanced recovery and physiotherapy protocol, and increased consumption of opioids and related side effects [64]. Hence, strategies have been sought to extend the benefits of single-shot PNBs beyond the maximum of 8–16 h. A continuous PNB involves the percutaneous insertion of a catheter adjacent to a peripheral nerve, plexus, or fascial plane, followed by the administration of LA through the catheter [64]. Such a procedure may involve problems such as inaccurate catheter tip placement and secondary block failure; catheter-related mechanical nerve irritation, catheter knotting, migration, obstruction or shearing, fluid leakage or inflammation at the insertion site of the catheter; bacterial catheter colonization; infusion pump malfunction; myonecrosis with repeated large boluses of bupivacaine; and LA systemic toxicity [64]. The use of "perineural adjuncts" is technically simple and effective alternative to the continuous PNBs in order to extend the benefits of single-shot PNBs. The term perineural adjuncts refers to the co-administration of pharmacological agent(s) with LA(s) around a peripheral nerve, plexus or fascial plane with the aim of affecting the characteristics of the resulting block [64]. Over time, the number of potential perineural adjuncts has increased to a wide variety of drugs.

Several drugs have been used to improve the quality and duration of block.

1. **Dexamethasone**: It is a potent long-acting glucocorticoid with minimal mineralocorticoid activity. It stimulates the glucocorticoid receptors located on the cell membranes of neurons after perineural administration, increasing the expression of inhibitory K^+ channels and thereby decreasing the excitability of and neuronal transmission in nociceptive unmyelinated C-fibers. It may be that its actions are mediated via localized vasoconstriction or systemic anti-inflammatory effects after absorption through the vasculature. Dexamethasone must be administered as a preparation without preservatives such as benzyl alcohol and propylene, both of which can cause neurolytic effects [64]. Studies have demonstrated that perineural dexamethasone was associated with an increase in the mean duration of analgesia, decrease in pain scores at rest and on movement, and reduction of cumulative morphine consumption at 24 hour [64].

2. **Clonidine and dexmedetomidine:** These are also useful adjuncts for PNB. As α_2-adrenoceptors are not located on the axons of peripheral nerves, the mechanism of action of α_2-adrenoceptor agonists after perineural administration is not related to these receptors. In the refractory phase of an action potential, hyperpolarization-activated cation currents normally restore the resting potential of the neuron, allowing restoration of functional activity [64].Clonidine and dexmedetomidine block the hyperpolarization-activated, cyclic nucleotide-gated channels responsible for these currents, maintaining the neuron in a hyperpolarized, thereby inhibiting conduction in Aδ and C-nerve fibers and producing analgesia. Clonidine could also work partially through localized vasoconstriction mediated through the lesser selective activity at α_1-adrenoceptors. Perineural clonidine and dexmedetomidine cause an increase in the mean duration of analgesia, sensory and motor block irrespective of whether intermediate-acting (lidocaine, mepivacaine, or prilocaine) or long-acting (bupivacaine or ropivacaine) LAs were injected [64]. They also increase the occurrence of adverse effects such as bradycardia, arterial hypotension, fainting or orthostatic hypotension, and sedation [64]. Furthermore, perineural dexmedetomidine was related to a decrease in the mean time to onset of sensory block and motor block.

3. **Adrenaline** is one of the oldest perineural adjuncts to LAs. It acts by decreasing the time to onset, increasing the duration of block characteristics, and delaying the systemic uptake of local anesthetic, thereby reducing the risk of LA systemic toxicity. It can also serve as a marker of intravascular injection. Its mechanism of action after perineural administration is thought to be related to vasoconstriction secondary to α_1-adrenoceptor stimulation. In a meta-analysis of five RCTs, perineural adrenaline was associated with an increase in the mean duration of analgesia by approximately 1 h [65]. However, adrenaline can lead to a significant decrease in blood flow to the peripheral nerve, particularly when administered in combination with LA, predisposing to neurotoxicity.

4. **Buprenorphine** is a partial MOP (μ) opioid receptor agonist and KOP (κ) opioid receptor antagonist, which has analgesic and antihyperalgesic properties [66]. Its mechanism of action after perineural administration is secondary to concentration-dependent block of voltage-gated sodium channels, inhibition of the generation of action potentials in a similar manner to LAs, and interaction with MOP opioid receptors on the axons of unmyelinated C fibers [64]. Perineural buprenorphine was associated with an increase in the mean duration of analgesia by approximately 8.5 h and a slightly longer duration of motor block of 13 min. Its main adverse effects were postoperative nausea and vomiting (PONV) and pruritus.

5. **Hyaluronidase** is an enzyme that can be administered in conjunction with LA to decrease the time to onset of ophthalmic blocks and provide improved akinesia and analgesia. It degrades hyaluronic acid, a glycosaminoglycan that attaches to proteoglycans in the orbital connective tissue and otherwise hinders the spread of LA [64].

6. **Sodium bicarbonate** can reduce the time to onset of neuronal block by alkalinization of the solution, increasing its pH closer to the p*K*a of the LA, and thus favoring the non-ionized form of the LA that is able to penetrate the peripheral nerve to reach its site of action [67].

7. **Magnesium** is an *N*-methyl-D-aspartate (NMDA) receptor antagonist that has been found to increase the excitation threshold in peripheral nerves, more so in myelinated Aβ than unmyelinated C-fibers. Its mechanism of action after perineural administration could be secondary to the effects of its positive divalent charge on the neuronal membrane or its role as a physiological calcium antagonist [64]. Perineural magnesium was associated with an increase in the mean duration of analgesia by approximately 2 h, duration of sensory block by 1.75 h and duration of motor block by 1.5 h. Perineural magnesium did not increase the risk of PONV [64].

Drugs such as fentanyl, morphine, ketamine, tramadol, midazolam, and neostigmine are not used as perineural adjuncts in PNBs because of conflicting or limited evidence and worries about their potential for adverse effects or neurotoxicity [64].

15. Non-pharmacological methods for acute pain

The non-pharmacological methods of pain management can be divided into physical interventions and psychological interventions. Physical/sensory interventions are patient-specific, they inhibit nociceptive input and pain perception. They include methods such as massage, positioning, rest, ice/heat therapy, acupuncture, TENS, accupressure, etc. [68]. The psychological interventions consist of therapies such as cognitive-behavioral therapy, mindfulness-based stress reduction, acceptance and commitment therapy, guided imagery, biofeedback, music therapy, and meditation etc. [69]. These can act as an important adjuvant for pain management. It has the advantage of being relatively inexpensive and safe. It helps decrease fear, distress, and anxiety and is convenient The non-pharmacological methods have significant and often enduring efficacy in pain management and can be employed alone or in combination with pharmacological methods [70]. A few of the common non-pharmacological techniques are discussed below.

1. **Massage:** It is manipulation applied on soft tissue with various techniques such as friction, percussion, vibration, and tapotement for recovery and supporting health [71]. It is done by pressing or kneading parts of the body especially joints and muscles with hands to reduce pain and decrease tension [71]. Massage can interrupt the patients' cycle of distress, it can increase the blood circulation as well as the lymphatic circulation, it can initiate an analgesic effect to the area being rubbed and decrease inflammation and edema. It can release spasm manually while increasing endogenous endorphin release and conflicting sensory stimuli that override pain signals. It can lead to relaxation of tense muscles and increase blood flow to the underlying tissues and decrease in pain.

2. Positioning: It is the most commonly employed non-pharmacological method of pain relief in postoperative period. It is the physical intervention that includes maintaining a proper body alignment to reduce stress and anxiety. Use of special beds, pillows and weight lifting are done. The benefits of positioning are prevention of bed ulcers, reduced risk of injuries, bed ulcers, relief of muscle pain, tension and discomfort, and improved blood circulation. Elevating extremities decreases pain and prevents edema [71].

3. Rest: It is useful for certain group of patients such as those with fractures, those receiving traction for back pain, etc. It should not be used as a sole method for pain management. It can decrease edema, when employed with proper positioning.

4. Hot and cold therapy: Hot and cold fomentation has the benefits of reduction in pain, anxiety, nausea, and heart rate in patients treated with active warming for pain related to mild trauma, cystitis, urolithiasis, and cholelithiasis. This is also indicated in muscle and joint pain, arthritis, back pain, etc. Hot therapy works by moving the reflex arcs that inhibits the pain by stimulating heat receptors in the skin and deeper tissues (gate control theory) and also reduces pain by vasodilatation effect [71]. It reduces striated muscle spasm by minimizing muscle spindle excitability and reducing tension in muscle trigger points. In painful joints, application of heat reduces the viscosity of synovial fluid, which alleviates painful stiffness and increases joint range [6]. Deep ultrasound therapy for tissues, which are 3–5 cm deep can increase the temperature of these areas and reduce pain by mechanism as explained before.

5. Benefits of hot application are it is inexpensive, easy-to-use with minimal side effects when used appropriately. Hot therapy is given by hot compresses, warm baths, paraphine usage, and surface application. Cold therapy: Can be done by application of cold temperature using cold gel package or ice package. Cold therapy works by increasing pain threshold, reduction of edema, and suppression of inflammatory process.

6. **Acupuncture**: The needle is put in specific region of the body, which stimulates the nerve [60]. Each needle will cause little to no discomfort and produces a small injury, which will stimulate the body and the immune system to increase the circulation, wound healing, pain modulation, and pain analgesia.

7. **Trans-electrical nerve stimulation (TENS)**: T.EN.S is an electric device used to treat pain. It is defined as applying electricity to the skin to manage pain. It is an electro-analgesia method. It consists of battery-powered unit and has two to four leads connected to sticky pads, which are positioned on the skin to cover or surround the painful area [71].

Trans-electrical nerve stimulation (TENS) and acupuncture may provide postoperative analgesia, decreased postoperative opioid requirements, reduced opioid-related side effects, and attenuate activation of sympathoadrenal system. In general, all of these techniques are relatively safe, noninvasive, and devoid of systemic side effects seen with other analgesic options [68–71]. Cognitive therapy and behavioral therapy may be efficacious in reducing pain and alleviating psychological factors associated with pain.

16. Considerations for acute postoperative control in specific patient populations

Opioid tolerant patients: These patients are chronically on opioid for preexisting pain or may be taking opioids for recreational purposes. Opioid tolerance is characterized by a decreased responsiveness to an opioid agonist such as morphine and is usually evident by the need to use increasing doses to achieve the desired effect [72]. Patients who are taking opioids for management of cancer pain or chronic non-cancer pain or who have an opioid addiction may become opioid-tolerant. Acute pain management in opioid-tolerant patients should ideally be done by a multidisciplinary team comprising pain specialists, physicians, psychologists, trained nursing staff, etc. A meticulous evaluation, proper coordination, and effective interdisciplinary communication are needed. So also, there should be effectual interaction between each discipline and the patient for a successful outcome. The aims of management in opioid-tolerant patients are to promote optimal perioperative analgesia, prevent withdrawal syndromes, and deal with any related social, psychiatric, and behavioral issues [73]. Patients with an opioid dependency have three challenges to effective pain management: : [i] opioid-induced hyperalgesia (OIH), resulting in increased pain sensitivity; [ii] opioid tolerance, leading to reduced efficacy of opioids used to treat pain; and [iii] opioid withdrawal, producing sympathetic stimulation and heightened stress responses if the usual opioids are not given [73]. There is a high prevalence of psychiatric disorders in those with drug dependence, with more than 50% of patients showing evidence of conditions such as anxiety disorders and affective disorders, including depression. Such comorbidities may further complicate patients' behavior and their interaction with staff while in the hospital [74].

Early identification through a careful assessment and history in patients with opioid tolerance is essential for adequate pain-management planning. Postoperative pain management should start at the time of preoperative assessment, even prior to admission, and should include appropriate discharge planning [72]. If opioid tolerance has not been identified preoperatively, it should be suspected if the following triad is present after surgery: 1) elevated pain scores, 2) high opioid use, and 3) low incidence of side effects (apart from sedation). A multimodal pain regimen with a combination of pharmacologic and non-pharmacologic approaches is ideal. Opioids are the drugs of choice for severe pain and are also useful to manage moderate pain. However, multimodal approach with acetaminophen, non-steroidal anti-inflammatory drugs (NSAIDs), and adjuvants such as ketamine also provides effective pain relief. Patients with opioid tolerance may require more opioids than opioid-naïve patients. The dose of opioids should be tailored as per the individual need of the patient so as to achieve adequate analgesia without causing harmful side effects, such as over-sedation or respiratory depression. "Opioid rotation" is the substitution with a different opioid when one opioid does not provide desired level of analgesia even with increasing doses. This may be employed as required in patients with opioid tolerance, as cross-tolerance is uncommon. The recommended approach for opioid rotation is to initially substitute with one-half to two-thirds equianalgesic opioid and then monitor for safety and effectiveness. One needs to exercise caution while switching from a long-acting opioid to a short-acting one as this may precipitate withdrawal symptoms in the patient [73].

Opioid-related side effects are less common in opioid-tolerant patients; however, if opioid therapy is selected as analgesia of choice in these patients, monitoring for side effects or complications related to opioid therapy is also important. The risk of adverse drug events is more if opioid dosage is increased rapidly, even if the patient is opioid-tolerant. In fact, opioid-tolerant patients are more susceptible to the sedative properties of opioids [73].

For opioid-tolerant patients, patient-controlled analgesia (PCA) offers a convenient method of delivery, as it minimizes the risk of under treatment, allows self-titration, and negates possible conflicts with nursing staff. Additionally, a retrospective study found that opioid-tolerant patients who had PCA were less likely to report adverse effects—with the exception of sedation—compared with the opioid-naïve group [72]. In order to calculate the PCA bolus dose and background infusion rate, an individual preoperative "fentanyl challenge" is done to the point of respiratory depression followed by pharmacokinetic modeling to predict intra and postoperative opioid requirements [72]. An alternative and simple method is to calculate the PCA bolus dose on the basis of the dose of long-term opioid already being taken. The use of PCA background infusions is to be avoided in the opioid-naïve, because of the increased risk of respiratory depression. However, in opioid-tolerant patients, the PCA infusion is used to deliver the equivalent dose of long-term oral opioid if oral administration is not possible. Various studies have shown that gabapentin and pregabalin, paracetamol, non-steroidal anti-inflammatory drugs, cyclooxygenase-2 inhibitors, and alpha-2 agonists all lessened the opioid tolerance [73].

Opioid withdrawal can occur in opioid-dependent patients receiving a reduced amount of their usual opioid or if an opioid antagonist is given. The patients may exhibit at least three of these signs and symptoms: dysphonic mood, nausea, vomiting, diarrhea, muscle aches, rhinorrhoea, lacrimation, pupillary dilation, piloerection, sweating, yawning, fever, and insomnia. These may impair social, occupational, and other important areas of functioning [73]. The central principle of withdrawal management is to prevent its development, providing more stability for patients and reducing psychological and physiological stress. Clonidine has long been used to manage opioid withdrawal symptoms [74]. The most commonly used drugs for OST (opioid substitution therapy) are sublingual buprenorphine and oral methadone. These drugs reduce the level of drug abuse and related behavior and provide stability to the drug users and their families. The duration of withdrawal suppression is about 24 hours, so the dose can be continued once a day or may be given in two or three divided doses [73]. The drugs used for OST will not provide analgesia, and hence, withdrawal prevention and analgesia provision should be considered as separate entities. Methadone may predispose patients to the ventricular arrhythmia, the torsades de pointes as it can cause prolongation of the corrected electrocardiographic QT interval. So appropriate monitoring is needed. When buprenorphine, which is a partial agonist with a high-binding affinity at the mu-opioid receptor, is used as OST at higher doses of 16–32 mg, there is minimum free receptor availability. In such cases, the additional pure opioid agonists including drugs such as heroin would provide no analgesic effect. Hence, buprenorphine should be stopped during perioperative period to allow receptor accessibility for opioids used for analgesia [73].

Patients with pain taking long-term opioids, those abusing heroin, and those on methadone and buprenorphine substitution therapy may develop hyperalgesia. Multimodal analgesia should be optimized by adding opioid-sparing analgesics such as paracetamol (acetaminophen), non-steroidal anti-inflammatory drugs, or cyclooxygenase-2 inhibitors, using local anesthetic regional techniques, whereas ketamine attenuates OIH in patients on long-term opioids. Studies have demonstrated that gabapentin and pregabalin reduce OIH in animal models, human volunteers, and patients [74]. Similarly, there is evidence that alpha-2 agonists—clonidine and dexmedetomidine—may also decrease OIH, whereas experimental results indicate that COX- 2 inhibitor can also impart this benefit [74].

Pediatric patients: Pediatric patients continue to be undertreated for acute pain. There is a common myth that pediatric patients do not feel pain or they do not remember the pain. Control of pain in pediatric patients is important because poor pain control may result in increased morbidity and mortality. Different treatment modalities have evolved, and multimodal analgesia has become the treatment of choice not only involving a pharmacological approach but also non-pharmacological approaches (e.g., regional analgesia, rehabilitation, cognitive behavioral therapy, virtual reality).

Special scales are available for children to self-report their pain. One important scale is Children and Infants Postoperative Pain Scale (CHIPPS) where scores of 0–2 are assigned as indicators of level of pain for crying, facial expression, posture of the trunk, posture of the legs, motor restlessness, etc. [12]. The other scales are Faces Pain Scale-Revised, pain word scale, Revised-Face Legs Activity Cry Consolability (r-FLACC), Premature Infant Pain Profile, Neonate Facial Coding system, Neonate Infant pain scale, Maximally Discriminative Facial Movement Coding System.

Oral and rectal route is preferred in children for administering analgesics [12]. Intramuscular injections are to be generally avoided for pain and fear associated with injection and unpredictable absorption of drug [12]. Regional nerve block, neuraxial blocks, peripheral nerve blocks, local infiltration analgesia with general anesthesia may improve postoperative pain management in pediatric patients. Intravenous patient controlled analgesia can be effectively used with prior education of patient about its use in children aged over 5–6 years [1].

Acetaminophen has antipyretic and anti-inflammatory properties. Its mechanism of action is through COX3 enzyme (inhibition of prostaglandin synthesis) inhibition, cannabinoid agonist, NMDA agonist, and activation of descending serotonergic pathways in CNS and via inhibition of prostaglandin synthesis [75]. NSAIDs are used commonly in pediatric population. Their use in pediatric population has demonstrated adequate pain control, opioid-sparing effect, and decrease in postoperative nausea vomiting [75, 76]. Use of ketorolac for pain control after tonsillectomy is associated with more risk of postoperative bleeding. However, that risk is counterbalanced with decreased PONV, sedation, and respiratory depression [75]. Gabapentinoids are not recommended in children for acute postoperative pain as per the current evidence [75]. Ketamine used in perioperative period in pediatric patients could have the potential of decreasing hyperalgesia, central sensitization, and reverse opioid tolerance [75]. The clinical scenarios where ketamine could be used are patients at high risk of developing postsurgical neuropathic pain, opioid-tolerant patients, patients who are more susceptible to develop opioid-related side effects, patients with chronic pain conditions, etc. Intravenous lidocaine should be avoided in patients weighing <40 kg [75]. Dexmedetomidine is useful adjunct to decrease postoperative pain with an opioid-sparing effect and decrease in emergence delirium [75].

Obese patients: These patients present various anatomic and pathophysiologic challenges in pain management. A major challenge is their altered pharmacokinetic profile, which accompanies physiologic changes in this population, which make obese patients more susceptible to respiratory depression and sleep apnea if opioids are used. The goal of pain management in such patients is provision of comfort, early mobilization, and improved respiratory function without causing respiratory compromise [26]. Recommendations are multimodal analgesic management, preference for regional techniques, avoidance of sedatives, noninvasive ventilation with supplemental oxygen, early mobilization, and elevation of the head.

17. Discussion

Optimal treatment of postoperative pain requires multidisciplinary approach and a dedicated team for providing a round-the-clock service [12]. Each surgical procedure produces varying degrees of pain. A comprehensive and effective pain management plan includes the appropriate care of individual patients' needs during the various stages of perioperative period. The patients and the caregivers should be educated about the importance of postoperative pain management. The acute pain teams should assess patients preoperatively and plan a pain management protocol. There should be regular assessment, treatment, and documentation of pain. The staff should be given training and continued education about physiology of pain, pathophysiology, pharmacology, monitoring routines, etc. All this is possible if an acute pain service is set up, which is a dedicated organization for acute pain management. Before establishing the acute pain service, an audit should be conducted for studying the effectiveness of the current pain management protocols, and later comparisons must be done after the establishment of pain service. Daily pain ward rounds should be started, which provides an ideal opportunity to teach service providers, address misconceptions, discuss pain-related issues with patients, and adopt prescription charts to improve pain control as needed. Various studies have shown improved pain scores after establishment of APS. The studies have shown that not only the newer techniques that improved postoperative pain but also the systematic and planned application of already existing ones [77].

18. Conclusion

Untreated postoperative pain can have untoward consequences not only on individual patient health but also adversely affects the health care system. Optimal pain management improves the quality of life, facilitates recovery, and decreases morbidity. A multimodal, evidence-based, and procedure-specific, individualized analgesic regimen with minimum side effects should be the standard of care. Such a regime is an integral part of ERAS, which facilitates the important ERAS milestones such as early mobilization and oral feeding. Assessment, documentation of pain and response to its treatment are vital for effective postoperative pain management. Patient-controlled intravenous and epidural analgesias have the advantages of superior pain relief and improved patient satisfaction. The regional techniques have become an integral part of pain management programs. The use of ultrasound-guided techniques has made the regional techniques hassle-free with potent analgesia and lesser possibility of complications. Besides the pharmacological methods, which are routinely used, non-pharmacological methods should also be integrated into the postoperative pain management plan. These techniques are relatively inexpensive and safe and help decrease fear, distress, and anxiety and can be instituted by the nursing staff as well as the patients' caretakers. The patients with special needs such as the opioid-tolerant patients, patients in extremes of age, and obese patients, etc., need a well-planned approach under the care of experienced and expert healthcare staff. The institutionalized and dedicated team approach for acute pain management in the form of Acute Pain Service will go a long way in incorporating all the above said principles, thus improving postoperative pain management and patient satisfaction.

Author details

Samina Khatib[1]*, Syed S.N. Razvi[2], Mudassir M. Shaikh[3]
and Mohammad Moizuddin Khan[4]

1 Department of Anesthesiology, Government Cancer Hospital, Aurangabad, Maharashtra, India

2 Department of Physiology, Parbhani Medical College, Parbhani, Maharashtra, India

3 Department of Anesthesiology, JIIU's Indian Institute of Medical Science and of Research, Maharashtra, India

4 Department of Physiology, College of Medicine, Dar-ul-Uloom University, Riyadh, Saudi Arabia

*Address all correspondence to: ssr.anesth@gmail.com

IntechOpen

© 2023 The Author(s). Licensee IntechOpen. This chapter is distributed under the terms of the Creative Commons Attribution License (http://creativecommons.org/licenses/by/3.0), which permits unrestricted use, distribution, and reproduction in any medium, provided the original work is properly cited.

References

[1] Vrooman BM, Richard WR. Morgan & Mikhail's Clinical Anaesthesiology. 6th ed. United States: McGraw-Hill Education; 2018

[2] Small C, Laycock H. Acute post-operative pain management. British Journal of Surgery. 2020;**107**(2):e70-e80

[3] Dolin SJ, Cashman JN, Bland JM. Effectiveness of acute-post-operative pain management. Evidence from published data. British Journal of Anesthesia. 2002;**89**(3):409-423

[4] Vijayan R. Managing acute pain in the developing world. PAIN: Clinical Updates. 2011;**19**:1-7

[5] Singh PK, Saikia P, Lahakar M. Prevalence of acute post-operative pain adults in patients in adult age-group undergoing inpatient abdominal surgery and correlation of intensity of pain and satisfaction with analgesic management: A cross-sectional single institute-based study. Indian Journal of Anaesthesia. 2016;**60**:737-743

[6] Warfield CA, Kahn CH. Acute pain management. Programs in U. S hospitals and experiences and attitudes among U. S. adults. Anesthesiology. 1995;**83**:1090-1094

[7] Mwashambwa MY, Isaya M, et al. Post-operative pain prevalence, predictors, management practices and satisfaction among operated cases at Regional Rferral Hospital in Dar es Salaam. Tanzania Tanzania Jourrnal of Health Rsearch. 2018;**v20i2**:10

[8] Apfelbaum JL, Chen C, Mehta SS, Gan TJ. Postoperative pain experience: Results from a national survey suggest postoperative pain continues to be undermanaged. Anesthesia and Analgesia. 2003;**97**:534-540

[9] Gramke HF, de Rijke JM, van Kleef M, Raps F, Kessels AG, Peters ML, et al. The prevalence of postoperative pain in a cross-sectional group of patients after day -case surgery in a university hospital. The Clinical Journal of Pain. 2007;**23**:543-548

[10] Sommer M, de Rijke JM, van Kleef M, Kessels AG, Peters ML, Geurts JW, et al. The prevalence of postoperative pain in a sample of 1490 surgical inpatients. European Journal of Anaesthesiology. 2008;**25**:267-274

[11] Couceiro TC, Valenca MM, Lima LC, de Menezes TC, Rapaso MC. Prevalence and influence of gender, age, and type of survey on postoperative pain. Revista Brasileira de Anestesiologia. 2009;**59**(3): 314-320

[12] Patel NB. Physiology of pain. In: Kopf A, Patel NB, editors. Guide to Pain Management in Low Resource Settings. e-book by International Association for the Study of Pain. 2010. pp. 13-18. Available from: www.iasp- pain.org/.../Guide_to_Pain_Management_in_Low-Resource_Settings.pdf

[13] Sharma RS, Das G. What is the minimum knowledge of pain medicine needed for other speciality. Journal on Recent Advances in Pain. 2018;**4**(1):32-35

[14] Brennan TJ. Acute pain: Pathophysiology and clinical implications. ASA Refresher Courses in Anesthesiology. 2010;**38**:8-15

[15] Ghori MK, Zhang Y, Sinatra RS. Pathophysiology of acute pain. In: Sinatra RS, de Leon Cassasola OA, editors. Acute Pain Management. 1st edn. New York: Cambridge University Press; 2009. pp. 21-32

[16] Rao M. Acute postoperative pain. Indian Journal of Anaesthesia. 2006;**50** (5):340-344

[17] Wu CL, Fleisher LA. Outcomes research in regional anesthesia and analgesia. Anesthesia and Analgesia. 2000;**91**(5):1232-1242

[18] Kissin I. Pre-emptive analgesia. Anaesthesiology. 2000;**93**(4):1138-1143

[19] Greenshields N, Mythen M. Enhanced recovery after surgery. Current Anesthesiology Reports. 2020; **10**:49-55. DOI: 10.1007/s40140-020-00372-y

[20] ERAS for Gastrointestinal Surgery Part 2: Consensus Statement for Anaesthesia Practice. Guidelines ERAS Society. Available from: http://erassociety.org [Accessed: July 22, 2022]

[21] Elzohry AAM, Foli AME. Basics of Acute Postoperative Pain. American International Journal of Multidisciplinary Scientific Research. 2018;**1**(2):19-23

[22] Twining J, Padula C. Pilot testing the clinically aligned pain assessment (CAPA) measure. Pain Management Nursing. 2019;**20**(5):462-467

[23] Breivik H, Borchgrevink PC, Allen SM. Assessment of pain. British Journal of Anaesthesia. 2008;**101**(1): 17-24

[24] Alderson S. Unrecognised, undertreated, pain in ICU—Causes, effects, and how to do better. Open Journal of Nursing. 2013;**03**:108-113. DOI: 10.4236/ojn.2013.31014

[25] Puntillo F, Giglio M, Varrassi G. The Routes of Administration for Acute Postoperative Pain Medication Pain Therapy. 2021;**10**(2):909-925

[26] De Andros J, Narachi P, Fischer HJB. General recmmendations for post-operative pain management. In: E-booklet Produced in Consulation with European Society of Regional Anaesthesia and Pain Therapy. Available from: www.anaesthesia-az.com. [Accessed: June 22, 2022]

[27] Horn R. Post-Operative Pain Control. Available from: https://www.statpearlSCom/Article Library/view article/27536

[28] Theinthong S, Niruthisard S, Ittichaikulthon W, et al. Clinical guidance for acute post-operative pain management 2019. The Royal College of Anasthesiologists of Thailand(RCAT) and the Thai Association for the study of Pain (TASP): Second edition. Thai Journal of Anesthesiology. 2020;**46**(1):47-70

[29] Perioperative Pain Management. Available from: https://www.mdanderson.org/documents/for-physicians/algorithms/clinical management/post-op-pain-web -algorithm.pdf

[30] Kim KH, Abdi S. Rediscovery of nefopam for the treatment of neuropathic pain. The Korean Journal of Pain. 2014;**27**(2):103-111

[31] Han C, Li X, Jiang H, et al. The use of gabapentin in the management of postoperative pain after total hip arthroplasty: A meta-analysis of randomised controlled trials. Journal of Orthopaedic Surgery and Research. 2016;**11**(1):79

[32] Pastino A, Lakra A. Patient controlled analgesia. In: StatPearls. Treasure Island (FL): StatPearls Publishing; 2022. Available from: https://www.ncbi.nlm.nih.gov/books/NBK551610/

[33] Carr A, Ferguson M. What is the evidence to support clonidine as an

adjuvant analgesic? Practical Pain Management. 2019;**19**(5)

[34] Joshi G, Gandhi K, Shah N, Gadsden J, Corman SL. Peripheral nerve blocks in the management of postoperative pain: Challenges and opportunities. Journal of Clinical Anesthesia. 2016;**35**:524-529

[35] Chang A, Dua A, Singh K, et al. Peripheral nerve blocks. In: StatPearls. Treasure Island (FL): StatPearls Publishing; 2022. Available from: https://www.ncbi.nlm.nih.gov/books/NBK459210/

[36] Zisquit J, Nedeff N. Interscalene block. In: StatPearls. Treasure Island (FL): StatPearls Publishing; 2022. Available from: https://www.ncbi.nlm.nih.gov/books/NBK519491/

[37] D'Souza RS, Johnson RL. Supraclavicular block. In: StatPearls. Treasure Island (FL): StatPearls Publishing; 2022. Available from: https://www.ncbi.nlm.nih.gov/books/NBK519056/

[38] Williams LM, Singh K, Dua A, et al. Infraclavicular nerve block. In: StatPearls. Treasure Island (FL): StatPearls Publishing; 2022. Available from: https://www.ncbi.nlm.nih.gov/books/NBK537016/

[39] Satapathy AR, Coventry DM. Axillary brachial plexus block. Anesthesiology Research and Practice. 2011;**2011**:5. DOI: 10.1155/2011/173796

[40] Neal J Gurkan Y. Cutaneous Blocks for the Upper Extremity –Landmarks and Nerve Stimulator Technique. Available from: https://www.nysora.com/techniques/upper-extremity/distal-nerves/cutaneous-blocks-upper-extremity/ [Accessed: July 30, 2022]

[41] Durrani MI, Dasgupta S. Radial nerve block. In: StatPearls. Treasure Island (FL): StatPearls Publishing; 2022. Available from: https://www.ncbi.nlm.nih.gov/books/NBK532951/

[42] Pester JM, Bechmann S, Varacallo M. Median nerve block techniques. In: StatPearls. Treasure Island (FL): StatPearls Publishing; 2022. Available from: https://www.ncbi.nlm.nih.gov/books/NBK

[43] Pester JM, Varacallo M. Ulnar nerve block techniques. In: StatPearls. Treasure Island (FL): StatPearls Publishing; 2022. Available from: https://www.ncbi.nlm.nih.gov/books/NBK459208/

[44] Polania Gutierrez JJ, Ben-David B. Lumbar plexus block. In: StatPearls. Treasure Island (FL): StatPearls Publishing; 2022. Available from: https://www.ncbi.nlm.nih.gov/books/NBK556116/

[45] Sykes Z, Pak A. Femoral nerve block. In: StatPearls. Treasure Island (FL): StatPearls Publishing; 2022. Available from: https://www.ncbi.nlm.nih.gov/books/NBK546704

[46] O'Reilly N, Desmet M, Kearns R. Fascia iliaca compartement block. British Journal of Anaesthesia and Education. 2019;**19**(6):191-197

[47] Yoshida T, Nakamoto T, Kamibayashi T. Ultrasound-guided obturator nerve block: A focused review on anatomy and updated techniques. BioMed Research International. 2017, 2017:9. DOI: 10.1155/2017/7023750

[48] Rodziewicz TL, Stevens JB, Ajib FA, et al. Sciatic nerve block. In: StatPearls. Treasure Island (FL): StatPearls Publishing; 2022. Available from: https://www.ncbi.nlm.nih.gov/books/NBK470391/

[49] Arnold C, Alvarado AC, Brady MF. Saphenous nerve block. In: StatPearls. Treasure Island (FL): StatPearls Publishing; 2022. Available from: https://www.ncbi.nlm.nih.gov/books/NBK536967/

[50] Berlioz BE, Bojaxhi E. PENG regional block. In: StatPearls. Treasure Island (FL): StatPearls Publishing; 2022. Available from: https://www.ncbi.nlm.nih.gov/books/NBK565870/. [Accessed: May 9, 2022]

[51] Feng W, Wenming M, Zhihui H. Analgesia effects of IPACK block added to multimodal analgesia regiments after total knee replacement: A systematic review of the literature and meta-analysis of 5 randomized controlled trials. Medicine. 2021;**100**(22):e25884

[52] Chakraborty A, Khemka R, Datta T. Ultrasound-guided truncal blocks: A new frontier in regional anaesthesia. Indian Journal of Anaesthesia. 2016;**60**(10):703-711. DOI: 10.4103/0019-5049.191665

[53] Karmakar MK. Thoracic paravertebral block. Anesthesiology. 2001;**95**(3):771-780

[54] Baxter CS, Singh A, Ajib FA, et al. Intercostal nerve block. In: StatPearls. Treasure Island (FL): StatPearls Publishing; 2022. Available from: https://www.ncbi.nlm.nih.gov/books/NBK482273/. [Accessed: July 26, 2022]

[55] Southgate SJ, Herbst MK. Ultrasound guided serratus anterior blocks. In: StatPearls. Treasure Island (FL): StatPearls Publishing; 2022. Available from: https://www.ncbi.nlm.nih.gov/books/NBK538476/. [Accessed: July 25, 2022]

[56] Battista C, Krishana S. Pectoralis nerve block. In: StatPearls. Treasure Island (FL): StatPearls Publishing; 2022

[57] Tran DQ, Bravo D, Leurcharusmee P, et al. Transversus Abdominis Plane Block. A narrative review. Anesthesiology. 2019;**131**(5):1166-1190

[58] Young MJ, Gorlin AW, Modest VE, et al. Clinical implications of the transvesus abdominis plane block in adults. Anesthesiology Research and Practice. 2012;**2012**:731645

[59] Kartalov A, Nn J, Kuzamanovsk B, et al. The effect of Rectus Sheath block as a supplement of general analgesia in adult patients undergoing umbilical hernia repair. Prilozi. 2017;**38**(3):135-142

[60] Tudor EC, Yang W, Brown R, Mackey PM. Rectus sheath catheters provide equivalent analgesia to epidurals following laparotomy for colorectal surgery. Annals of the Royal College of Surgeons of England. 2015 Oct;**97**(7):530-533

[61] Dhanjal S, Tonder S. Quadtratus lumboram block. In: Statpearls. Treasure Island (FL): Statpearls Pblishing; 2022. Available from https://www.ncbi.nlm.nih.gov/books/NBK 537212/ [Accessed: August 22, 2022]

[62] Krishnan S, Cascella M. Erector spinae plane block. In: StatPearls. Treasure Island (FL): StatPearls Publishing; 2022. Available from: https://www.ncbi.nlm.nih.gov/books/NBK545305/. [Accessed: April 30, 2022]

[63] Khedkar SM, Bhalerao PM, Yemul-Golhar SR, Kelkar KV. Ultrasound-guided ilioinguinal and iliohypogastric nerve block, a comparison with the conventional technique: An observational study. Saudi Journal of Anaesthesia. 2015;**9**(3):293-297

[64] Desai N, Albrecht E, El-Boghdadly K. Perineural adjuncts for peripheral

nerve block. BJA Education. 2019;**19**(9): 276-282

[65] Tschopp C, Tramèr MR, Schneider A, Zaarour M, Elia N. Benefit and harm of adding epinephrine to a local anesthetic for neuraxial and locoregional anesthesia: A meta-analysis of randomized controlled trials with trial sequential analyses. Anesthesia and Analgesia. 2018;**127**(1):228-239

[66] Schnabel A, Reichl SU, Zahn PK, et al. Efficacy and safety of buprenorphine in peripheral nerve blocks. A meta-analysis of RCTs. European Journal of Anaesthesiology. 2017;**34**(9):376-586

[67] Brummett CM, Brian W. Additives to local anaesthetics for peripheral nerve blocks. International Anesthesiology Clinics. 2011;**49**(4):104-116

[68] Geziry AE, Toble Y, Kadhi FA, Nobani MPMA. Non-pharmacological pain management. In: Shallik NA, editor. Pain Management in Special Circumstances. London: IntechOpen; 2018. DOI: 10.5772/intechopen.79689. Available from: https://www.intechopen.com/chapters/62969 [Accessed: August 03, 2022]

[69] Nasiri M, Le-Wendling L, Ihnatseka B Y. Emerging Techniques in Acute Pain Medicine. ASRA Pain Medicine Practice Management. Available from: https://www.asra.com/nes/-pubication/asranewsletter/feb2020 [Accessed: August 3, 2022]

[70] Bushnell MC, Frangos E, Madian N. Non –pharmacological treatment of pain. Grand challenge and future oppurtunities. Frontiers in Pain Research. 2021. DOI: 10.3389/fpain.2021.696783

[71] Demir Y. Non-pharmacological therapies in pain management. In: Racz GB, Noe CE, editors. Pain Management - Current Issues and Opinions. London: IntechOpen; 2012. DOI: 10.5772/30050. Available from: https://www.intechopen.com/chapters/26152 [Accessed: August 3, 2022]

[72] Morgan MM, Christie MJ. Analysis of opioid efficacy, tolerance, addiction and dependence from cell culture to human. British Journal of Pharmacology. 2011;**164**(4):1322-1334

[73] Adesoye A, Duncan N. Acute pain management in patients with opioid tolerance. US Pharm. 2017;**42**(3):28-322

[74] Quinlan J, Cox F. Acute pain management in patients with drug dependence syndrome. PAIN Reports. 2017;**2**(4):e611. DOI: 10.1097/PR9.0000000000000611

[75] Eduardo V, Rivera G, Gonzalez V. Current trends and new strategies in acute post-operative pain management in children. Medical Research Archives. 2021;**9**(9). DOI: 10.18103/mra.v9i9.2539

[76] Huxtable CA, Roberts LJ, Somogyl AA, et al. Acute pain management in opioid-tolerant patients: A growing challenge. Anaesthesia and Intensive Care. 2011;**39**(5):804-823

[77] Gould TH, Crosby DL, Harmer M, Lloyd SM, Lunn JN, Rees GA, et al. Policy for controlling pain after surgery: Effect of sequential changes in management. BMJ. 1992;**305**(6863): 1187-1193

Section 7

Neuroanesthesia

Chapter 11

Updates in Neuroanesthesia

Christian N. Schill, Rebecca E. Bates, Troy D. Lovett and Isha Kaza

Abstract

Providing anesthesia care to neurosurgical and neurocritical care patients presents unique challenges to the anesthesiologist. Over the last century, anesthetic care for such patients has become a robustly studied field, with tools and techniques to keep patients safe and comfortable in the perioperative period. A review of the major updates and considerations for perioperative care for awake craniotomies, thrombectomy for stroke, and endoscopic neurosurgery is critical for the anesthesiologist. Additionally, newly developed enhanced recovery after surgery procedures have improved patient experiences and outcomes after both cranial and spinal neurosurgery. Finally, post-operative delirium is a major neurologic complication in elderly patients undergoing all types of procedures which all anesthesiologists should be well versed in. Here, such topics are reviewed with a focus on recent updates to the literature which are important for clinical practice.

Keywords: neuroanesthesia, intraoperative brain mapping, thrombectomy, enhanced recovery after surgery, neurotoxicity, perioperative delirium

1. Introduction

From Henry Cushing in the early 20th century to Jane Matjasko in the 1980s, over the last century anesthesia for neurosurgical patients has advanced enormously through the work of many brilliant physicians. What was once a field that posed enormous difficulty for anesthesiologists and surgeons alike, has become robustly studied and an established subspecialty of anesthesiology. Anesthesiologists now have a range of tools at their disposal to ensure patient safety during cranial or spinal procedures, can develop plans to keep patients awake during intracranial surgery for brain mapping and language center preservation, and can provide enormous benefits in the intensive care unit for the neurosurgical patient. Here, a discussion of some of the more recent advances in neuroanesthesiology is reviewed.

2. Methods

Research presented in this chapter was collected via a relevant literature search and review. Online databases and search engines including Pubmed.gov and GoogleScholar were utilized to search out peer-reviewed articles relating to each of the major topics discussed. Keywords included but were not limited to: "awake craniotomy", "intraoperative brain mapping", "Anesthesia for Thrombectomy", "ERAS for craniotomy", "ERAS for spinal surgery", and "postoperative delirium". Published articles including original research, case reports, and reviews were all included. Articles with key and up-to-date information were selected and compiled and major take-aways across the articles were synthesized and included in this chapter. The majority of topics were chosen based on the topics of major reviews or landmark studies published between 2019 and 2022.

3. Updates to neuroanesthesia: cranial procedures

3.1 Anesthesia considerations during asleep craniotomy

A craniotomy is an extraordinarily common neurosurgical procedure in which portions of the skull are removed in order to gain access to the intracranial vault [1]. Traditionally, this procedure is performed with the patient asleep under general anesthesia for the duration of the operation. This can be a component of a larger procedure such as tumor resection or can be the primary procedure being performed such as in patients with brain swelling and refractory increased intracranial pressure (ICP). Other indications can include clipping of large ruptured or unruptured aneurysms when endovascular therapy is not indicated, hematoma evacuation, tissue biopsy, and debridement of an abscess [1]. In cases where the bone flap removed is not immediately placed back after the procedure, often in cases of brain swelling after TBI or massive stroke, the procedure is called a craniectomy. Cranioplasty to replace the bone flap can be done once the swelling has subsided.

3.1.1 Preoperative assessment

In the case of craniotomy, in addition to traditional pre-anesthesia work ups, establishing the neurological status of a patient and individualizing their premedication regimen are key pre-operative steps to ascertain. Determining a baseline neurological status for all neurosurgical patients is critical as this helps delineate whether deficits present upon the patient awakening from surgery were present prior to surgery or appeared after [1]. Establishing their Glasgow Coma Scale score, whether they have signs of elevated intracranial pressure, or if they have any focal neurological deficits are all key to establishing prior to surgery so that changes can be detected post-operatively [1]. In terms of premedication, whether the patient takes anticonvulsants and has a history of seizures is important to determine. For most procedures, pre-medication with daily anti-epileptic drugs (AEDs) is appropriate [2]. If the patient is undergoing resection of epileptic foci, the use of benzodiazepines should be avoided. However, more unclear, and individualized is whether the patient should take their regular anticonvulsants on the morning of epilepsy surgery [2]. Different institutions will have variable procedures regarding AEDs, but consultation with the patient's neurologist, neurosurgeon, and institutional procedures should be done to determine whether the patient takes AEDs prior to epilepsy surgery [2]. If the patient takes regular steroids, stress dose steroids should be administered as well prior to surgery.

3.1.2 Intraoperative considerations

Patients are positioned on the operating table in a variety of ways depending on which region of the skull is being removed. Patients may be prone, supine, lateral, semi-lateral, or even in a sitting position [1]. In most cases, the head is immobilized utilizing head pins attached to a Mayfield apparatus which pierce the skin, galea aponeurosis, and the skull itself and hold the head in a fixed position throughout the procedure [1]. Often a dose of propofol, opioids, or local lidocaine is administered just prior to pinning as this can induce hemodynamic responses including hypertension and tachycardia just as incisions or other painful stimuli do. Additionally, it is important that pressure points throughout the body and regions associated with peripheral nerve compression are padded as many neurosurgical procedures take long periods of time and patients can develop compressive neuropathies and skin pressure injuries [1]. Ocular injury from cleaning solutions and other surgical fluids can be avoided by placing an adhesive over the eyes just after anesthesia is induced.

Monitoring craniotomy patients intraoperatively is a very individualized job and should be planned on a patient-by-patient basis. In most cases, an arterial line is needed. Accurate monitoring of blood pressure is paramount in neurosurgical patients, as blood pressure can be reflective of intracranial pressures and high blood pressure increase the risk of intracranial bleeding after surgery [1]. In patients undergoing craniotomy after traumatic brain injury (TBI) often intracranial pressure (ICP) monitoring may be critical. In those patients, they may have an external ventricular drain (EVD) in place or will have one placed during the procedure which will allow for continuous ICP monitoring [3].

Anesthetics generally do not have a major effect on ICP or will actually promote brain relaxation, with the exception possibly of ketamine [4]. This means most typical choices for induction, such as propofol and opioids work well to induce general anesthesia in most craniotomy patients. Some studies have reported that ketamine induces an increased ICP, while others have shown no changes or even decreases in ICP after its use [5]. While ketamine's use remains controversial in the literature, avoiding its use in most craniotomy patients is advisable. Total IV anesthesia (TIVA) is primarily maintained in craniotomy with propofol (50–100 μg/kg/minute), a short-acting opioids such as remifentanil (0.1–0.2 μg/kg/minute), and dexmedetomidine 90.1–0.3 mcg/kg per hour) [6]. Note that doses of propofol and opioids should be titrated based on the patient's age and other medical conditions that may affect their ability to metabolize the anesthetics.

Somatosensory Evoked Potentials (SSEP) and Motor Evoked Potentials (MEP) are monitoring steps often taken during craniotomies to establish the location of the primary motor and somatosensory cortices [1]. Often these are used when resection will include resection of the brain tissue and function to avoid or minimize damage to brain tissue involved in motor and sensory functions. With SSEP, peripheral nerves, most often the ulnar, median, and tibial nerves, are stimulated and the regions of the brain that become electrically active on EEG as a result help the surgeon determine the boundaries of the primary somatosensory cortices [1, 7]. MEP on the other hand includes electrical or magnetic stimulation of the brain surface and records muscular responses throughout the body so as to delineate the boundaries of the primary motor cortex [1, 8]. If MEP is required, neuromuscular blockers can be used during intubation, but are not used in the maintenance of anesthesia afterward, as MEP monitoring requires muscles to contract in response to cerebral stimulation [1, 8].

3.1.3 Postoperative care

In the postoperative period, a neurologic exam should be performed once the patient is awake enough to follow commands and once the neuromuscular block has been completely reversed [1]. If the patient underwent an infratentorial craniotomy, there is a higher risk of damage to the cranial nerves which innervate the reflexes of the airway, such as the vagus nerve [9]. In such patients, extubation may be delayed until the patient is awake enough for the cough reflex to be tested [9]. The patient will need to undergo serial neurologic exams by the nursing team and the neurointensivist during recovery. While somewhat controversial, most craniotomy patients, even those without complications, should be admitted to the ICU [10]. As such, opioids for pain control should be titrated to maximize pain control but not to depress the patient's ability to cooperate with a neurologic exam. Additionally, blood pressure should be maintained below 160 mmHg systolic as pressures greater than that are associated with a higher risk of postoperative intracranial bleeds [11]. Both beta-blockers such as labetalol and calcium channel blockers like nicardipine can be used if medication is needed to reduce the patient's pressures.

3.1.4 Complications

Craniotomy complications are numerous including seizures, subdural hygroma, and increased intracranial pressure [1]. If a seizure occurs during a craniotomy and the dura is open, the first line treatment is the application of sterile iced saline to the brain surface by the surgeon [12]. If the seizure continues, a dose of midazolam (1 mg or 2 mg IV) or propofol (10 mg or 20 mg IV) can be administered to abort the seizure [1]. Prevention of brain herniation in those who have suffered TBI with rising ICP is critical. If an EVD is in place, the first line treatment for high ICP is CSF drainage from the EVD [13]. Other methods of lowering ICP could include hyperventilating the patient, sedation to reduce cerebral metabolism, elevation of the head of the bed, and in critical situations, IV mannitol or hypertonic saline [13]. Subdural hygroma refers to a collection of cerebral spinal fluid in the subdural space secondary to tears in the arachnoid membrane [13]. Such collections can increase in size and cause mass effects on the brain, causing focal neurologic findings and CSF density fluid on CT or MRI [14]. If symptomatic, treatment could include burr hole drainage, placement of a subdural drain, and in recurrent or severe cases repeat craniotomy and the placement of a subdural-peritoneal shunt [14]. If developing after craniectomy, cranioplasty is the definitive treatment for hygroma [14].

3.2 Anesthesia considerations during awake craniotomy for intraoperative brain mapping

Over the last 40 years, intraoperative cortical and subcortical brain mapping has led to major improvements in both recurrence-free survival and postoperative outcomes in patients undergoing resective brain surgery [15]. The primary goal of mapping is to identify and preserve tissue associated with speech and motor function while also ensuring adequate margins during mass resection [15]. This often includes waking a patient after a successful craniotomy in order to ask the patient a series of questions to test speech and cognitive function while brain regions are stimulated. Such methods have been enhanced and supported by advances in anesthesiology [15]. This poses unique challenges to the anesthesiologist and preparation is paramount. Here, the major considerations for the anesthesiologist caring for a patient undergoing intraoperative brain mapping with awake craniotomy are reviewed through the entire perioperative period.

3.2.1 Preoperative assessment

A key first step in the preparation for surgery is the pre-operative assessment of each surgical candidate. An awake craniotomy can create enormous anxiety and some patients may be unable to undergo this type of procedure. Additionally, if the patient cannot cooperate with the surgeon's commands due to altered mental status, baseline aphasia, or confusion, an awake craniotomy is contraindicated [15]. Patients who may be more difficult and necessitate consideration of other alternative methods include those patients with uncontrolled seizures, a history of anesthesia emergence delirium, obstructive sleep apnea, patients which may present a challenging airway, and those with GERD [15]. Prior to surgery, the anesthesiologist should discuss with the patient what an awake craniotomy entails. Discussion of possible complications and adverse events should be discussed, as well as the testing that they will undergo while the surgeon operates.

Consideration regarding the type of procedure and why it is performed should also inform the anesthesiologist's premedication of the patient. Patients who are undergoing surgical resection of epileptogenic brain foci should not be premedicated with benzodiazepines as this will hinder the identification of target regions by suppressing epileptiform activity [2]. If the patient takes daily steroids or anti-hypertensives those should also be given on the day of surgery.

3.2.2 Intraoperative anesthesia

Anesthetic strategies for patients undergoing intraoperative mapping can range from the use of an "awake-asleep-awake" strategy to conscious sedation [15]. In the former, patients are placed under general anesthesia for the initial craniotomy, awakened for mapping, and then are placed back under general anesthesia for the resection of the tumor and cranioplasty. In conscious sedation, the patient is sedated but arousable throughout the surgery but the depth of sedation can vary throughout [15]. General anesthesia methods require the establishment of an airway, but in awake craniotomy using an endotracheal tube is difficult, as the patient must be extubated when they are awakened for monitoring [15]. Some anesthesiologists still prefer to use endotracheal intubation, but supraglottic airways and laryngeal mask airways are other viable options during deep sedation [15]. One major benefit of this strategy is that general anesthesia allows for more control of the blood carbon dioxide levels and encourages brain relaxation, which is beneficial during the resection of highly vascular tumors or large deep-seated tumors such as those found in the insula [15].

The major concern of the general anesthesia pathway is the need for airway management which may include inducing coughing, distress, and aspiration while emerging from anesthesia mid-operation. Conscious sedation alleviates this concern as the goal is to avoid the use of airway management by avoiding oversedation [15]. However, oversedation and airway obstruction remain a concern if a fine balance is not found between sedation and airway patency. While these two plans have variable strengths and weaknesses, meta-analyses comparing these two have failed to find major differences in postoperative outcomes, so planning and shared decision-making between the surgeon, the patient, and the nursing team are important, as both methods are appropriate for most patients [15].

In terms of the medications used to induce anesthesia, historically propofol and midazolam have been used in patients who are undergoing awake craniotomy [16]. Propofol is rapid in its onset and offset and can be used to titrate sedation and rapid awakening, Midazolam also has long been used as an anxiolytic during awake sedation

Anesthetic	Dosage regimen	Indications and considerations
Propofol	CS drip: 20–50 μg/kg/minute	For CS regimens, dosages can be titrated so the patient is arousable but drowsy
	GA drip: 50–100 μg/kg/minute	Respiratory depression should be monitored
Remifentanil	CS drip: 0.01–0.06 μg/kg/minute	Respiratory depression should be monitored
	GA drip: 0.1–0.2 μg/kg/minute	While transitioning to awake phase, continued low-dose remifentanil can maintain analgesia
Dexmedetomidine	CS drip: 0.3–0.5 μg/kg/minute	Less respiratory depression than propofol
Midazolam	Pre-op: 1–2 mg IV bolus	Pre-op can be used as an anxiolytic, unless performing epilepsy surgery
Sevoflurane	GA: <0.5 MAC	Rapid onset and rapid clearance allow for rapidly inducing GA and rapidly awakening the patient

CS, conscious sedation, GA, general anesthesia, MAC, minimum alveolar concentration.

Table 1.
Anesthetics typically utilized for awake craniotomy [16].

but cannot be used in patients undergoing epilepsy surgery [16]. Dexmedetomidine is a newer agent recently approved by the FDA for use in awake craniotomy in 2008 [16]. This can be used as an anxiolytic and as a sedative and is associated with fewer respiratory side effects as compared to propofol [15]. The dosages and onset times for key drugs used during awake craniotomy are given in **Table 1**.

For CS regimens, low-dose propofol and remifentanil drips are often given simultaneously, unless respiratory depression necessitates the use of dexmedetomidine [16]. For GA regimens, propofol and remifentanil can also be used, as well as inhaled agents, such as sevoflurane, with IV remifentanil [16].

Key procedures to perform prior to craniotomy include placement of an arterial line, a central venous catheter, and a foley catheter [15]. For intraoperative monitoring, body temperature surveillance is crucial; if the patient begins to shiver, brain mapping will become extremely difficult. The threshold for shivering in most unanesthetized adults is 35.5°C, but this threshold can be lowered by inhaled anesthetics and opioids [17]. Typically, maintaining a patient's core body temperature above this threshold will prevent shivering. The addition of dexmedetomidine or ondansetron to the anesthesia regimen may reduce shivering, but body temperature monitoring remains paramount [17]. Keeping the room warm, warm IV fluids, and utilizing forced air warming blankets are standard methods that are also employed to maintain normal body temperature in surgical patients.

Among those undergoing awake craniotomy, scalp blocks can be particularly helpful in reducing patient discomfort during and after craniotomy [15, 18]. This is especially important in those undergoing awake sedation. These blocks can either be performed by targeting specific nerves innervating the scalp, most often the zygomaticotemporal, supraorbital, auriculotemporal, lesser occipital, and greater occipital nerves [18]. Scalp blocks can also be done by creating a circumferential block around the surgical field subdermally. Neurosurgeons or anesthesiologists can perform this technique by injection of a long-lasting local anesthetic, usually 2 mL of 0.5% bupivacaine, with effects lasting up to 8 hours after injection [18].

In these procedures, the patient will be awakened after the craniotomy is complete and the brain surface is exposed. A grid will be placed on the brain surface to allow the surgeons to keep track of regions of tissue and their effects on the patient's speech and motor capabilities. Before the patient is awakened, MEP and SSEP are typically used to identify the sensory and motor cortices, as this method can be used in anesthetized patients [1]. After being awakened, a bipolar stimulator is then used to stimulate various brain regions with varying amounts of current while the patient is shown a series of cue cards displaying words and imagery [15, 19]. The patient is instructed to read and name the objects on each card out loud. Often the cards will contain widely recognizable objects such as a ball or a tree. The surgeon stimulates various brain regions while listening for changes in the patient's speech patterns as they read each of the cards [15, 19]. Changes include total speech arrest, dysnomia, semantic errors, and phonological paraphasia [1, 15]. Each of these speech errors correlates to the afterdepolarization of a key region of the eloquent brain and by identifying the region responsible for each of these functions, the surgeon can spare this tissue during resection. For example, total speech arrest correlates to the primary speech area in the frontal operculum whereas dysnomia (the inability to name

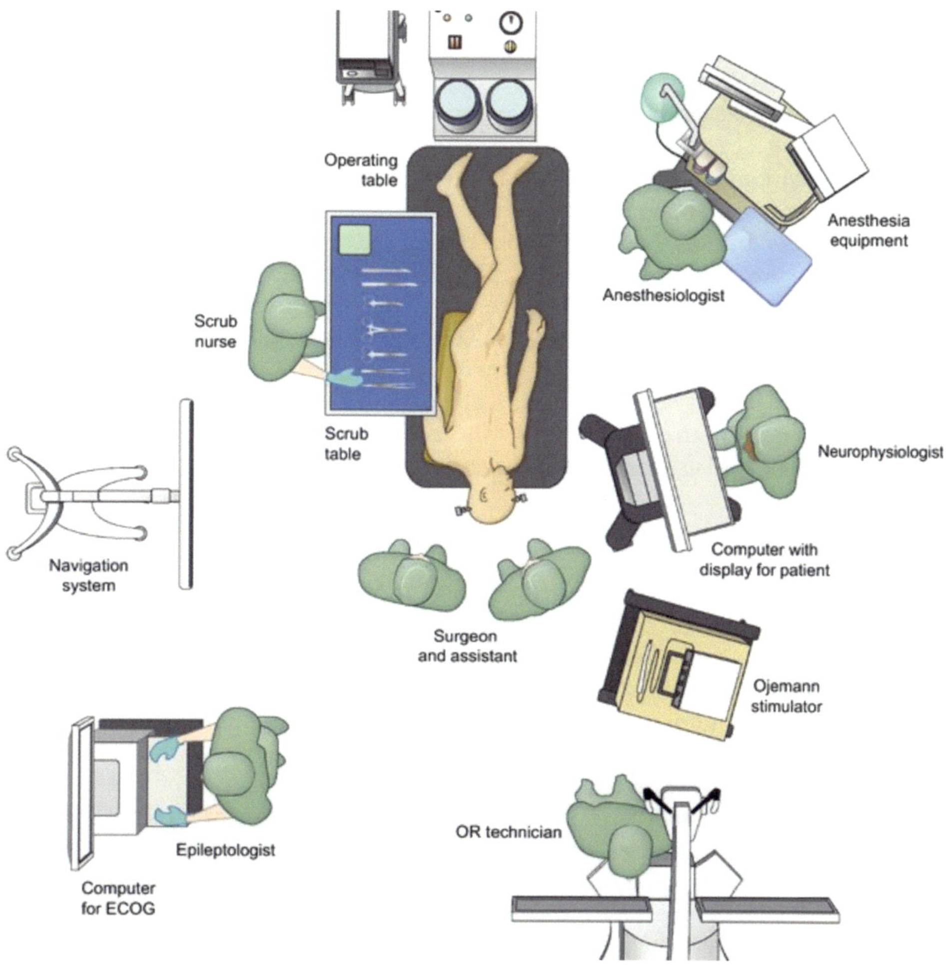

Figure 1.
Room set up and patient positioning for awake craniotomy. Note the display within the patient's field of view and the surgical team at the head of the bed. Typically, anesthesiology will be at the head of the patient's bed, but in the case of a craniotomy, the neurosurgeon must be at the patient's head [19].

objects) typically is associated with the posterior, inferior frontal gyrus, and inferior parietal and temporal regions [1]. **Figure 1** shows a schematic of what an awake craniotomy may look like in terms of room set up and patient positioning.

3.2.3 Post-operative care

Post-op care for patients after awake procedures is fairly standard. In fact, patients who underwent awake craniotomy for resections had better outcomes than those who underwent general anesthesia for the duration of their resection [20]. Nursing should perform neurological exams on the patient every 1 to 2 hours while the patient is inpatient post-operatively. Neurologic exams in these patients should always include pupillary light reflex exam, cranial nerve assessment, testing of the extremity muscles for new focal or global weakness, and cognitive status [15]. There are currently no major differences between postoperative care in patients who had "asleep-awake-asleep" or who had conscious sedation [15]. Key considerations are maintaining a target blood pressure of 150–160 for most patients, as uncontrolled hypertension is associated with longer hospital stays and a higher risk of intracranial bleeds [21]. Special care should be taken to monitor for surgical site infections, brain herniation, intracranial bleeds, hydrocephalus, and seizure, as these are common complications post-craniotomy. Like asleep craniotomy, awake craniotomy patients should be admitted to the ICU post-operatively.

While most craniotomies come with numerous risks and complications, awake craniotomy in particular comes with some specific concerns. Seizure for example is a risk of all craniotomies, but in particular risk of seizure is particularly high during stimulation for brain mapping purposes [22]. Most are focal and brief and do not pose a major risk to the patient [22]. In the case of patients who are undergoing monitored anesthesia care and are not intubated, risks for airway complications including hypoventilation leading to hypercarbia are of particular concern [15]. Hypercarbia can contribute to brain swelling as well. If the patient is to deeply be sedated and not respirating well on their own, medications should be backed off and the patient should be aroused and asked to breathe deeply until blood gases normalize [15].

3.3 Cerebral aneurysm procedures

While the treatment of unruptured cerebral aneurysms is controversial, neurosurgeons still intervene on those aneurysms whose risk of rupture is high. Generally, aneurysms between 7 mm and 10 mm are considered high risk, but a multitude of factors including morphology and regional anatomy are considered [1]. While in some cases open craniotomy and aneurysmal clipping cannot be avoided, endovascular interventions became another standard therapy for aneurysms in the 1990s [1]. This includes access to the cerebral vasculature via the advancement of a catheter that entered the vascular system at another site (femoral artery or radial artery) [1]. Once the aneurysm is reached, titanium coils are inserted into the aneurysm lumen where a thrombus forms around the coils, filling the space within the outpouching [23]. Advances in this technique have included the use of balloons and stents to aid in coil insertion and more recently the use of flow diverters. Flow diverters are mesh-like stents that are placed into the parent vessel to redirect blood flow along the original path of the parent artery while stagnating flow into the aneurysm itself [23]. This causes shrinkage and thrombosis of the aneurysm and remodeling of the artery [23].

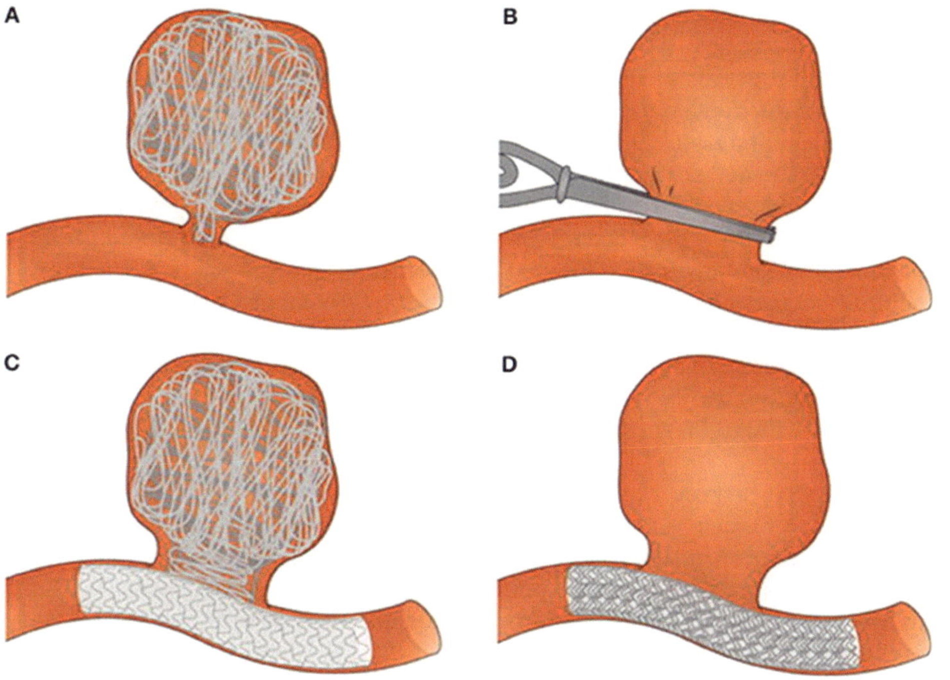

Figure 2.
Treatment strategies for unruptured intracranial aneurysms. (A) Depicts endovascular coiling embolization alone, (B) depicts aneurysmal clipping, (C) depicts stent placement and coil embolization combined, and (D) depicts the use of a flow diverter alone [24].

As compared to traditional coiling techniques, flow diversion is associated with lower rates of aneurysm recurrence and higher rates of successful occlusion [23]. While these diverters have become a widely accepted method of endovascular treatment for aneurysms very recently, their role in the treatment of ruptured aneurysms or aneurysms which would typically be treated by craniotomy and clipping is yet to be determined. **Figure 2** shows an image of some of the key treatment strategies for intracranial aneurysms.

While every aneurysm warrants individual assessment, some factors can delineate whether a ruptured aneurysm is an ideal candidate for endovascular treatment or for open craniotomy. Emergent craniotomy for rupture aneurysms used to be the standard of care, but recently endovascular treatment has become more utilized in emergent cases as well [25]. Ideal candidates for endovascular treatment after rupture include elderly patients, with aneurysms smaller than 15 mm, those with aneurysmal necks less than 4 mm wide, those found in the posterior circulation and those with major medical comorbidities [25]. Those which may be more ideal for open surgery include aneurysms in younger patients, diameters greater than 15 mm or very small aneurysms, those arising from the middle cerebral artery, those with complex aneurysmal neck anatomy or fusiform shape, fear that the patient cannot cooperate with diligent follow up [25]. It is also worth noting that studies have found higher rates of recurrence in ruptured aneurysms which undergo endovascular coiling as compared to those which underwent surgical repair [25]. As such, follow-up is critical, particularly in the 6 months after an endovascular repair of a ruptured aneurysm [25].

3.3.1 Preoperative assessment

Like most intracranial surgeries, neurological assessment should be performed prior to anesthesia induction for endovascular coiling procedures. This should include a neurologic exam including assessing whether the patient is alert and oriented, the function of the cranial nerves, and sensation and motor function of all the extremities. This allows for tracking of neurologic status post-operatively and better identification of postoperative complications. Baseline blood pressure should be determined for the patient and determination if pre-medication for blood pressure management will be needed [24]. In a more emergent situation, such as endovascular treatment of a ruptured aneurysm, these are the two most important steps to take in the pre-operative assessment. More careful examination can be performed for the treatment of unruptured aneurysms.

3.3.2 Intraoperative considerations

Endovascular therapy is generally performed under general anesthesia and includes catheter access to the cerebral vasculature from another access site. During these procedures prevention of hypertensive responses to components of the procedure such as foley catheter insertion, intubation, or incision should be avoided [24]. High blood pressures increase the risk of aneurysmal rupture intraoperatively, so small doses of opioids (for example fentanyl 3 μg/kg) are given just prior to intubation and incision to prevent hemodynamic responses. An arterial line should be placed for blood pressure monitoring and typically systolic blood pressure should not rise above 120 mmHg [24]. If the patient has hypertension or pressures are running higher than intended, using a beta-blocker or calcium-channel-blocker like nicardipine may help manage blood pressure.

3.3.3 Complications of endovascular coiling and post-operative care

In the event that the patient's aneurysm has ruptured and subarachnoid hemorrhage has developed, it is key to maintain higher pressures than in unruptured patients to ensure cerebral perfusion is maintained in the face of vasospasm, but not to exceed pressures of 160 mmHg so as to protect the patient from re-bleeding [26]. Vasospasm is a major complication after intracranial hemorrhage and can result in ischemia to affected brain regions. Treatment with nimodipine (often 60 mg every 4 hours) is standard of care in such patients with subarachnoid hemorrhage [27]. Nimodipine is a calcium channel blocker that induces vasodilation in the cerebral blood vessels [27]. Heparin is also usually dosed before the procedure and hourly throughout, but it is important to be prepared to rapidly reverse heparin if an intracranial bleed should occur so having protamine (50 mg) available to rapidly administer is wise. Protamine is the reversal agent for Heparin and can be used in the case of a bleed to rapidly reverse Heparin's effects. To assess for complications, post-operatively, serial neurological exams should be performed by the nursing team and the neurointensivist. Again, opioid pain control should be titrated so as to ensure full neurologic exams can still be performed as needed.

3.4 Endoscopic neurosurgery

Another recent and major advancement in cranial neurosurgery is the use of endoscopic navigation, which allows the surgeon to reach and operate in deep-seated regions of the brain without extensive dissection [28]. Such techniques allow for advanced skull base tumor resections, ventriculostomy, intraventricular tumor resections, and sellar tumor resections using only burr hole-sized craniotomies [28]. The ability for extensive tumor resection with minimal manipulation of healthy brain tissues thereby reducing post-operative complications [28]. The angled optics that endoscopy allows also offers particular advantages to the neurosurgeon. Accessing some sites in the intracranial vault to perform microscopic neurosurgery is difficult and requires a large craniotomy, such as the cerebellopontine angle [28]. However,

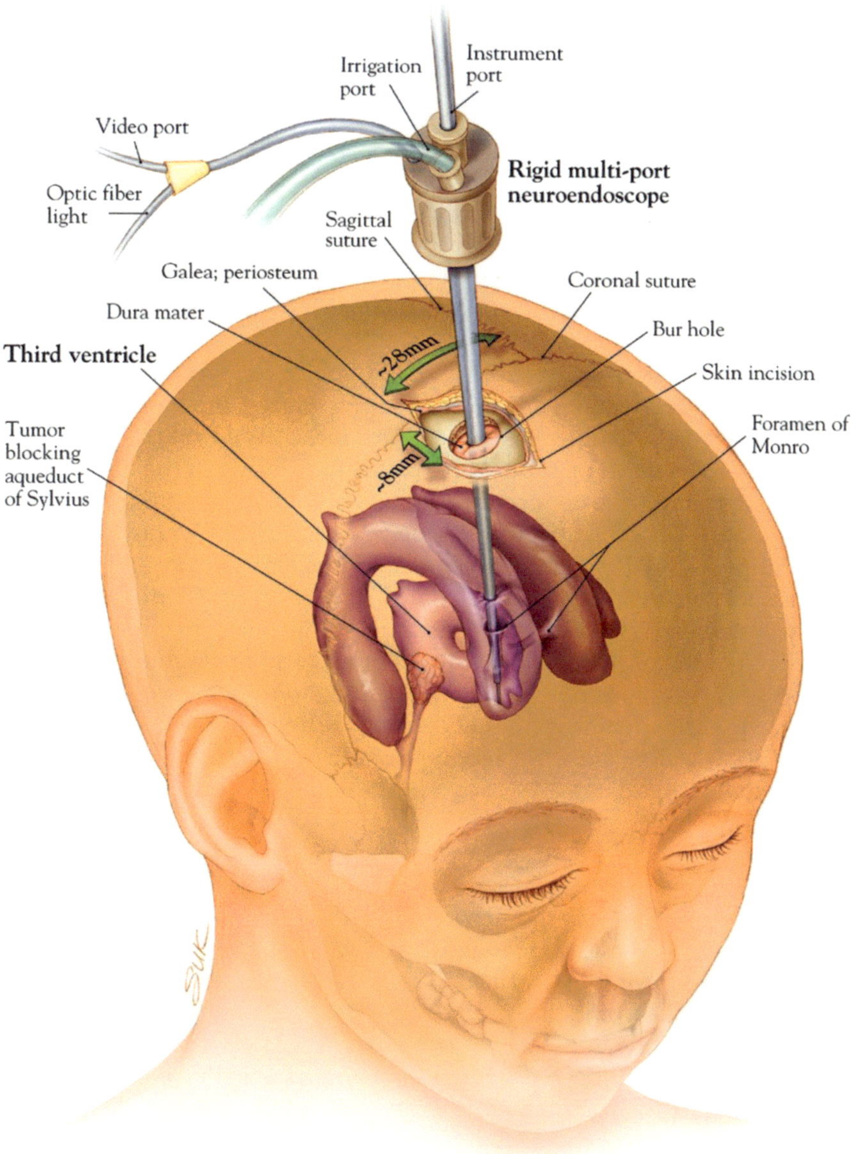

Figure 3.
Endoscopic neurosurgery for ventricular tumor resection schematic. Shown here is an example of an endoscopic cranial procedure. A key-hole-sized craniotomy is made in the skull and an endoscope is advanced into the ventricles so that microscopic resection can be done [28].

with angled optics offered by the endoscope, such tumors in precarious positions can be reached without aggressive dissection [28]. However, it is important to note that the use of minimally invasive neurosurgery is elective in nature and the surgeon's comfort in removing a particular tumor or cyst via this method will determine if a patient is eligible for a minimally invasive approach. Such methods are still being studied for a variety of new procedures and are likely to become more widely used in the future. **Figure 3** shows an example schematic of an endoscopic neurosurgical procedure.

3.4.1 Preoperative assessment

Pre-operative assessment for endoscopic neurosurgery is very similar to assessments for other cranial procedures. Always perform a pre-operative neurological assessment, assess the patient's baseline intracranial pressure, and get accurate baseline blood pressure. This allows for adequate intraoperative and postoperative monitoring for complications. The neurologic status of these patients will vary greatly. Some may have neurologic symptoms due to hydrocephalus if an intraventricular tumor is obstructing cerebrospinal fluid flow or is asymptomatic with normal neurologic status.

3.4.2 Intraoperative considerations and complications

General anesthesia remains the method of choice for patients undergoing endoscopic cranial procedures. Unlike most procedures, the unique challenge to the anesthesiologist of endoscopic procedures is the need for accurate and constant monitoring of intracranial pressures [28]. Due to working in the still enclosed space of the cranium with endoscopy, fluid irrigation used throughout the procedure, especially in the ventricular system, can contribute to rapid increases in intracranial pressure [28]. Rapid changes in ICP may not induce the traditional changes associated with the Cushing triad, so monitoring ICP directly and continuously during such procedures is critical [28]. Such monitoring can be done by insertion of a Codman Microsensor through the working channel of an endoscope and allows for continuous ICP monitoring throughout the procedure and while irrigating in the ventricular system [29]. Arterial lines should always be placed in these patients as well to allow for blood pressure monitoring and rapid identification of cerebral ischemia.

3.5 Anesthesia for thrombectomy in acute ischemic stroke

Although stroke mortality has declined over the last decade, ischemic stroke remains one of the top 20 leading causes of death and long-term disability in the United States [30]. Prior to 2015, the only reperfusion therapy with proven efficacy in these patients was thrombolysis with intravenous alteplase (tPA). As a result of a number of successful randomized-controlled trials, the AHA/ASA Stroke guidelines were updated in 2015 to reflect the addition of endovascular thrombectomy (EVT) to the standard of care for acute ischemic stroke due to large vessel occlusion [31]. This revolutionary approach dramatically improved neurological recovery and functional outcomes in these patients. Despite the success and impact of EVT in this setting, the optimal anesthetic strategy for this procedure remains controversial. In this section, preoperative considerations, anesthetic strategy recommendations, and possible complications of EVT will be discussed.

3.5.1 Preoperative planning

Both tPA administration and endovascular thrombectomy are time-limited interventions; the patient must have a last known normal of less than 4.5 and 6 hrs, respectively. Due to the time restrictions, rapid identification and emergent management of acute ischemic stroke are critical and around-the-clock intervention must be available, including the ability to transfer to a facility with appropriate staffing and equipment. As a result, most hospitals have instituted Stroke Alert Protocols to expedite the assessment of hospitalized patients with changes in neurological status [32].

Stroke alerts immediately notify appropriate providers, including neurology, interventionalists, and nursing. Initial management is with emergency non-contrast CT imaging of the brain to assess for hemorrhage prior to tPA administration. Once the patient is determined to be eligible, tPA should be administered even if endovascular treatment is being considered. EVT is indicated when the cause of stroke is deemed to be the occlusion of a large cerebral artery in the anterior circulation and the procedure can be initiated within the 6-hour window of symptom onset. For stroke patients entering the emergency room, the goal for "door-to-needle time" is less than <60 min. In practice, less than one-third of the patients meet this goal [33].

As soon as the need for thrombectomy is confirmed, goals for the procedure need to be addressed between the surgeon and anesthesiology team regarding hemodynamic monitoring and anesthetic approach. In terms of monitoring, blood pressure, heart rate, electrocardiogram, oxygen saturation, and end-tidal carbon dioxide concentration should be continuously monitored throughout the procedure. Invasive arterial blood pressure or blood pressure cycling as frequently or more frequently than every 3 minutes should be employed. Intraoperatively, systolic blood pressure should be maintained between 140- and 180-mm Hg with diastolic blood pressures <105 mm Hg [34]. In the following section, anesthetic strategies for EVT are explored.

3.5.2 Anesthetic strategies

The anesthetic strategies used in EVT include general anesthesia, conscious sedation, and local anesthesia. General anesthesia involves full airway control and the option for neuromuscular blockade; in this state, patients are unconscious, unarousable, and paralyzed. Conscious sedation results in a depressed level of consciousness but allows the patient to protect their own airway, and in certain settings, respond to commands. Local anesthesia is done at the arterial access site and has no effect on the patient's level of consciousness. There are a number of presumed advantages and disadvantages to each strategy when it comes to acute ischemic stroke (**Table 2**) [35].

One of the proposed advantages of general anesthesia is the ability to achieve full paralysis. In theory, this would be expected to increase the chances of successful recanalization and reduce the risk of distal embolization and vessel injury. Additionally, the added airway protection would be beneficial in cases where the patient begins to deteriorate. Possible disadvantages include the significant hemodynamic changes that occur with intubation and induction, and the added time and personnel required to accomplish general anesthesia.

Compared to general anesthesia, conscious sedation is theoretically more cost-effective, as less medication is required, and critical care time can be minimized by avoiding intubation. More importantly, this strategy offers the ability to perform neurologic assessments intraoperatively. The main disadvantage is the potential for airway compromise, and especially in stroke patients, an elevated risk for aspiration.

	General anesthesia	Conscious sedation	Local anesthesia
Advantages	Use of paralytic = little to no patient movement Avoid potential urgent/emergent intubation Airway protection Pain control	Enables intraprocedural neurologic assessment Lower cost (less staffing, equipment, and monitoring) Decreased critical care time	Enables intraprocedural neurologic assessment Lower cost (less staffing, equipment, and monitoring) Decreased critical care time
Disadvantages	Hemodynamic changes w/ induction and intubation Potential for delayed time to recanalization Additional staff required (nursing, anesthetics, ICU)	Lack of airway protection, increased risk of aspiration	Lack of airway protection Aspiration is possible, but mental status is less impacted compared to conscious sedation

Table 2.
Proposed advantages and disadvantages of anesthetic strategies in acute ischemic stroke [35].

The advantages and disadvantages of conscious sedation mirror those of local anesthesia. The main difference is that local anesthesia should pose a lower risk of aspiration since it does not alter the patient's level of consciousness. While these are some of the proposed theories used to argue which strategy is optimal, the answer continues to remain unclear.

A number of large observational retrospective studies have been conducted over the past decade to assess the differences in clinical outcomes between these anesthetic strategies in acute ischemic stroke. Initial nonrandomized studies were in favor of conscious sedation and local anesthesia, suggesting increased adverse outcomes associated with general anesthesia. In more recent years, the data has continued to reveal mixed results. A major multicenter retrospective study in 2021 showed improved functional outcomes and reduced complications and mortality with conscious sedation compared with general anesthesia [33]. Other studies conducted around the same time period showed no difference in outcomes or mortality between these strategies [34]. When comparing local anesthesia to CS and GA, some studies report improved functional outcomes, while others reveal worsened outcomes or no difference at all [36].

To date, five single-center randomized clinical trials have been published comparing the use of general anesthesia to conscious sedation during endovascular thrombectomy. The first was the SIESTA (Sedation versus Intubation for Endovascular Stroke Treatment) trial which found no difference between strategies in the change in NIHSS at 24 hours, but patients managed with GA were significantly more likely to achieve functional independence at 3 months [37]. The ANSTROKE (Anesthesia During Stroke Trial) found no significant difference in neurologic outcomes at 3 months [38]. The GOLIATH trial (General Or Local anesthesia in Intra Arterial Therapy) revealed final infarct volume was significantly lower in the GA, inferring the possibility of higher rates of successful recanalization with GA. Additionally, the GA group had better functional outcomes at 3 months [39]. In Beijing, an RCT called the CANVAS (Choice of ANesthesia for EndoVAScular Treatment of Acute Ischemic Stroke) trial was conducted and found functional outcomes at 3 months were similar between groups and the difference in mortality (GA 5%, CS 30%) was insignificant.

Most recently, Ren et al. found no significant difference in functional outcomes or mortality at discharge or 3 months post-stroke in AIS patients [40]. Secondary outcome analysis revealed significantly more stable hemodynamics and a lower incidence of pneumonia in the CS group.

Thus far, no RCTs exist that include local anesthesia as a comparator arm and meta-analyses of observational studies have failed to show differences in functional outcomes with LA compared to CS and GA. Some of these studies show evidence of shorter door-to-needle time in patients and less intraprocedural hypotension, which are important considerations for functional outcomes [41].

By and large, the optimal anesthetic approach for patients undergoing EVT in acute ischemic stroke therapy remains unclear. Large, multicenter RCTs are warranted comparing LA, CS, and GS with strict blood pressure targets and use of the standardized anesthetic agents to minimize confounding variables. Due to the lack of consensus and the existence of widely contradictory evidence, interventionalists should be advised to choose their anesthetic approach based on their professional experience pending the publication of more conclusive evidence [41]. Regardless of the approach, keeping open communication between the interventionalist and the anesthesiologist is key. Coordinating patient plans and ensuring timely and efficient line placement requires that channels of communication remain open.

3.5.3 Potential complications of EVT

With the success of EVT and its integration into the standard of care for AIS, there are still a number of potential complications that exist intra- and postoperatively. Awareness of these complications is crucial for quick recognition and management when one arises and additionally allows for preventative measures to be taken. Hemorrhagic complications including symptomatic intracranial hemorrhage (sICH), subarachnoid hemorrhage (SAH), and vessel perforation are some of the more serious problems that can occur [34]. sICH is typically a result of hemorrhagic transformation within infarcted brain parenchyma while SAH can be a direct result of traction created by the device used for clot retrieval. Arterial perforation is a rare, but grave complication, leading to poor functional outcomes in up to 75% of cases and a mortality rate greater than 50% [34]. Reported in less than 5% of patients undergoing EVT in large, randomized trials, most perforations occur when crossing the occlusion site or with deployment or retrieval of the stent retriever device. Coiling, balloon devices, or more invasive neurosurgical techniques can be used, but the main supportive measure that can be taken from a Neuroanesthesia standpoint is the temporary reduction of blood pressure until the bleeding is controlled [34].

Another possible complication of EVT is vasospasm. Vasospasm can be induced as a result of mechanical irritation of the vessel wall during catheter or guidewire manipulation [34]. Due to impacts on cerebral blood flow, vasospasm can result in unrecognized residual thrombus and vessel wall irregularities after thrombectomy. These are predictors of early reocclusion and associated with unfavorable outcomes [34]. If recognized intraoperatively, a calcium blocker such as nimodipine can be administered (0.5–1 mg/500 mL infusion), either as a bolus or continuously through the flushing line of the guiding catheter. It is important to note that the administration of nimodipine can result in systemic hypotension, which should be avoided in AIS patients during EVT. Close monitoring of the blood pressure and correction to systolic pressures between 140 and 180 mmHg should be prioritized.

The last major potential complication is embolization, either distal to the initial infarct or to new vascular territories [34]. This typically occurs iatrogenically, with the fragmentation of the original clot during retrieval. Incidence is reported to be around 5%. If new clinical deficits would be reasonably expected as a result, management is with further EVT of the new lesion. The potential of the clinical benefit must outweigh the risk of prolonging the procedure. If EVT is not possible or contraindicated, intra-arterial thrombolysis could be considered.

4. Updates to neuroanesthesia: spinal procedures

Spinal Neurosurgery makes up the majority of the procedures performed by most neurosurgeons. Improving technologies have allowed for more precise surgeries with improving patient outcomes. CT navigation, for example, has become a broadly used technology to allow for more precise placement of screws during spinal fusion surgery. Placement of spinal pedicle screws is done in a broad range of procedures and previously surgeons had to insert these screws using only C-arm fluoroscopy assistance. However, due to the close proximity to the dura, spinal cord, nerve roots, and blood vessels, screw misplacement can cause a multitude of complications that remain relatively common [42]. CT navigated tools, however, use CT scans of the patient's spine to build a three-dimensional map of vertebrae and can display the trajectory of a screw in 3-D space [42]. This method has been shown to be accurate and has low rates of screw misplacement. Other methods to increase screw placement accuracy have also included robot-assisted procedures and even augmented reality-guided screw placement.

While deep brain stimulators for various neurologic disorders including Parkinson's disease, essential tremor, and dystonias, have been used for some time, spinal stimulators have also recently become an option available for patients with a myriad of spinal diseases including sciatica, neuropathy, radiculopathy, complex regional pain syndrome, phantom limb pain, and even complications of multiple sclerosis [43]. The stimulator's electrodes are placed epidurally and, by inducing electrical stimulation of the spinal cord, actually modulate the neural activity being relayed to the brain, masking pain transmission [43]. Patients first undergo a trial period for about a week where a temporary stimulator device is inserted in the outpatient office to see how well the stimulator reduces the patient's pain. If the patient reports a greater than 50% reduction in pain, permanent stimulator placement is indicated. For permanent stimulator implantation, patients must undergo surgery wherein the stimulator and battery are placed under the skin of the upper buttock and using fluoroscopic guidance, each electrode is inserted into the epidural space. Typically, this is performed with conscious sedation with titrated propofol or dexmedetomidine and local anesthesia at sites of incision, but general anesthesia may also be appropriate for some patients.

Minimally invasive spine surgery is also rapidly advancing. Microdiscectomy for example is an option for those with herniated intervertebral discs which require surgical intervention. Previously, discectomies required large incisions with major disruptions of the paraspinal muscles in order to access the spinal canal and included removal of the entire disc. With microdiscectomy, smaller incisions are used to gain a window into the spinal canal and then remove only the portions of the disc that are herniated and causing nerve compression [44]. Multiple methods have been developed to accomplish microdiscectomy including midline discectomy, tubular microdiscectomy, and even endoscopic microdiscectomy. With endoscopic approaches, a small endoscope is advanced through a very small incision into the spinal canal and along with CT-guidance techniques, the endoscope is used to direct the operation with minimal disruption of paraspinal muscles, minimal dural dissection, minimal facet dissection, and minimal blood loss [44]. Such minimally invasive procedures also mean discectomy no longer necessitates general anesthesia. Rather, local anesthesia and conscious sedation is now an option for these procedures. Minimally invasive and endoscopic spine surgery is associated with shorter hospitalizations, faster recovery, and less postoperative pain during recovery [44].

5. Enhanced recovery after surgery protocols in neurosurgery

A relatively new concept in anesthesiology, Enhanced Recovery After Surgery (ERAS) Protocols first emerged in the 1990s for colonic and rectal resections [45]. Some of the earliest studies of ERAS protocols for craniotomy and spinal fusion would come out in the early 2000s and slowly evidence has been built for the dramatic outcomes that ERAS protocols can provide [46]. As consensus is reached on the benefits of ERAS protocols, it is key that anesthesia and neurosurgical departments everywhere begin adopting practices that are well-established in the literature. ERAS protocol development for cranial neurosurgery has lagged behind spinal neurosurgery significantly. While there are few published full ERAS protocols for craniotomy, many studies have been published in the last decade with similar core elements with significant improvement in patient satisfaction and clinical outcomes. ERAS protocols for spinal neurosurgery have been well established and have excellent data supporting the utilization of key practices in the perioperative period to optimize patient satisfaction and clinical outcomes. **Table 3** summarizes some key evidenced based practices which are supported across studies for both cranial and spinal neurosurgery.

Some notable elements specific to craniotomy include the utilization of local anesthetics to perform scalp blocks and minimization of the surgeon's manipulation of brain tissue. A 2019 randomized control trial by Yang et al. of patients undergoing

Pre-operative interventions	Intraoperative interventions	Postoperative interventions
Identification of the right patients for fast-track and minimally invasive surgery Patient education about the perioperative experience, what symptoms and side effects to expect Preoperative carbohydrate loading and nutritional assessment Smoking and alcohol abstinence Mechanical thromboembolism prophylaxis In patients with a seizure history, seizure prophylaxis	Regional or scalp blocks Hypothermia avoidance Minimization of patient or time Avoidance of tissue drains Use of absorbable sutures Minimization of brain tissue manipulation Antibiotic prophylaxis (Cefazolin 1 hour before incision) Post-operative nausea and vomiting assessment and management	Avoidance of ICU admission Early extubation prior to PACU Early mobilization Early fluid de-escalation Resume solid food intake early Early removal of urinary catheters Early removal of arterial lines Post-operative nausea and vomiting assessment and management Post-operative brain imaging within the first 24 hours to rule out bleeding and edema Standardized discharge instructions

Table 3.
Summary of some major ERAS practices for craniotomy and spinal surgery that are supported in the literature.

craniotomy for aneurysm repair compared effects of scalp block with injection of ropivacaine versus standard IV analgesia [47]. They found reductions in postoperative scalp inflammation, blood loss during scalp incision, and better control of postoperative pain as compared to a control group [45]. Minimally invasive techniques for neurosurgical diseases are few and far between, but some patients can be treated through keyhole incisions for some cysts and tumors. A retrospective study of patients elected for minimally invasive surgery found that, unlike typical craniotomy, the vast majority of the complications occurred within hours of the procedure, not days [48]. They suggested that rapid discharge within a day of minimally invasive procedures with minimal manipulation of the brain tissue is appropriate due to the low risk of postoperative complications [49].

Additionally, the use of seizure prophylaxis in neurosurgical patients is somewhat controversial, with some critics citing the low doses of anti-seizure medications often used for prophylaxis as not enough to significantly reduce the seizure threshold. Recent systematic reviews of studies exploring the use of antiepileptic drugs to prevent craniotomy-associated seizures have all found minimal evidence to support this practice and agree that a large, randomized trial would be needed to better establish evidence-based guidelines for seizure prophylaxis [49].

Open spinal fusion and removal of spinal tumors are typically perceived by patients as large open procedures with a long recovery and rehabilitation timelines. ERAS protocols, however, have reduced the psychologic, physical, and economic impacts of such life-changing procedures. A consensus statement in ERAS protocols for open spinal surgery was recently published in 2021 by the ERAS Society which outlines the evidence for each practice and their recommendations for perioperative medicine [50]. Taken together, an amalgam of these practices can be applied on an institution-by-institution basis.

More spine-specific interventions could include the use of liposomal bupivacaine or other regional blocks specifically for the treatment of postoperative pain in spinal surgery. Liposomal bupivacaine is included as a strong recommendation by the ERAS Society, but it should be noted that the data supporting its use is relatively weak. A number of studies have attempted to show its effectiveness on postoperative opioid utilization, reduction of adverse reactions, and infection rates [51, 52]. Consistently, these studies have failed to show significant evidence that its use reduces any of these outcomes. As such, further studies into other methods of local analgesia should be performed. Institutions should examine the most up-to-date studies to decide whether to implement regional analgesia in their ERAS protocols.

6. Postoperative delirium

Delirium is defined as an acute deterioration of cerebral function that clinically presents as changes in mental status [53]. In the perioperative setting, delirium presents significant clinical and economic challenges. Patients may experience extended hospital stays and mortality rates of up to 10%, especially within the geriatric population [54]. The occurrence of perioperative delirium also yields a remarkable financial burden. One prospective cohort study analyzed perioperative data from patients undergoing major surgery at Harvard-affiliated hospitals. Their work revealed 25% of 497 eligible patients in the study experienced delirium with an average unadjusted healthcare cost of $146,358 while the cost of care for those without delirium was $94,609 [55]. The economic and clinical burdens of perioperative delirium exemplify the necessity for implementing preventative measures along with risk stratification. Here the diagnosis, risk factors, and management of perioperative delirium will be discussed while also addressing the most current methods of clinical management and risk reduction.

6.1 Epidemiology

The incidence of delirium has long been associated with the geriatric patient population. Recent literature suggests the rate of postoperative delirium among those aged 60–70 is roughly 10–20% [56]. Emergency surgery is associated with a significantly higher risk of postoperative delirium (20–45%) when compared to elective (2.5–3%) and truncal surgery (10–20%) [50]. In addition, hospital stays on average are prolonged by 2–3 days [55].

6.2 Diagnosis

The current gold standard for the diagnosis of delirium technically requires the presence of a psychiatrist to use the Diagnostic and Statistical Manual of Mental Disorders, Fifth Edition (DSM-5). Patients can present with an array of symptoms including alterations in their awareness, disturbances in their ability to maintain and shift attention, disorientation, difficulty with speech, misidentification of people and objects, and pathognomonically fluctuations in the severity of these cognitive symptoms over time. Diagnosis is tricky, as this presents typically in elderly patients who may have underlying cognitive impairment at baseline. In the postoperative period, emergence delirium is a common phenomenon that presents as agitation or excessive somnolence as the patient awakens from general anesthesia and is temporary and rapidly resolves as they awaken. If it persists after the patient is awakened and is taken to the PACU, diagnosis at this stage becomes key.

To effectively diagnose delirium, a patient's mental status/arousal must be determined. The Richmond Agitation Sedation Scale (RASS) and the Sedation Agitation Scale (SAS) are commonly used scoring systems [53]. However, recent work suggests that the Confusion Assessment Method (CAM) is the most effective tool for delirium evaluation without the need for a psychiatrist present at the bedside. The CAM evaluates various traits of delirium including altered mental status requiring monitoring, acute onset, fluctuations in behavior, and disorganized thinking [56]. In 2014, the CAM-S was developed as an addition to the original CAM scoring tool with the primary goal of determining delirium severity in a quantitative approach [57]. It is not a diagnostic tool but can be used in conjunction with CAM for a complete assessment. **Figure 4** shows the CAM tool that may be used in a PACU setting to assess a patient's mental status. Versions of this tool have also been developed for the ICU or to be done rapidly in a setting like PACU, such as the 3-D CAM which is a 3-minute version of the tool. Preoperative screening for neurocognitive disorders is not typical in most centers and often pre-existing cognitive disorders can be missed by the surgical and anesthesia teams. However, such practices like obtaining a baseline cognitive exam or CAM could result in the more effective diagnostic value of these tools.

6.3 Risk factors

There is a myriad of factors involved in the development of delirium. Recent literature suggests categorizing risk factors as those preceding or directly causing the onset

Feature	Severity Score		
Scoring the CAM-S: Rate each symptom of delirium listed in the CAM as absent (0), mild (1), marked (2). Acute onset or fluctuation is rated as absent (0) or present (1). Add these scores into a composite. Higher scores indicate more severe delirium.			
	Not Present	**Present (mild)**	**Present (marked)**
1. ACUTE ONSET & FLUCTUATING COURSE	0	1	
2. INATTENTION	0	1	2
3. DISORGANIZED THINKING	0	1	2
4. ALTERED LEVEL OFCONSCIOUSNESS	0	*vigilant/lethargic:* 1	*stupor or coma:* 2
5. DISORIENTATION	0	1	2
6. MEMORY IMPAIRMENT	0	1	2
7. PERCEPTUAL DISTURBANCES	0	1	2
8. PSYCHOMOTOR AGITATION	0	1	2
9. PSYCHOMOTOR RETARDATION	0	1	2
10. ALTERED SLEEP-WAKE CYCLE	0	1	2
Short Form SEVERITY SCORE:	Add the scores in rows 1-4. Range is 0-7.		
Long Form SEVERITY SCORE:	Add the scores in rows 1-10. Range is 0-19.		

Figure 4.
Confusion assessment method [58].

of delirium. Older age, male sex, low pre-operative hematocrit, diabetes, preexisting cognitive impairment, and previous history of delirium are all factors that increase the risk of developing delirium [59]. Substances such as alcohol, recreational drugs, and steroids can lead to altered mental status and eventually delirium. Preventing delirium in the intraoperative setting provides a unique challenge to anesthesiologists, as patients may experience acute changes in hemodynamics due to the pharmacologic properties of volatile anesthetics and narcotics administered. Specifically, one clinical trial assessed postoperative delirium in patients receiving light versus heavy anesthesia. The depth of anesthesia was determined using the bispectral index (BIS). For reference, the BIS ranges from 0 (flatline EEG) to 100 (response to normal voice). Patients undergoing anesthesia with a BIS 35 had a 28% incidence of postoperative delirium compared to 19% of patients with a BIS of 50 [60]. This study suggests patients under deeper anesthesia tend to suffer a higher incidence of postoperative delirium. The necessity for maintaining an appropriate dose of anesthetics has been outlined by the American Society of Anesthesiology Brain Health Initiative, providing evidence-based guidelines for anesthesia providers to follow as reference. These guidelines will be succinctly described in the following section.

6.4 Management and risk reduction

Current literature suggests risk scales or scores are not well-studied or effective tools for guiding providers to appropriate management of postoperative delirium. Rather, success in treatment has been found with the mitigation of underlying precipitating risk factors. Managing postoperative pain, for instance, with epidural analgesia has been associated with a lower risk of delirium [51]. The departure from narcotic pain management in the postoperative setting may prove efficacious in preventing delirium in the future, especially with the increasing popularity of regional anesthesia implementation. Recently dexmedetomidine has revealed promising results with regard to preventing the onset of delirium postoperatively. In one 2019 study, dexmedetomidine treatment in the postoperative setting reduced levels of the inflammatory cytokine interleukin-6, improved MMSE scores, and decreased the development of delirium. It is important to mention that dexmedetomidine is not currently recommended for critically ill patients as advised by the Society of Critical Care Medicine as it has provided little benefit in this demographic [56].

Outside of dexmedetomidine use, the American Society of Anesthesiologists (ASA) Perioperative Brain Health Initiative reviewed the literature on perioperative delirium management released from 2010 to 2019. After considerable filtering, six management options were chosen as recommendations for use among anesthesiologists and their care teams. For patients at risk for developing delirium, the ASA recommends providing baseline cognitive screening, education for providers on delirium, adequate pain control, avoiding the use of antipsychotics and benzodiazepines, and screening in the perioperative setting for noticeable symptoms. In addition, non-pharmacologic methods are encouraged including patient mobilization, communication, and orientation, similar to the current methods used for preventing delirium in the inpatient setting [58].

Following pre-procedure consent, a preoperative cognitive assessment is recommended for developing an understanding of the relative risk of developing delirium for any given patient. A variety of mental status exams such as the MMSE and MoCA are recommended by literature supporting the Brain Health Initiative, specifically. Though, CAM and 3-D CAM have also been used in studies for pre-operative assessment. If patients are determined to have a moderate-high risk of developing delirium, anesthesiologists may take a different approach to perioperative management. For example, providers can consider avoiding medications such as benzodiazepines or reduce doses of narcotics used for pain control and sedation [61].

Providing informed consent to patients about delirium also provides an essential commodity—time. Following an operative procedure, some patients that develop delirium may experience cognitive changes for days, weeks, or even months. The ability of these patients to perform cognitively demanding tasks such as balancing a checkbook and paying bills may be hindered. Therefore, providing timely consent grants patients time to prepare for rehabilitation and support with their family and loved ones in the instance they develop postoperative delirium, improving their long-term clinical outcomes. Anesthesiologists are presented with a unique challenge when following this tenant of care, however. Most patients meet their anesthesiologists and are given consent on the day of their procedure [61]. It may be beneficial for anesthesia providers to meet with patients and families in the postoperative setting to assure adequate resources are in place in the setting of suspected delirium.

Provider education on delirium should include not just the physicians, but also nurse anesthetists, respiratory therapists, and nursing staff who may be caring for the patient in the OR or the PACU. They should also be prepared to recognize signs of cognitive disturbance and relay their concerns to the anesthesiologist or surgeon so that prompt assessment and management can occur.

As the patient is wheeled into the operating room and placed on the table, the anesthesiologist obtains access to a myriad of drugs. Unfortunately, many pharmacological interventions can potentiate the risk of developing delirium in the post-operative setting including benzodiazepines, first-generation antihistamines,

Medication or Class of Medication	Examples	Rationale for Avoiding
First-generation antihistamines	Diphenhydramine	Central anticholinergic effects
Phenothiazine-type antiemetics	Prochlorperazine, promethazine	Central anticholinergic effects
Antispasmodics/anticholinergics	Atropine, scopolamine	Central anticholinergic effects
Antipsychotics (first and second generation)	Haloperidol	Risk of cognitive impairment, delirium, neuroleptic malignant syndrome, tardive dyskinesia
Benzodiazepines	Midazolam, diazepam	Risk of cognitive impairment, delirium
Corticosteroids	Hydrocortisone, methylprednisolone	Risk of cognitive impairment, delirium, psychosis
H_2-receptor antagonists	Ranitidine	Risk of cognitive impairment, delirium
Metoclopramide		Extrapyramidal effects
Meperidine		Neurotoxic effects
Skeletal muscle relaxants	Cyclobenzaprine	Anticholinergic effects

Abbreviation: H_2, histamine 2 receptor.

Figure 5.
Medications that increase the risk of postoperative delirium [61].

corticosteroids, and several others illustrated in **Figure 5** [61]. Avoiding these medications can help to reduce the risk of postoperative delirium. It is also recommended to utilize age-adjusted minimum alveolar concentration (MAC) fractions when providing anesthetic management to geriatric patients. For reference, the MAC is the volume of inhaled anesthetic required to prevent motor response in 50% of patients undergoing surgical stimuli. The MAC tends to decrease in patients with age as much as 6% per decade following the age of 30. It is also essential to recall the most commonly used volatile anesthetics have particularly narrow therapeutic indexes [61]. These factors exemplify the necessity for careful maintenance of anesthetic agents during the management of geriatric patients due to the high risk of overdose and potential postoperative delirium.

Finally, screening during the recovery period by members of the team should be implemented as a routine part of the post-operative process. Assessing pain levels, assessing orientation, and reorienting the patient, if need be, and mobilizing the patient early should all be a part of the recovery protocol for high-risk patients to both monitor and prevent postoperative delirium from occurring. Re-orienting the patient regularly is a key treatment in the inpatient setting and could be implemented as a regular part of PACU care for elderly patients.

7. Discussion

As neurosurgery advances, so does the practice of the anesthesiologists who work alongside them. To best serve neurosurgical patients, anesthesiologists must stay abreast of the options available to their patients. Additionally, anesthesiologists often may be the only physician to see the patient before their procedure on the day of surgery, and being able to answer their questions about the procedure and what their experience will be like in the OR is key. Therefore, updates in surgical techniques and the technologies utilized in the OR are important to understand. The advances discussed thus far are reshaping neurosurgery toward an ever more precise and ever-safer process for patients. On the horizon are newer tools for the anesthesiologist and new procedures that may even expand the gamut of diagnoses treated by the neurosurgeon. Here are reviewed some of those tools and procedures which the anesthesiologist should watch for in the literature.

There has been a resurgence of the study of surgery in the treatment of psychiatric disorders. Deep brain stimulation has become a widely used method of treating tremors from Parkinson's disease and essential tremors which are refractory to medical therapy. While not yet common practice, research into the expansion of the use of deep brain stimulators and neuromodulators to treat medication-refractory depression, anxiety, schizophrenia, and obsessive-compulsive disorder is showing great promise [62]. Deep brain stimulation (DBS) utilizes electrodes that when implanted in regions of the brain can stimulate those regions and functionally and reversibly ablate them [62]. Advances in functional neuroimaging such as functional MRI and PET have helped identify dysfunctional brain regions common among those with similar diagnoses and given evidentiary basis for ablative neurosurgery to treat these disorders. Examples of major brain targets supported across studies include the genu of the corpus callosum in major depressive disorder and schizophrenia and the medial cingulate cortex [62].

Currently, clinical trials are ongoing surrounding the use of neuromodulation for each of these disorders with preliminary results being largely promising. Treatment of some disorders is still very early and is not yet beyond the case report level of evidence. Case reports have reported a small number of patients with opioid use disorder who have not had relapses after DBS implants into the nucleus accumbens [63]. However, much more extensive work must be published before this becomes a realistic option for substance use disorders. For the anesthesiologist, relying on the knowledge and experience gained since DBS has been done for other disorders t0 ensure patients remain safe and comfortable while undergoing these new treatments. Such procedures are performed under either monitored anesthesia care or under general anesthesia or at some intuitions deep brain electrodes are placed under MAC and pulse generators are implanted under general anesthesia [64]. Similar protocols would be applied to these treatment options. However, since they are so new, anesthesia protocols specific for the placement of these stimulators have yet to be developed and published. However, as studies are published and this topic is explored further, the anesthesiologist should stay abreast of the advances and be ready to alter practice as we learn more about these procedures and how to best serve these patients.

Advances in therapy for spinal injury may also begin the change the way neurosurgeons and intensivists address traumatic spinal injury and how anesthesiologists care for such patients intraoperatively. Acutely, hypothermia induced either by cold IV saline or local cooling during spinal decompression has been shown to improve functional outcomes in animal models in preliminary studies in the late 60s but little traction was gained in the clinical world after these studies were published. However, following the successful treatment of NFL player Kevin Everett with cooling therapy in the field after a devastating C4 spinal cord injury leaving him paralyzed from the neck down, the clinical literature has begun to examine the possibility of utilizing systemic cooling or localized cooling intraoperatively to improve patient outcomes [65]. While the majority of the research currently is pre-clinical, some small cohort studies have also been published on the topic and so far, the data has largely been supportive of some degree of clinically significant improvement [65]. However randomized clinical trials with large sample sizes are still required before this becomes a regular part of clinical practice.

Finally, emerging tools in monitoring may also lead to new methods for monitoring cerebral blood flow both in the operating room and the intensive care unit utilizing Near-Infrared Spectroscopy (NIRS). NIRS uses changes in photon phases as they pass through tissues and reflect moving blood cells to construct temporal measurements of the amount of red blood cell movement through vasculature [66]. This method can actually detect changes far below the skin surface and could allow for non-invasive bedside monitoring of cerebral blood flow intraoperatively or in the ICU [66]. Interestingly, early studies also have used this method for measuring intracranial pressure and hemoglobin concentrations in non-human subjects [66]. Early studies have supported proof of concept for using these monitors for noninvasive ICP and CBF monitoring but clinical studies have yet to be undertaken to support the clinical efficacy of this method in practice. However, if implemented, neurointensive monitoring of cerebral blood flow and intracranial pressure would become far easier and allow for quicker clinical decision-making in patients with rising ICP or experiencing cerebral ischemia.

8. Conclusions

The anesthesiologist is faced with many challenges in caring for patients undergoing brain or spinal surgery. Facing these challenges with the most up-to-date evidence is critical for excellent clinical practice. Newly developed ERAS protocols and image-guided, minimally invasive cranial and spinal procedures have minimized postoperative pain and shortened hospital stays. New flow diversion stent technology for the endovascular treatment of cerebral aneurysms is improving our control of unruptured aneurysms and in the future may impact our treatment of ruptured cerebral aneurysms as well. The use of spinal stimulators is expanding to include relief of radicular and neuropathic pain.

Many uncertainties still abound in neuroanesthesia, despite the recent advances in the literature. At these unsure junctures, shared decision-making with the patient and the rest of the care team becomes key. In the future, much work will need to be done to delineate which anesthetic techniques most benefit patients for procedures like awake craniotomy and embolectomy. We also expect future work to shine more light on the management of perioperative delirium and the steps that can be taken to prevent it. On the horizon are new treatments for psychiatric disorders, acute treatment of spinal trauma, and noninvasive methods of cerebral blood flow monitoring are on the horizon. Such tools will expand the purview of the neurosurgeon and neuroanesthesiologist into the treatment of psychiatric disorders and will offer new tools to better treat the patients they typically serve in the OR and beyond.

DOI: http://dx.doi.org/10.5772/intechopen.109004

Author details

Christian N. Schill[1]*, Rebecca E. Bates[2], Troy D. Lovett[2] and Isha Kaza[3]

1 Department of Research and Innovation, St. Luke's University Health Network, Bethlehem, PA, USA

2 Department of Anesthesiology, St. Luke's University Health Network, Bethlehem, PA, USA

3 Department of Cognitive Science, Case Western Reserve University, Cleveland, OH, USA

*Address all correspondence to: christian.schill@temple.edu

IntechOpen

© 2022 The Author(s). Licensee IntechOpen. This chapter is distributed under the terms of the Creative Commons Attribution License (http://creativecommons.org/licenses/by/3.0), which permits unrestricted use, distribution, and reproduction in any medium, provided the original work is properly cited.

References

[1] Greenberg M. Handbook of Neurosurgery. 9th ed. New York: Thieme; 2020

[2] Bindra A, Tripathi M. Anesthesia for epilepsy surgery in children. In: Rath GP, editor. Fundamentals of Pediatric Neuroanesthesia. Singapore: Springer; 2021. DOI: 10.1007/978-981-16-3376-8_28

[3] Muralidharan R. External ventricular drains: Management and complications. Surgical Neurology International. 2015;**6**:S271-S274

[4] Petersen KD, Landsfeldt U, Cold GE, et al. Intracranial pressure and cerebral hemodynamic in patients with cerebral tumors: A randomized prospective study of patients subjected to craniotomy in propofol-fentanyl, isoflurane-fentanyl, or sevoflurane-fentanyl anesthesia. Anesthesiology. 2003;**98**(2):329-336. DOI:10.1097/00000542-200302000-00010

[5] Wyte SR, Shapiro HM, Turner P, Harris AB. Ketamine-induced intracranial hypertension. Anesthesiology. 1972;**36**(2):174-176. DOI:10.1097/00000542-197202000-00021

[6] Cole C, Gottfried O, Gupta D, Couldwell WT. Total intravenous anesthesia: Advantages for intracranial surgery. Operative Neurosurgery. 2007;**61**(5):369-378. DOI: 10.1227/01.neu.0000303996.74526.30

[7] Toleikis J. American Society of Neurophysiological Monitoring. Intraoperative monitoring using somatosensory evoked potentials. A position statement by the American Society of Neurophysiological Monitoring. Journal of Clinical Monitoring and Computing. 2005;**19**(3):241-258. DOI: 10.1007/s10877-005-4397-0

[8] Macdonald DB. Intraoperative motor evoked potential monitoring: Overview and update. Journal of Clinical Monitoring and Computing. 2006;**20**(5):347-377. DOI: 10.1007/s10877-006-9033-0

[9] Cai Y, Zeng H, Shi Z, Shen J, Lei Y, Chen B, et al. Factors influencing delayed extubation after infratentorial craniotomy for tumor resection: A prospective cohort study of 800 patients in a Chinese neurosurgical center. Journal of International Medical Research. 2013;**41**(1):208-217

[10] Rhondali O, Genty C, Halle C, et al. Do patients still require admission to an intensive care unit after elective craniotomy for brain surgery? Journal of Neurosurgical Anesthesiology. 2011;**23**(2):118-123. DOI: 10.1097/ANA.0b013e318206d5f8

[11] Basali A, Mascha E, Kalfas I, Schubert A. Relation between perioperative hypertension, and intracranial hemorrhage after craniotomy. Anesthesiology. 2000;**93**:48-54. DOI: 10.1097/00000542-200007000-00012

[12] Sartorius CJ, Berger MS. Rapid termination of intraoperative stimulation-evoked seizures with application of cold Ringer's lactate to the cortex. Technical note. Journal of Neurosurgery. 1998;**88**(2):349-351. DOI: 10.3171/jns.1998.88.2.0349

[13] Rangel-Castilla L, Gopinath S, Robertson CS. Management of intracranial hypertension. Neurologic Clinics. 2008;**26**:3. DOI: 10.1016/j.ncl.2008.02.003

[14] Salunke P, Garg R, Kapoor A, Chhabra R, Mukherjee KK. Symptomatic

contralateral subdural hygromas after decompressive craniectomy: Plausible causes and management protocols. Journal of Neurosurgery. 2015;**122**(3):602-609. DOI: 10.3171/2014.10.JNS14780

[15] Lee CZ, Poon CCM. An update of neuroanesthesia for intraoperative brain mapping craniotomy. Neurosurgery. 2022;**90**(1):1-6. DOI: 10.1093/neuros/nyab022

[16] Stevanovic A, Rossaint R, Veldeman M, Bilotta F, Coburn M. Anaesthesia management for awake craniotomy: Systematic review and meta-analysis. PLoS One. 2016;**11**(5):e0156448

[17] Alfonsi P, Nourredine K, Adam F, Chauvin M, Sessler D. Effect of postoperative skin-surface warming on oxygen consumption and the shivering threshold. Anaesthesia. 2003;**58**:1228-1234. DOI: 10.1046/j.1365-2044.2003.03444.x

[18] Osborn I, Sebeo J. "Scalp block" during craniotomy: A classic technique revisited. Journal of Neurosurgical Anesthesiology. 2010;**22**(3):187-194

[19] Gogos A, Young J, Morshed R, Hervey-Jumper S, Berger M. Awake glioma surgery: Technology, evolution, and nuances. Journal of Neuro-Oncology. 2020;**147**(3):515-524. DOI: 10.1007/s11060-020-03482-z

[20] Shlobin NA, Rosenow JM. Nonopioid postoperative pain management in neurosurgery. Neurosurgery Clinics of North America. 2022;**33**(3):261-273. DOI: 10.1016/j.nec.2022.02.004

[21] Zhang K, Geld A. Awake craniotomy: Indications, benefits, and techniques. Colombian Journal of Anesthesiology. 2018;**46**(2):46-51. DOI: 10.1097/CJ9.0000000000000045

[22] Nossek E, Matot I, Shahar T, et al. Intraoperative seizures during awake craniotomy: Incidence and consequences: Analysis of 477 patients. Neurosurgery. 2013;**73**(01):135-140

[23] Dabhi N, Sarathy D, Snyder MH, Kellogg RT, Park MS. Flow diverter devices for treatment of intracranial aneurysms in small parent vessels—A systematic review of literature. World Neurosurgery. 2022;**162**:183.e7-194.e7. DOI: 10.1016/j.wneu.2022.02.034

[24] Perrone R, Malek A, Watnick T. Vascular complications in autosomal dominant polycystic kidney disease. Nature Reviews Nephrology. 2015;**11**:589-598. DOI: 10.1038/nrneph.2015.128

[25] Abecassis IJ, Zeeshan Q, Ghodke BV, Levitt MR, Ellenbogen RG, Sekhar LN. Surgical versus endovascular management of ruptured and unruptured intracranial aneurysms: Emergent issues and future directions. World Neurosurgery. 2020;**136**:17-27. DOI: 10.1016/j.wneu.2019.12.127

[26] Calviere L, Gathier CS, Rafiq M, et al. Rebleeding after aneurysmal subarachnoid hemorrhage in two centers using different blood pressure management strategies. Frontiers in Neurology. 2022;**13**:836268. DOI: 10.3389/fneur.2022.836268

[27] Laskowitz DT, Kolls BJ. Neuroprotection in subarachnoid hemorrhage. Stroke. 2010;**41**(10 Suppl):S79-S84. DOI: 10.1161/STROKEAHA.110.595090

[28] Rigante L, Borghei-Razavi H, Recinos P, Roser F. An overview of endoscopy in neurologic surgery. Cleveland Clinic Journal of Medicine. 2019;**86**(10):16ME-24ME. DOI: 10.3949/ccjm.86.me.18142

[29] Vassilyadi M, Ventureyra EC. Neuroendoscopic intracranial pressure monitoring. Child's Nervous System. 2002;**18**(3-4):147-148. DOI: 10.1007/s00381-001-0549-9

[30] Tsao CW, Aday AW, Almarzooq ZI, et al. Heart disease and stroke statistics—2022 update: A report from the American Heart Association [published correction appears in circulation. 2022 Sep 6;146(10):e141]. Circulation. 2022;**145**(8):e153-e639. DOI: 10.1161/CIR.0000000000001052

[31] Powers WJ, Derdeyn CP, Biller J, et al. 2015 American Heart Association/American Stroke Association focused update of the 2013 guidelines for the early management of patients with acute ischemic stroke regarding endovascular treatment: A guideline for healthcare professionals from the American Heart Association/American Stroke Association. Stroke. 2015;**46**(10):3020-3035. DOI: 10.1161/STR.0000000000000074

[32] Del Brutto VJ, Ardelt A, Loggini A, et al. Clinical characteristics and emergent therapeutic interventions in patients evaluated through the in-hospital stroke alert protocol. Journal of Stroke and Cerebrovascular Diseases. 2019;**28**(5):1362-1370. DOI: 10.1016/j.jstrokecerebrovasdis.2019.02.001

[33] Politi M, Kastrup A, Marmagkiolis K, Grunwald IQ, Papanagiotou P. Endovascular therapy for acute stroke. Progress in Cardiovascular Diseases. 2017;**59**(6):534-541. DOI: 10.1016/j.pcad.2017.03.004

[34] Talke PO, Sharma D, Heyer EJ, Bergese SD, Blackham KA, Stevens RD. Republished: Society for Neuroscience in Anesthesiology and critical care expert consensus statement: Anesthetic management of endovascular treatment for acute ischemic stroke. Stroke. 2014;**45**(8):e138-e150. DOI: 10.1161/STROKEAHA.113.003412

[35] Harrison EL, Hill MD. Is general anesthesia for endovascular thrombectomy helpful or harmful? Canadian Journal of Neurological Sciences. 2021;**49**:1-15. DOI: 10.1017/cjn.2021.218

[36] Feil K, Herzberg M, Dorn F, et al. General anesthesia versus conscious sedation in mechanical thrombectomy. Journal of Stroke. 2021;**23**(1):103-112. DOI: 10.5853/jos.2020.02404

[37] Schönenberger S, Uhlmann L, Hacke W, et al. Effect of conscious sedation vs general anesthesia on early neurological improvement among patients with ischemic stroke undergoing endovascular thrombectomy: A randomized clinical trial. JAMA. 2016;**316**(19):1986-1996. DOI: 10.1001/jama.2016.16623

[38] Löwhagen Hendén P, Rentzos A, Karlsson JE, et al. General anesthesia versus conscious sedation for endovascular treatment of acute ischemic stroke: The AnStroke trial (Anesthesia during stroke). Stroke. 2017;**48**(6):1601-1607. DOI: 10.1161/STROKEAHA.117.016554

[39] Simonsen CZ, Yoo AJ, Sørensen LH, et al. Effect of general anesthesia and conscious sedation during endovascular therapy on infarct growth and clinical outcomes in acute ischemic stroke: A randomized clinical trial. JAMA Neurology. 2018;**75**(4):470-477. DOI: 10.1001/jamaneurol.2017.4474

[40] Ren C, Xu G, Liu Y, Liu G, Wang J, Gao J. Effect of conscious sedation vs. general anesthesia on outcomes in patients undergoing mechanical thrombectomy for acute ischemic stroke:

A prospective randomized clinical trial. Frontiers in Neurology. 2020;**11**:170. DOI: 10.3389/fneur.2020.00170

[41] Pilgram-Pastor SM, Piechowiak EI, Dobrocky T, et al. Stroke thrombectomy complication management. Journal of NeuroInterventional Surgery. 2021;**13**(10):912-917. DOI: 10.1136/neurintsurg-2021-017349

[42] Gubian A, Kausch L, Neumann JO, et al. CT-navigated spinal instrumentations—Three-dimensional evaluation of screw placement accuracy in relation to a screw trajectory plan. Medicina. 2022;**58**(9):1200. DOI: 10.3390/medicina58091200

[43] Perez J. Spinal cord stimulation. Neurología. 2019;**37**:586-595. DOI: 10.1016/j.nrleng.2019.05.007

[44] Debono B, Wainwright TW, Wang MY, et al. Consensus statement for perioperative care in lumbar spinal fusion: Enhanced recovery after surgery (ERAS®) society recommendations. Spine Journal. 2021;**21**(5):729-752. DOI: 10.1016/j.spinee.2021.01.001

[45] Hagan M, Remacle T, Leary O, et al. Navigation techniques in endoscopic spine surgery. BioMed Research International. 2022;**2022**. DOI: 10.1155/2022/8419739 [Online]

[46] Ljungqvist O, Scott M, Fearon KC. Enhanced recovery after surgery: A review. JAMA Surgery. 2017;**152**(3): 292-298

[47] Stumpo V, Staartjes VE, Quddusi A, et al. Enhanced recovery after surgery strategies for elective craniotomy: A systematic review. Journal of Neurosurgery. 2021;**135**(6):1857-1881. DOI: 10.3171/2020.10.JNS203160

[48] Yang X, Ma J, Li K, et al. A comparison of effects of scalp nerve block and local anesthetic infiltration on inflammatory response, hemodynamic response, and postoperative pain in patients undergoing craniotomy for cerebral aneurysms: A randomized controlled trial. BMC Anesthesiology. 2019;**19**(1):91. DOI: 10.1186/s12871-019-0760-4

[49] Sughrue ME, Bonney PA, Choi L, Teo C. Early discharge after surgery for intra-axial brain tumors. World Neurosurgery. 2015;**84**(2):505-510. DOI: 10.1016/j.wneu.2015.04.019

[50] Youngerman BE, Joiner EF, Wang X, et al. Patterns of seizure prophylaxis after oncologic neurosurgery. Journal of Neuro-Oncology. 2020;**146**(1):171-180. DOI: 10.1007/s11060-019-03362-1

[51] Puffer RC, Tou K, Winkel RE, Bydon M, Currier B, Freedman BA. Liposomal bupivacaine incisional injection in single-level lumbar spine surgery. Spine Journal. 2016;**16**(11):1305-1308. DOI: 10.1016/j.spinee.2016.06.013

[52] Grieff AN, Ghobrial GM, Jallo J. Use of liposomal bupivacaine in the postoperative management of posterior spinal decompression. Journal of Neurosurgery: Spine. 2016;**25**(1):88-93

[53] Rengel K, Pandharipande P, Hughes C. Postoperative delirium. La Presse Médicale. 2018;**47**(4):53-64. DOI: 10.1016/j.lpm.2018.03.012

[54] Jin Z, Hu J, Ma D. Postoperative delirium: Perioperative assessment, risk reduction, and management. British Journal of Anesthesia. 2020;**125**(4):492-504. DOI: 10.1016/j.bja.2020.06.063

[55] Gou RY, Hshieh TT, Marcantonio ER, et al. SAGES study group. One-year Medicare costs associated with delirium in older patients undergoing major elective surgery. JAMA Surgery.

2021;**156**(5):430-442. DOI: 10.1001/jamasurg.2020.7260

[56] Migirov A, Chahar P, Maheshwari K. Postoperative delirium and neurocognitive disorders. Current Opinion in Critical Care. 2021;**27**(6):686-693. DOI: 10.1097/MCC.0000000000000882

[57] Inouye SK, Kosar CM, Tommet D, Schmitt EM, Puelle MR, Saczynski JS, et al. The CAM-S: Development and validation of a new scoring system for delirium severity in 2 cohorts. Annals of Internal Medicine. 2014;**160**:526-533

[58] Inouye SK. The CAM-S Training Manual and Coding Guide. Boston: Hospital Elder Life Program; 2014

[59] Albanese AM, Ramazani N, Greene N, Bruse L. Review of postoperative delirium in geriatric patients after hip fracture treatment. Geriatric Orthopaedic Surgery & Rehabilitation. 2022;**13**:21514593211058947. DOI: 10.1177/21514593211058947

[60] Evered L, Chan M, Han R, et al. Anethesthic depth and delirium after major surgery: A randomized clinical trial. British Journal of Anesthesia. 2021;**127**(5):704-712. DOI: 10.1016/j.bja.2021.07.021

[61] Berger M, Schenning K, Brown C, Deiner S, Whittington R, Eckenhoff R. Best practices for postoperative brain health: Recommendations from the fifth international perioperative neurotoxicity working group. Anesthesia and Analgesia. 2018;**127**(6):1406-1413

[62] De Jesus O, Fogwe DT, Mesfin FB, et al. Neuromodulation surgery for psychiatric disorders. In: StatPearls [Internet]. Treasure Island, FL: StatPearls Publishing; 2022 [Updated: 29 August 2022]

[63] Holewijn RA, Verbaan D, van den Munckhof PM, et al. General anesthesia vs local anesthesia in microelectrode recording-guided deep-brain stimulation for Parkinson disease: The GALAXY randomized clinical trial. JAMA Neurology. 2021;**78**(10):1212-1219. DOI: 10.1001/jamaneurol.2021.2979

[64] Zhu R, Zhang Y, Wang T, Wei H, Zhang C, Li D, et al. Deep brain stimulation of nucleus accumbens with anterior capsulotomy for drug addiction: A case report. Stereotactic and Functional Neurosurgery. 2020;**98**(5):345-349

[65] Ransom S, Brown N, Pennington Z, Lakomkin N, Mikula A, Bydon M, et al. Hypothermia therapy for traumatic spinal cord injury: An updated review. Journal of Clinical Medicine. 2022;**11**:1585. DOI: 10.3390/jcm11061585

[66] Relander F, Ruesch A, Yang J, et al. Using near-infrared spectroscopy and a random forest regressor to estimate intracranial pressure. Neurophotonics. 2022;**9**(4):045001. DOI: 10.1117/1.NPh.9.4.045001

Section 8

Psychiatric Medicine

Chapter 12

Anesthetic Concerns in Psychiatric Disease

Maria Martinez-Baladejo, Franzes Anne Z. Liongson, Dustin Wong, Christina Spoleti, Diyor Suyumov, Sanjay V. Menghani, Christopher McCarthy, Alec James Divito, Shani Varghese Daniel, Shilpa Salpekar, Rina Bhalodi, Maaz Siddiqui and Christine Marchionni

Abstract

As the prevalence of mental health illnesses rises worldwide, the use of psychotropic medications follows. Undoubtedly, many patients using psychotropic medications will undergo procedures requiring anesthesia both in the operating room and outside of it. This chapter focuses on psychotropic medications that may complicate the surgical and postoperative course of patients undergoing anesthesia. Toward this aim, we performed a literature review using targeted key terms. Relevant articles were cited, and findings are summarized in this narrative review. We begin with discussing psychotropic medication pharmacology, drug-drug interactions, and side effects, emphasizing their interaction with anesthetic agents. We summarize the current recommendations for managing these medications in the perioperative period. In the discussion section, we focus on highlighting future directions for the intersection between psychotropic medications and anesthesia. Overall, we provide insight into the perioperative management of patients taking psychotropic medications, the point of intersection between the fields of psychiatry and anesthesia.

Keywords: antidepressants, antipsychotics, anxiolytics, stimulants, substances, ketamine, dexmedetomidine, samidorphan, lumateperone, medication-assisted treatments, herbal supplements

1. Introduction

As of 2022, an estimated nearly one billion people around the globe carry a diagnosis of at least one mental health condition or substance dependence disorder [1]. Focusing on the United States, there has been an increase of psychiatric disease prevalence over the last 30 years [2]. Subsequently, there has been a rise in the consumption of psychotropic medications with the greatest increase seen for antidepressants, which are commonly long-term medications [3]. This fact is supported by a study in 2017 finding that in a sample of surveyed patients taking psychotropic medications, 84.3% responded that they had taken their medication for at least 3 years [4].

Given the increase in mental health disorders and subsequent rise in utilization, we expect an increased number of patients presenting for outpatient or inpatient procedures requiring anesthesia. Some of these drugs, if taken in conjunction with sedatives, can have dangerous interactions, and some of these interactions can be life threatening. Thus, anesthesiologists and anesthesia professionals must be informed of the potential side effects, drug-drug interactions, and management of these drugs in the perioperative setting. Furthermore, if discontinued, various psychotropic medications will cause withdrawal symptoms and can impact the patient's well-being and management.

This chapter describes the most used psychotropic medications and herbal supplements used by psychiatric patients. In addition to more commonly known medications, newer agents are discussed, such as dexmedetomidine, the combination of olanzapine and samidorphan, and lumateperone. In the sections that follow, pharmacology, side effects, and drug-drug interactions are discussed and recommendations during the perioperative period from relevant societies and governing bodies.

2. Antidepressants

Depression is one of the most prevalent mental health disorders in the United States. In 2020, an estimated 21.0 million adults in the United States had at least one major depressive episode, roughly 8.4% of all U.S. adults [5]. Per the Diagnostic and Statistical Manual of Mental Disorders (DSM-5), a major depressive episode is defined as a period of at least 2 weeks of experiencing depressed mood or loss of interest or pleasure and symptoms of affected sleep, eating, energy, concentration, or self-worth without the root cause stemming from a medical illness, substance use disorder, or medication [6]. Of those with major depressive episodes, an estimated 66% of U.S. adults received treatment in 2020 [5]. Treatment of depression includes medications, non-pharmaceutical modalities such as electroconvulsive therapy (ECT), or a combination of both. Five major classes of antidepressants include selective serotonin reuptake inhibitors (SSRIs), serotonin and norepinephrine reuptake inhibitors (SNRIs), tricyclic antidepressants (TCAs), monoamine oxidase inhibitors (MAOIs), and atypical antidepressants. Though the primary mechanism of action is relatively known for each of these medication classes, off-target and secondary mechanisms are relatively unknown despite significant investigation. The effectiveness of these medications requires both downregulation of synaptic receptors and activation of secondary messengers to cause a response over the course of time. The process is not immediate, supporting why antidepressants may take two or more weeks for patients to notice clinical improvements [7].

2.1 Selective serotonin reuptake inhibitors

SSRIs are first-line treatment for depression and anxiety and the most widely prescribed class of antidepressants, with examples that include citalopram, escitalopram, fluoxetine, fluvoxamine, paroxetine, and sertraline. The drug is popularly used because it has little effects on the adrenergic, cholinergic (except paroxetine), or histaminergic systems, which minimize its side effect profile by almost exclusively blocking presynaptic reuptake of serotonin to allow increased serotonin levels [8]. Two newer medications, vortioxetine and vilazodone, are considered SSRIs but are hypothesized to also block serotonin uptake through direct modulation of various serotonin receptors. SSRIs should not be stopped perioperatively to avoid discontinuation syndrome. Careful consideration should be taken when monitoring for serotonin syndrome (SS), a life-threatening drug reaction that can lead to autonomic dysfunction (symptoms of hyperthermia, tachycardia, labile blood pressure, diarrhea) and can cause seizures, rhabdomyolysis, renal failure, arrhythmia, coma, and potentially death. Serotonin syndrome can occur when serotonin levels are increased, such as changes in dosages or introducing a new serotonergic agent. Recommendations to avoid pethidine/meperidine, tramadol, pentazocine, and dextromethorphan should be taken to reduce serotonin syndrome risks [8]. Of note, SSRIs are metabolized and interact with the CYP-450 enzymes. Thus, special consideration should be taken when prescribing antiarrhythmics, benzodiazepines, and neuromuscular blocking medications in patients who are taking SSRIs. Some SSRIs are inhibitors of CYP2D6, such as escitalopram, fluoxetine, sertraline, paroxetine, and citalopram [9]. Fluvoxamine and fluoxetine inhibit CYP2C19, while fluvoxamine inhibits CYP1A2 [9]. Finally, QT prolongation can occur (particularly with citalopram) and can affect platelet function resulting in abnormal bleeding [10].

2.2 Serotonin-norepinephrine reuptake inhibitors

The mechanism of action for SNRIs is through inhibiting the reuptake of both serotonin and norepinephrine in the synaptic cleft while minimizing effects to other neurotransmitters. This class includes desvenlafaxine, duloxetine, levomilnacipran, milnacipran, and venlafaxine. SNRIs should not be stopped perioperatively to avoid discontinuation syndrome. Primarily due to their norepinephrine reuptake inhibition, SNRIs can cause tachycardia and hypertension and may require tighter blood pressure control. SNRIs can also cause side effects of sexual dysfunction, mydriasis, urinary constriction, dry mouth, dizziness, and sedation. Like SSRIs, SNRIs have a potential of causing serotonin syndrome and are linked with inhibition of platelet aggregation. It is recommended to avoid pethidine/meperidine, tramadol, pentazocine, and dextromethorphan to reduce serotonin syndrome risks [8]. Likewise, venlafaxine inhibits the CYP-450 enzymes, but desvenlafaxine (active metabolite) will not [10]. Thus, it is important to keep this fact in mind when prescribing antiarrhythmics, benzodiazepines, and neuromuscular blocking medications during anesthesia in patients who are taking SNRIs.

2.3 Tricyclic antidepressants

Tricyclic antidepressants (TCAs) are relatively older antidepressants, having been discovered earlier than SSRIs and the newer SNRIs. TCAs are so named after their chemical structure containing three rings. Specific medications in the TCA class include amitriptyline, amoxapine, doxepin, desipramine, nortriptyline, protriptyline, imipramine, and trimipramine. TCAs act on roughly five different neurotransmitter pathways, but receive its antidepressant effects by blocking serotonin and norepinephrine reuptake in presynaptic terminals [11]. Attached to its ring structure is either a secondary amine (desipramine, nortriptyline, protriptyline) that causes greater norepinephrine uptake blockade or tertiary amine (amitriptyline, clomipramine, doxepin, imipramine, trimipramine) that causes greater serotonin reuptake blockade.

Since these medications are also competitive antagonists of alpha-1 adrenergic, alpha-2 adrenergic, muscarinic, and histaminergic receptors, they can lead to unwanted side effects of dizziness, memory impairment, and drowsiness among other symptoms [12].

Though TCAs have displayed efficacy in treating depression (arguably equivocal efficacy to SSRIs), their side-effect profile has dissuaded many providers from using them first line. One of the feared complications with TCAs includes cardiac conduction changes that include QT prolongation, Torsade de Pointes, and sudden cardiac death [13]. Special consideration and caution should be taken when prescribing sympathomimetics (such as ketamine, ephedrine, or metaraminol) in patients taking TCAs to avoid hypertensive crises. TCAs are also known to reduce seizure threshold, and when taken in combination with tramadol, clomipramine, and maprotiline, they may place patients at higher risk for seizures [14, 15]. Notably, TCAs can have sedative properties (particularly amitriptyline and doxepin), which may augment anesthetic sedatives. Abruptly discontinuing the medication can lead to rhinorrhea, muscle aches, chills, and malaise [14]. In *in vitro* studies, TCAs have shown mild inhibitory effects on the CYP450 enzymes CYP1A2, CYP2D6, and CYP2C19 [16]. Interaction with CYP1A2 can cause a theoretical alteration in clearance rate of ropivacaine, a local anesthetic, but this interaction has not been studied extensively clinically [17]. CYP2D6 causes activation of anesthetic medications such as codeine and tramadol to their active form and, if disrupted, can lead to less pain control [18]. CYP2C19 enzymes can affect the clearance of diazepam, which is commonly utilized perioperatively [19]. These interactions are important to keep in mind when a patient taking TCAs is to undergo anesthesia for an upcoming procedure.

2.4 Monoamine oxidase inhibitors

Monoamine oxidase inhibitors (MAOIs) are a relatively older class of antidepressants. They are not used as commonly in clinical practice in comparison with SSRIs or SNRIs due primarily to their side effect profile. Monoamine oxidases are enzymes that break down serotonin and norepinephrine. Inhibition of these enzymes leads to a reduced decline in serotonin and norepinephrine levels. MAOIs can be reversible (moclobemide) or irreversible (phenelzine, tranylcypromine, isocarboxazid). If an irreversible MAOI binds, the enzyme is permanently inactivated, leading to prolonged effects; therefore, more caution should be taken with individuals on irreversible MAOIs before initiating anesthesia.

The primary anesthesia concern for patients taking MAOIs is concern for hypertensive crisis as sympathomimetics like phenylephrine or ketamine can precipitate these crises. Additionally, meperidine and dextromethorphan should be avoided for patients on MAOIs as it can precipitate a serotonergic crisis due to synergistic inhibition of serotonin reuptake [15]. The MAOI phenelzine can prolong neuromuscular blockade and should be cautioned with administration of succinylcholine. The benefits and risks should be weighed when deciding between discontinuing MAOIs, but are often discontinued perioperatively and would recommend a 2-week washout prior [8]. MAOIs are also known to interact with several liver enzymes, most notably CYP3A4 and CYP2C19 [20]. As mentioned above, interactions with anesthetic medications may occur with CYP2D6 (codeine and tramadol), CYP1A2 (ropivacaine), and CYP2C19 (diazepam) [17–19].

2.5 Atypical antidepressants

There are several antidepressants used in clinical practice that are not part of the other classic families, as they have alternative mechanisms of action. Three of these atypical antidepressants are mirtazapine, trazodone, and bupropion.

Mirtazapine has both 5-HT2 and 5-HT3 antagonistic effects, which provides both anxiolytic and antiemetic properties. It also has antihistaminic properties that help with insomnia at low doses and commonly utilized is its side effect to increase appetite and promote weight gain. Mirtazapine may also help postoperative nausea and vomiting [21]. It is also extensively metabolized by CYP2D6, CYP3A4, and CYP1A2 [22].

Trazodone blocks serotonin reuptake, histamine, and alpha-1-adrenergic receptors; therefore, it is used as an antidepressant but also commonly as a sleep agent. Trazodone has a risk of QT prolongation and can lead to excess somnolence during procedures and, however, can be continued perioperatively [23].

Bupropion inhibits dopamine and norepinephrine, and has a chemical structure similar to amphetamines. It increases risk of seizures and neuroleptic malignant syndrome [24]. Notably, atypical antidepressants do not significantly interact with epinephrine and can be perioperatively continued [25].

2.6 Ketamine

Ketamine was first synthesized in the 1960s and initially approved as an anesthetic agent. Though ketamine continues to be used in treatment-refractory migraines and acutely agitated patients, it was recently approved for antidepressant use with potent anti-suicidal effects [26]. Esketamine, the S-enantiomer of ketamine, is clinically indicated for adults with major depressive disorder with or without acute suicidal ideation or behavior [27]. It functions as a glutamate N-methyl-D-aspartate (NMDA) receptor antagonist. Ketamine has sedative, anesthetic, amnesia, and analgesic properties [28, 29]. Ketamine may also interact with other medications utilized in the psychiatric patient and have lower efficacy as an antidepressant, notably the mood stabilizer lamotrigine [30]. The mechanism of action of lamotrigine is believed to be inhibition of sodium and calcium channels in presynaptic neurons and decreased glutamine, and increased GABA release. The decreased glutamate release can reduce ketamine anesthetic response in patients [31].

Anesthetic providers should carefully screen patients for ketamine prescription or recreational use and confirm with primary/consulting teams whether ketamine was used during patient care. It is important to accurately determine the overall amount of ketamine administered to avoid ketamine poisoning. High doses may cause an increase in systemic and pulmonary artery pressure, increase in cardiac outpatient, tachycardia, and respiratory arrest [28].

2.7 Discontinuation syndrome

When preparing for the use of anesthetics, abruptly discontinuing a patient's antidepressants can result in discontinuation syndrome or withdrawal symptoms. Rarely do symptoms become serious but discontinuing antidepressants with anticholinergic effects can lead to symptoms of cholinergic rebound, such as nausea, vomiting, abdominal cramping, sweating, headache, and muscle spasms. Discontinuing MAOIs can result in flu-like symptoms, dysphoria, restlessness, tachycardia, hypertension, and a delirium-like state. Discontinuing serotoninergic antidepressants may cause dizziness, weakness, nausea, headache, lethargy, insomnia, anxiety, poor concentration, and paresthesia [32]. Because the discontinuation symptoms may be worse than possible interactions with anesthetics, the recommendations provided can help guide individuals in the discussion of risks and benefits for each of their medications.

Please refer to Summary Table for a summarized view of side effects and recommendations at the end of the chapter.

3. Anxiolytics

Anxiolysis is of particular concern both to psychiatrists and to anesthesiologists. In practice, both specialties share several medications that they can prescribe to achieve this desired effect in their patients. Perhaps the most historically used anxiolytics are the benzodiazepines. In addition to benzodiazepines, other anxiolytics include buspirone and hydroxyzine, among others.

3.1 Benzodiazepines

Several examples of medications within the benzodiazepine class include alprazolam, chlordiazepoxide, clonazepam, clorazepate, diazepam, estazolam, flunitrazepam, flurazepam, loflazepate, lorazepam, midazolam, oxazepam, quazepam, temazepam, and triazolam. Benzodiazepines work primarily as positive allosteric modulators on the gamma amino butyric acid (GABA)-A receptor, which is a chloride channel [33, 34]. This association between benzodiazepines and the $GABA_A$ receptor has been well established, so much so that before known as $GABA_A$, this receptor was known as the "benzodiazepine receptor" [35]. The receptor itself is a pentamer of two alpha, two beta, and a gamma subunit. Benzodiazepines are allosteric modulators, which bind to the extracellular domain making the receptor adopt the pore conformation. Additional receptor subtypes confer differential responsivity to benzodiazepines [35].

Beyond anxiolysis, benzodiazepines are used for other reasons in anesthesia. Notable is their use as amnestic and premedication for procedures, from those requiring general anesthesia to procedures of shorter duration. Benzodiazepines are thought to impair memory formation by impairing new information acquisition [36]. A meta-analysis found that for general anesthesia and general anesthesia with inhalational maintenance, benzodiazepine premedication seemed to have a protective role in preventing implicit memory formation. However, the result was not significant for benzodiazepine premedication and general anesthesia with intravenous maintenance. The reason may be that the intravenous maintenance administration of propofol is already impacting memory and confounding the effect [37]. During surgery, benzodiazepines reduce awareness compared to thiopental, ketamine, and placebo [38]. A meta-analysis found that while benzodiazepines do increase time to recover, time to discharge is unaffected while the incidence of postoperative side effects is reduced. Psychological outcomes are not significant [39]. It is important to mention that the benzodiazepines triazolam, alprazolam, brotizolam, and midazolam are primarily metabolized by CYP3A4 [40]. As mentioned above, specific antidepressants like MAOIs and mirtazapine are metabolized by CYP3A4, leading to a potential interaction between benzodiazepine administration in the perioperative period and home antidepressant use.

Two additional considerations for the use of benzodiazepines in anesthesia are the treatment of serotonin syndrome and perioperative alcohol withdrawal. Benzodiazepine infusions are used to prevent rhabdomyolysis in serotonin syndrome-associated increased muscle tone [41]. Intravenous benzodiazepines are used for acute withdrawal syndrome in the perioperative context; it is important that the anesthetist distinguishes the syndrome from delirium, which is notably not treated with benzodiazepines [42].

3.2 Remimazolam

A relatively new benzodiazepine, remimazolam, was approved for use by the United States Food and Drug Administration (FDA) in 2021 and its effects in the perioperative setting are less studied. Remimazolam is a rapidly metabolized benzodiazepine with high organ-independent elimination clearance and no active metabolites. Remimazolam does not seem to have a prolonged sedative effect. It was shown to be non-inferior to midazolam for providing adequate sedation when co-administered with opioids, and non-inferior to propofol for induction and maintenance of general anesthesia [43]. It has smaller effects on the respiratory and circulatory systems than propofol and midazolam, and may be a potentially safer option for pediatric, geriatric, and obese populations and those with multiple comorbidities. However, additional work is needed to determine safety of long-term use and use in ICU sedation, and to determine optimal dosing for specific indications [44, 45].

3.3 Benzodiazepine-associated risks and adverse events

Benzodiazepines are associated with some risks in anesthesia, for short and long term. In immediate use, emergent agitation, allergy, and paradoxical reaction should be kept in mind. Paradoxical reactions occur at a frequency of $<1\%$ and are possibly associated with alcohol use. This phenomenon is thought to be caused by genetic predisposition due to $GABA_A$ subunit expression generating heterogeneous receptor isoforms [46]. Considering emergence agitation, benzodiazepine premedication increases the risk of emergence agitation and may be a greater risk in patients with long-term benzodiazepine use [47]. Also considering patients with long-term benzodiazepine use, it was shown that the amount of propofol required for intravenous sedation was significantly lower in those with long-term benzodiazepine use compared to the control; this finding was not influenced by preoperative oral benzodiazepine administration on the day of procedure [48]. Finally, benzodiazepine allergy is exceedingly rare and difficult to assess due to the likelihood of multiple other exposures occurring. If a benzodiazepine allergy is documented, alternatives for anxiolysis and sedation do exist [49].

A 2022 study discussed the important consideration for abuse potential. First, general anesthesia was associated with new postoperative benzodiazepine use that occurred 90–180 days post-surgery. General anesthesia was also more associated with new postoperative benzodiazepine use than neuraxial anesthesia. Perioperative benzodiazepine use was associated with postoperative persistent benzodiazepine use. Additionally, 15.2% and 4.9% of patients with new benzodiazepine prescriptions continued to use benzodiazepines for 1 and 8 years after, respectively. Additional risk factors for new postoperative use of benzodiazepines were orthopedic surgery, pre-existing malignancy, anxiety disorder, concurrent systemic steroid use, postoperative complications, and admission to ICU, among others [50].

3.4 Considerations for the geriatric population

There is no formal defining age of "geriatric" or "elderly." Study designs may define onset as early as 50 years, however 65 years is frequently seen. The American Geriatric Society Beers Criteria recommend that elderly patients avoid benzodiazepines in the treatment of insomnia due the risks of cognitive impairment and falls [51]. Although the risks of benzodiazepine use in the elderly are common knowledge, their use remains disproportionately high in the elderly. In a United States national survey, prevalence of benzodiazepine use in non-institutionalized adults was 3.8%, while in a Dutch survey of the elderly, prevalence approached 8% [52]. One systematic review measured the prevalence of potentially inappropriate prescription (PIP; percentage of cohort taking at least one potentially inappropriate medication) of multiple drug classes in elderly patients with dementia. The authors found the most prescribed potentially inappropriate medications were anxiolytic-hypnotic and anticholinergic medications. Rates of anxiolytic-hypnotic use ranged from 5 to 38% [53]. One meta-analysis associated their use with falls in the elderly and found an odd ratios of 2.00 for short-acting benzodiazepines, 2.16 for long-acting, and 1.67 for any benzodiazepine use compared to elderly patients not taking benzodiazepines [54]. Therefore, continued work to publicize the danger of benzodiazepine use in the geriatric population is indicated.

3.5 Non-benzodiazepine anxiolytics

In addition to benzodiazepines, buspirone and hydroxyzine are used as anxiolytics. Buspirone is a serotonin 1A preceptor partial agonist that is effective in treating generalized anxiety disorder but is not first line [55]. Buspirone is thought to be safe intraoperatively but should be avoided in the context of administration with meperidine or tramadol due to a theoretical risk of serotonin syndrome [56, 57]. Hydroxyzine is an antihistamine medication with anxiolytic and sedative effects [58]. Hydroxyzine has been studied in the context of preventing preoperative anxiety in the pediatric population but has been shown to have limited resulting efficacy [59]. It has been FDA approved for perioperative sedation, but it has been largely replaced by alternative agents for this purpose.

4. Mood stabilizers

Bipolar disorder is a chronic psychiatric illness characterized by episodes of alternating mania or hypomania and depression, or mixed features of depression and mania. The lifetime prevalence is estimated to be approximately 3–7% and annual incidence of 3–10 cases per 100,000 population [60]. The diagnosis of Bipolar I Disorder is made if there is any lifetime episode of mania, whereas Bipolar II Disorder is diagnosed if there is at least one lifetime episode of hypomania and one lifetime episode of depression. Many patients with bipolar disorder are treated with mood stabilizers which can affect preoperative, perioperative, and postoperative outcomes. Some of the medications interact with the commonly used anesthetic agents and require a decision whether they need to be continued or held prior to a surgical procedure. There are many mood stabilizers on the market today, including lithium, antipsychotics, and anti-epileptic Drugs (AEDs) such as valproic acid, carbamazepine, and lamotrigine. This section will focus on lithium and AEDs as they are the most commonly used mood stabilizers.

4.1 Lithium

Lithium is commonly used as a first-line mood stabilizer in people suffering acute manic episodes in bipolar disorder, as well as mixed and depressive episodes. Its exact mechanism of action is uncertain but is believed to affect multiple molecular pathways involved in neurotransmission. Lithium enters cells, modifies sodium transport in nerve and muscle cells, and impacts secondary messenger systems *via* inhibition of inositol monophosphate (IMP), which affects phosphatidylinositol and neurotransmission. It also decreases protein kinase C, which alters gene expression involved in neurotransmission [61].

Lithium has a narrow therapeutic index, ranging from 0.6 mmol to 1.2 mmol/L. Dosing is guided by plasma lithium levels. Above 1.5 mmol/L concentration, lithium induces dose-related intoxication, including tremors, vomiting, confusion, diarrhea, increased deep tendon reflexes, hypotension, seizures, and death [62]. As it is renally excreted, plasma lithium levels are sensitive to changes in patient's renal function and volume status. Medications that affect renal function, such as diuretics, angiotensin-converting enzyme inhibitors, and non-steroidal anti-inflammatory drugs, can increase lithium concentration and lead to toxicity [63]. For these reasons, caution must be taken pre- and postoperatively to monitor patient's volume status and renal function.

Ideally, patients on lithium therapy should have lithium discontinued at least 48–72 hours prior to a surgical procedure owing to its half-life off 24–36 hours [8]. As lithium does not have discontinuation side effects, it is safe to discontinue abruptly. For anesthesia purposes, administration of lithium prolongs depolarization and polarization phase of neuromuscular blockade by acting additively with depolarizing neuromuscular agents and synergistically with non-depolarizing neuromuscular agents. [63] As a result, it can prolong neuromuscular blockade [64, 65]. As a precaution, all patients treated with lithium undergoing neuromuscular blockage should be monitored appropriately.

4.2 Valproic acid

Valproic acid is a commonly prescribed anti-epileptic agent used for mood stabilization alone or with another medication to treat manic, mixed, or depressive episodes of bipolar disorder. It exerts its anti-seizure activity by blocking voltage-gated sodium channels, thereby decreasing the frequency of neuronal firing [66]. It also increases levels of GABA in the CNS. Side effects can include sedation, tremors, dizziness, thrombocytopenia, elevated liver enzymes. Serious side effects include Steven Johnson Syndrome, hyponatremia, syndrome of inappropriate anti-diuretic hormone release (SIADH), encephalopathy, and coma. Abrupt discontinuation can cause withdrawal seizures [66].

In general, valproic acid (VPA) can be continued peri-operatively for patients treated with bipolar disorder and does not need to be stopped, although it can interact with anesthetic agents. Some research shows that VPA is highly plasma protein bound and presence of other highly protein bound medications can increase free VPA plasma concentrations [67]. Certain highly protein bound anesthetics such as propofol can have their levels increased in the presence of VPA [68]. Similarly, VPA can decrease clearance of propofol by competing for the same liver enzymes (CYP3A4) that metabolize them [69, 70]. Another consideration is increased bleeding risk, which is thought to be caused by platelet dysfunction and associated decrease in platelet count, fibrinogen, protein C, factor VII, and factor VIII [67]. It is therefore recommended to assess preoperative bleeding risk and to obtain baseline hemostasis and coagulation factors such as bleeding time, platelet count, Prothrombin Time (PT), Activated Thromboplastin Time (aPTT), von Willebrand factor, and fibrinogen.

4.3 Carbamazepine

Carbamazepine is another AED that is used as a mood stabilizer to treat manic or mixed episodes of bipolar disorder. Carbamazepine exerts its effect primarily *via* binding and inactivation of voltage-gated sodium channels, thereby decreasing neuronal action potential and neurotransmission. Side effects of carbamazepine include dizziness, sedation, dry mouth, ataxia, nausea, and vomiting. Serious side effects include hyponatremia, agranulocytosis, hepatotoxicity, confusion, and serious dermatologic reaction [71].

Carbamazepine can be continued perioperatively. But it is a strong cytochrome p450 inducer. Medications that use CYP450 can have their levels reduced in the presence of carbamazepine, including neuromuscular blocking agents. Specifically, the duration of effect of non-depolarizing aminosteroid neuromuscular blockers such as vecuronium is shortened [15]. Therefore, neuromuscular blockade may need to be administered more frequently or at a higher dose. A structurally similar mood stabilizer, oxcarbazepine, is associated with lesser CYP450 induction and is considered safer in terms of interactions (refer to Summary Table section for preoperative recommendations) [72].

4.4 Lamotrigine

Lamotrigine is another mood stabilizer found to be effective in treating depression associated with bipolar disorder [73]. Its mechanism of action is not entirely clear but is believed to stabilize presynaptic neuronal membrane *via* blockade of voltage gated sodium channels and decrease the release of excitatory neurotransmitters such as glutamate. Side effects include visual disturbance, headaches, dizziness, tremors, agitation, and in rare cases, serious dermatological side effects such as Steven Johnson Syndrome [74].

In general, lamotrigine can be continued and does not need to be held for surgery or anesthesia. However, some data suggest that the dissociative effects of ketamine anesthetic can be decreased in the presence of lamotrigine since ketamine's dissociative effects are thought to be due to augmentation of glutamate neurotransmission [75]. The implication of this effect is important to consider since ketamine is commonly used as a procedural anesthetic.

Medications used to treat bipolar disorder can be safely continued perioperatively but sometimes pose a challenge to potential drug-drug interactions. Of the mentioned medications, it is recommended that lithium be discontinued prior to procedures requiring anesthesia or sedation, and appropriate patient monitoring is important if the decision is made to continue lithium.

The summary of side effects and recommendations can be found in the Summary Table at the end of the chapter.

5. Antipsychotics

Approximately 0.25–0.64% of people living in the United States have schizophrenia and related disorders, which are characterized by psychosis [76–78]. Psychosis itself is characterized by the presence of hallucinations, delusions, or both in such a way that disrupts a patient's capacity to meet the ordinary demands of life [79]. Antipsychotics, classified as first-generation antipsychotics (FGAs), and second-generation antipsychotics (SGAs), are pharmacologic treatment options for bipolar disorder, acute psychosis, psychotic disorders such as schizophrenia, agitation, and schizoaffective disorder. In this section, we will briefly discuss FGAs and SGAs, their mechanism of action, adverse effects, and considerations for anesthesia or perioperative use.

5.1 First- and second-generation antipsychotics

The proposed mechanism of action of antipsychotics is post-synaptic blockade of dopamine D2 receptors in the brain. Adverse effects in this medication class include tardive dyskinesia (TD), extrapyramidal symptoms (EPS), hyperprolactinemia, neuroleptic malignant syndrome (NMS), weight gain, insulin resistance, QT prolongation, and sudden death, among others. Many of these agents are metabolized *via* the cytochrome P450 (CYP450) system, so drug-drug interactions and altered plasma medication levels when used in individuals with altered hepatic function or with agents that act on the CYP450 system. Of note, CYP gene polymorphisms can alter metabolism of antipsychotics. For example, individuals with CYP-2D6, a cytochrome gene polymorphism, are slow metabolizers and typically have higher plasma levels of antipsychotics, which lead to increased risk of more severe adverse effects [80].

First-generation antipsychotics (neuroleptics, conventional or typical antipsychotics, FGAs) include fluphenazine, haloperidol, loxapine, perphenazine, pimozide, thiothixene, trifluoperazine, chlorpromazine, and thioridazine. Although the agents in this class act *via* D2 dopamine blockade, they vary based on their effects on neuronal 5-HT2, alpha-1 sympathetic, histamine, and anticholinergic receptors, which can correspond to the differences in their adverse effect profiles as seen in **Table 1**.

Second-generation antipsychotics (atypical antipsychotics, SGAs) include aripiprazole, asenapine, brexpiprazole, cariprazine, clozapine, iloperidone, lumateperone, lurasidone, olanzapine, paliperidone, pimavanserin, quetiapine, risperidone, and ziprasidone. Generally preferred over FGAs due to their side effect profile seen in **Table 1**, most medications in this class of antipsychotics differ from FGAs due to their increased affinity for serotonin 5HT2 receptors relative to dopamine D2 receptors. Decreased risk of EPS in SGAs compared to FGAs is thought to be due to 5HT2 activity.

In the perioperative setting, the adverse effect profile of antipsychotic medications should be considered. The four key adverse effects in focus are anticholinergic effects, orthostatic hypotension, QT prolongation, and sedation. Direct inhibition of the cardiac delayed potassium rectifier channels is the proposed mechanism for the increased risk of QT prolongation, Torsade de Pointes, and sudden death with all antipsychotics [81]. Thioridazine and quetiapine are the FGA and SGA, respectively, associated with the highest risk of QT prolongation. Olanzapine, an SGA, has been suggested to cause some of the least changes in QTc [82]. When preparing for anesthesia clearance, a

	Anticholinergic effects	Orthostatic hypotension	QTC prolongation	Sedation
First-generation antipsychotics (GFA, typical, conventional)				
Chlorpromazine	↑↑	↑↑	↑↑	↑↑
Fluphenazine	↑	↑	↑	↑
Haloperidol	↑	↑	Oral: ↑ IV:↑↑	↑
Loxapine	↑	↑	—	↑
Perphenazine	↑	↑	—	↑
Pimozide	↑	↑	↑	↑
Thioridizine	↑↑	↑↑	↑	↑↑
Thiothixene	↑	↑	—	↑
Trifluoperazine	↑	↑	—	↑
Second-generation antipsychotics (SGA, atypical)				
Aripiprazole	↑	↑	—	↑
Asenapine	↑	↑	↑	↑
Brexipiprazole	↑	↑	—	↑
Cariprazine	↑	↑	—	↑
Clozapine	↑↑	↑↑	↑	↑↑
Iloperidone	↑	↑↑	↑	↑
Lumateperone	↑	↑	—	↑
Lurasidone	↑	↑	—	↑
Olanzapine	↑	↑	↑	↑↑
Paliperidone	↑	↑	↑	↑
Pimavanserin	↑	↑	↑	↑
Quetiapine	↑	↑	↑	↑↑
Risperidone	↑	↑	↑	↑
Ziprasidone	↑	↑	↑↑	↑

In this table, the "↑" sign is used to signify mild- to moderately increased risk of side effect. The "↑↑" sign is used to signify severely increased risk of side effect. The "-" is used to indicate no clinically significant increased risk.

Table 1.
Side effect profile of antipsychotics.

standard pre-operative electrocardiogram (ECG) is recommended to determine if a patient has prolonged QTc [15]. Since many antipsychotics cause sedation due to H1 receptor antagonism, a decreased anesthetic requirement may be considered during surgery. Chlorpromazine and thioridazine are the most sedating of the FGAS, and clozapine and olanzapine are the most sedating of the SGA. In general, SGAs are typically less sedating than FGAs and would be preferable when planning for anesthetic intervention [83].

First- and second-generation antipsychotics should be continued in the perioperative setting in order to avoid exacerbation of underlying psychiatric disorder, postoperative delirium, and discontinuation syndrome as described in Section 5.2. Due to the effects of antipsychotics on blood pressure, seizure threshold, and temperature regulation, enflurane should be avoided due to increased risk of hypotension, arrhythmias, and seizures if used concurrently [84].

5.2 Discontinuation syndrome

Dopamine blockade from antipsychotics over a prolonged period of time can cause hypersensitivity of dopamine receptors. When the dopamine antagonists are abruptly stopped, the body's own physiologic dopamine can cause overstimulation of these receptors, causing the symptoms of withdrawal. Thus, to discontinue the use of antipsychotics, the recommendation is to taper them off gradually over at least 6–12 months. Abrupt discontinuation of first- or second-generation antipsychotics can cause tachycardia, anxiety, diaphoresis, insomnia, dyskinesia, hyperkinesia, myalgia, dry mucus membranes, in addition to GI symptoms such as nausea, vomiting, diarrhea, and abdominal pain [85]. These symptoms can last up to one to 4 weeks, and the only way to prevent them is to slowly taper the dose of antipsychotics if cessation is required [86].

5.3 Postoperative concerns

There are postoperative concerns with continued use and abrupt cessation of antipsychotics. Antipsychotics have been implicated in causing paralytic ileus due to the drugs' anticholinergic and noradrenergic effects. In a database review of 26,720 patients, one study showed statistical significance in clozapine causing postoperative ileus [85] which can be concerning especially in patients with schizophrenia due to potential decreased pain awareness and subsequent decreased awareness of symptoms that lead to ileus. Also, antipsychotic drugs can increase risk of hypotension due to α-adrenergic blockade. Of the FGAs, thioridazine and chlorpromazine are most commonly associated with postoperative hypotension [81, 87]. Conversely, abrupt discontinuation of antipsychotics can increase incidence of delirium and further supports recommendations to continue this medication perioperatively [88].

5.4 Neuroleptic malignant syndrome

Neuroleptic malignant syndrome (NMS) is a life-threatening neurological emergency associated with antipsychotic use during which decreased serotonin inhibition and dopaminergic blockade in the anterior hypothalamus led to sympathetic dysregulation [87, 88]. The clinical picture consists of hyperthermia, muscle rigidity, altered mental status, motor abnormalities (bradykinesia), and autonomic dysfunction (blood pressure and heart rate lability) [89]. Although commonly associated with use of FGAs such as haloperidol or fluphenazine, all neuroleptic drugs have been implicated, including low-potency drugs such as chlorpromazine [90, 91]. NMS has also been seen with use of antiemetic medications such as metoclopramide or promethazine [92–94]. Frequently seen following medication initiation or dosage changes, NMS can also occur up to several weeks after starting treatment NMS can persist a week after the causal agent has been discontinued [95–97]. Although most patients with NMS are young adults, the syndrome has been described in all age groups from 0.9 to 78 years, and age is not considered a risk factor for its development, although infection, severe trauma, and surgery may precipitate NMS [98].

It is important to distinguish the clinical presentation of NMS from malignant hyperthermia (MH) and serotonin syndrome (SS). MH can be distinguished by two primary features in clinical history: spasms in the masseter muscles with the administration of succinyl choline, as its earliest indicator. Subsequently, the development of tachypnea, tachycardia, increased carbon dioxide concentrations, and acidosis occur during the induction or maintenance of anesthesia [99]. This causes hyperthermia and cyanosis, which can lead to stiffness and rhabdomyolysis [95]. If left untreated or misdiagnosed, MH can be fatal. NMS can also be confused with serotonin syndrome (SS), but they can be differentiated by onset time. SS starts within hours or a day of initiation or dose change of the drug, while NMS typical symptoms progress over one to three days and have a later onset (1–44 days) compared to SS [100, 101]. The pathophysiology of NMS, MH, and SS is different. Misdiagnoses and, subsequently, mistreatments can be prevented with a detailed medical history. See **Table 2** for a more detailed evaluation of NMS in contrast to malignant hyperthermia and SS.

6. Stimulants

Central nervous system (CNS) stimulants comprise a drug class that causes excitation of the cerebral cortex, brain stem, and spinal cord [102]. This drug class is widely used in the clinical setting and is also often used recreationally. Stimulants are commonly used in the clinical setting for attention deficit hyperactivity disorder, depression, chronic fatigue, and narcolepsy. Stimulants can cause side effects such as euphoria, anxiety, insomnia, psychosis, and seizures.

Recent evidence supports that approximately 17.2 million American adults or 6.6% of the American adult population used prescription stimulants from 2015 to 2016 [103]. Commonly used stimulants include amphetamines, caffeine, cocaine, methylphenidate, and modafinil. As a drug class, stimulants are considered to have high potential for misuse due to their euphoric properties [104]. In fact, there were 1.1 million users of recreational stimulants among persons 12 years or older in the United States as of 2010 [105]. Due to the prevalence of stimulant use in the population, it is probable that some of the individuals who use stimulants, prescription or recreational, will undergo anesthesia. Subsequently, it is imperative that practitioners understand how to manage the pharmacologic interactions and effects of stimulants with anesthetics to ensure optimal care.

6.1 Amphetamines

Amphetamines are synthetic methylphenethylamine derivatives that act by inhibiting monoamine reuptake by the norepinephrine transporter (NET) and the dopamine active transporter (DAT), reversing their normal activity and increasing neurotransmitter displacement from neuronal vesicles in the cortex, motor nuclei, and reticular-activating system [106]. Acute stimulant intoxication results in sympathetic activation including agitation, hypertension, hyperthermia, tachycardia, and tachypnea [107]. Methylenedioxymethamphetamine, MDMA or ecstasy, is a stimulant that may present with a toxidrome or fever, hyponatremia, rhabdomyolysis, renal injury, and liver injury [108].

This group includes mixed amphetamines, methamphetamine ("crystal meth"), and MDMA. MDMA also is a weak agonist of the 5-hydroxytryptamine/serotonin 1A (5-HT1A) receptor, which may be responsible for its hallucinogenic properties [106].

	Neuroleptic malignant syndrome	Malignant hyperthermia	Serotonin syndrome
Associated drugs	First-generation antipsychotics, antiemetic drugs	Administration of inhaled anesthetics (ex: halothane, isoflurane, sevoflurane, desflurane) with or without succinylcholine	Combination of any of the following: SSRI's, SNRI's, MAOI's, TCA's, Linezolid, oxycodone, morphine
Mechanism of action	Unknown but likely dopamine receptor blockade (hypothalamic dopamine blockade leading to dysautonomia and nigrostriatal dopamine blockage leading to parkinsonian-type symptoms)	Dihydropyridine (DHP) receptors and Ryanodine (RYP) receptors within the muscle cells normally regulate the movement of calcium into the intracellular space. In MH-susceptible patients, there is a mutation in the DHP or RYP1receptors, and thus unregulated movement of calcium from the sarcoplasmic reticulum. The accumulation of calcium causes the classic symptoms.	Serotonin Syndrome (SS) results from the concomitant use of drugs that have the net effect of increasing serotonin release (stimulation of the post-synaptic 5-HT1A and 5-HT2A)
Symptoms	Classic Tetrad: fever, rigidity, mental status change, autonomic instability Later onset-days	Sustained muscle contractions causing muscle rigidity, tachycardia, tachypnea, hyperthermia	Hyperthermia, hyperreflexia, clonus Earlier onset-within hours
Diagnosis	Clinical with history of antipsychotics or other associated medications	Clinical diagnosis, also suspect with hypercarbia, when the end-tidal CO_2 continues to increase despite increasing minute ventilation	Clinical diagnosis can use the Hunter Toxicity Criteria Decision Rules: must have the presence of a serotonergic agent and have one of the following: • Spontaneous clonus • Inducible clonus plus agitation or diaphoresis • Ocular clonus plus agitation or diaphoresis • Tremor plus hyperreflexia • Hypertonia plus temperature above 38°C PLUS ocular clonus or inducible clonus
Lab findings	Elevated CK, leukocytosis, low serum iron, hypocalcemia, hyperkalemia	Hypercarbia, mixed respiratory/metabolic acidosis, hyperkalemia, myoglobinuria	Leukocytosis, elevated CPK, decreased serum bicarbonate
Treatment	1. Stop offending agent 2. Supportive Care 3. If severe manifestations, dantrolene, benzodiazepines, bromocriptine, or amantadine	Dantrolene ASAP—it binds to ryanodine receptors to stop the release of calcium, acts as a skeletal muscle relaxant. Treat electrolyte abnormalities, institute cooling, cardiovascular support Make sure to take a good family history to prevent an episode.	1. Stop offending agent 2. Supportive Care 3. Sedation with benzodiazepines to control agitation, which can worsen the muscle contractions/hyperthermia 4. If nothing helps, use Cyproheptadine, a 5-HT1A, and 5-HT2A antagonist

Table 2.
Comparison of neuroleptic malignant syndrome, malignant hyperthermia, and serotonin syndrome.

As a group, amphetamines lead to euphoria, wakefulness, increased concentration, and tachycardia. Prescription amphetamines are commonly used for attention deficit hyperactivity disorder and narcolepsy [102]. They may also be used for appetite suppression, depression, or management of Parkinson's disease symptoms. Some physiologic effects of amphetamines include increased systolic and diastolic blood pressure, weak bronchodilation properties, and respiratory stimulation [109].

6.2 Methylphenidate

Methylphenidate is a synthetic piperidine derivative that is thought to stimulate CNS activity through inhibiting dopamine and norepinephrine reuptake, thus increasing their quantities in the extra neuronal space [102]. This medication leads to increased attention and wakefulness. Prescription methylphenidate is commonly used for attention deficit hyperactivity disorder and narcolepsy. Adverse drug reactions include psychosis, anxiety, difficulty sleeping, palpitations, and mydriasis. In setting of overdose, methylphenidate can lead to delirium, hyperthermia, rhabdomyolysis, convulsions, and coma [110].

6.3 Modafinil

Modafinil is a synthetic benzhydryl sulfinyl compound that is thought to increase dopamine neurotransmission through DAT inhibition, although the mechanism is unclear [102]. The compound appears to have affinity for norepinephrine and serotonin receptors, to promote histamine and orexin release, and to act as a partial agonist at the D2 receptors. This medication causes wakefulness and is commonly used for the treatment of narcolepsy. Modafinil is an inducer of CYP3A4, CYP1A2, and CYP2B6 as well as a potent suppressor of CYP2C19 and CYP2C9, so caution should be maintained in patients for drug interactions associated with the pharmacokinetic profile of the medication [111].

6.4 Caffeine

Caffeine is a methylated xanthine alkaloid derived from *Coffea* plant seeds (coffee beans), *Camellia sinesis* leaves (tea), and the kola nut. It acts as an adenosine receptor antagonist and as a phosphodiesterase inhibitor (PDEi). Caffeine causes improved concentration and reduced fatigue. Caffeine is often used recreationally in the form of coffee or tea to increase energy levels, focus, and attention. Clinical uses of caffeine include the treatment of apnea of prematurity in newborns [102]. There is evidence that caffeine may provide symptomatic relief of post-dural puncture headache, although the evidence is limited and does not decrease the number of patients who need an epidural blood patch [112].

6.5 Anesthetic considerations

Repeated or chronic use of stimulants has been reported to blunt dopamine neurotransmission in the striatum through depletion of catecholamine receptor storage, a mechanism that may be responsible for increasing the reward threshold and driving drug consumption of stimulants [113]. This attenuation of dopaminergic signaling has been demonstrated even after longer periods of withdrawal [114, 115]. Reduced endogenous catecholamine stores produce a blunted physiologic and sympathetic response to hypotension associated with anesthetic use [113].

It is worth noting that the blunted response associated with stimulant use may cause limited to poor response to sympathomimetic medication in patients. Ephedrine is noted to have a reduced pressor response in patients with chronic stimulant use, although it is traditionally used as a first-line agent for intraoperative hypotension [116]. Due to the altered pressor response after stimulant use, direct-acting vasopressor agents such as epinephrine and phenylephrine are recommended for intraoperative management of refractory hypotension or bradycardia in patients using stimulants [113].

Although the literature is unclear as to whether stimulants should be discontinued prior to surgery to improve patient outcomes, there are case reports supporting that patients on stimulants maintained cardiac and hemodynamic stability intraoperatively with general anesthesia [116].

For a summary of the side effects and recommendations, please refer to the Summary Table at the end of the chapter.

7. Recreational substances

Substance use disorder is defined as an individual's inability to control their use of these substances, legal or illegal. Substance use disorders have an estimated prevalence of 13.24% (43.63 million) of the population aged 12 years or greater in the United States per the 2020 National Survey on Drug Use and Health [117]. In addition, there are individuals who use substances recreationally without meeting criteria for substance use disorder. Commonly used recreational substances include tobacco, alcohol, benzodiazepines, opioids, cocaine, amphetamines, marijuana, hallucinogens, and inhalants. These substances affect the physiologic status of a patient and can interact with other medications, notably anesthetic agents.

Preoperatively, providers should assess patients for substance use, emphasizing the questions asked are to provide better and safer care to the patient and not to judge [108]. Urine drug screens and other toxicology screens are helpful to determine the presence of one or more substances pre-operatively/pre-procedurally. Screening should be utilized in the unconscious patient, altered patient, and in those patients with clinical symptoms consistent with substance intoxication or withdrawal.

7.1 Tobacco

Tobacco contains thousands of ingredients including nicotine and carbon monoxide. Nicotine activates nicotinic cholinergic receptors resulting in sympathetic stimulation. This stimulation can cause an increase in heart rate, blood pressure, and respiratory rate. Carbon monoxide binds hemoglobin with increased affinity compared to oxygen. This binding creates carboxyhemoglobin, lowers stores of oxyhemoglobin, and results in decreased tissue oxygenation [118]. Long-term smoking is associated with chronic obstructive pulmonary disease (COPD), coronary artery disease (CAD), peripheral vascular disease (PVD), and stroke.

Pulmonary system effects which are important to consider peri- and intraoperatively are increased airway irritability and decreased mucociliary clearance. Smoking also increases the risk of postoperative complications including pulmonary complications of laryngospasm, pneumonia, respiratory failure, impaired tissue oxygenation, and impaired wound healing. Smoking cessation is encouraged prior to elective surgery, with a minimum recommendation of 72 hours before surgery with significant pulmonary benefit seen with cessation 4–8 weeks before surgery [118].

7.2 Alcohol

Alcohol is a central nervous system depressant believed to act at GABA-A receptors. Acute intoxication causes disinhibition, impaired motor control, and altered mentation. Alcohol can delay gastric emptying time and therefore increase the risk of aspiration. Chronic use is associated with gastritis, cirrhosis, chronic pancreatitis, Wernicke's encephalopathy, Wernicke-Korsakoff Syndrome, and cardiac beriberi [118].

Anesthetic requirements are decreased during acute alcohol intoxication due to CNS depression. Conversely, anesthetic requirements tend to be higher in chronic alcohol use disorder patients due to alcohol inducing liver enzymes. Aspiration risk is increased in acute intoxication and chronic use. Chronic users have increased airway colonization of pathologic bacteria which increases their risk for pneumonia [119]. Dehydration, cardiomyopathy, and decreased adrenocortical response to stress from chronic alcohol use may result in hypotension [108]. Thiamine (vitamin B1) and folate (vitamin B9) replacement should be initiated in alcohol use disorder patients.

Alcohol withdrawal is potentially life threatening with seizure and delirium tremens as possible effects. Withdrawal symptoms can begin within 12–24 hours following discontinuation, with seizures possible 24–48 hours after discontinuation, and delirium tremens possible after 48–72 hours after discontinuation. Symptoms can be mild to severe and can vary from autonomic symptoms to delirium tremens. Some mild symptoms include diaphoresis, palpitations, headaches, nausea, vomiting, and anorexia. More severe symptoms include tachycardia, hypertension, anxiety, insomnia, tremors, hallucinations, and hyperreflexia [120]. Alcoholic hallucinosis may present with intact consciousness, but the patient may experience auditory, visual, or tactile hallucinations and delusional thinking. Delirium tremens, on the other hand, may present with altered mental status, hallucinations, psychomotor agitation, and autonomic instability.

Treatment of alcohol withdrawal symptoms may include tapers of benzodiazepines, phenobarbital, or gabapentin. Alcohol withdrawal seizures are treated with intravenous benzodiazepines. The preferred benzodiazepines for the treatment are lorazepam, oxazepam, and temazepam. These are selected over other benzodiazepines due to their decreased hepatic metabolism. Importantly, supportive care is recommended, including hydration and electrolyte repletion. Folate and thiamine supplementation is also recommended, and for patients with Wernicke encephalopathy, high-dose thiamine should be initiated [42, 121].

Alcohol cessation before anticipated or elective surgery is recommended at least 1–2 weeks before surgery. Evidence demonstrates some organ dysfunction improves after the 1–2 weeks from cesation and that intervention programs starting 3–8 weeks prior to surgery significantly reduce the incidence of postoperative complications [122].

7.3 Cocaine

Cocaine is a naturally occurring benzoic acid ester derived from *Erythroxylon* coca leaves that acts as a dopamine, norepinephrine, and serotonin reuptake inhibitor

[102]. At high concentrations, cocaine can also inhibit voltage-gated sodium and potassium channels. This substance is a stimulant with vasoconstrictor and anesthetic properties. Peak effects of cocaine occur in 1–5 minutes, and the half-life is 60–120 minutes. Intoxication can lead to complications including hyperthermia, severe cardiovascular events such as hypertension, arrhythmias, myocardial infarction, prothrombotic events, coronary artery dissection, aortic dissection, heart failure, and cardiomyopathy [123]. Typically used recreationally, it leads to euphoria, perceptual disturbances, and convulsions and can also cause confusion and coma. In the United States, there are approximately 5 million people who use cocaine regularly. Cocaine addiction develops due to psychological and physiological tolerance, and rapid discontinuation of use results in drug craving, depressive symptoms, and fatigue.

Due to possible unopposed alpha-adrenergic receptor activation in combination with effects of cocaine, beta-blocker use is contraindicated in patients with acute cocaine toxicity due to unopposed alpha-adrenergic stimulation, coronary vasoconstriction, reduced nitric oxide production, and increased endothelin-1 levels [31, 123]. It is recommended to utilize nitric oxide mediated vasodilators, calcium channel blockers, and non-selective beta-blockers to manage hemodynamic instability in acute cocaine intoxication [31]. Acute intoxication causes sympathetic stimulation and may result in increased anesthetic requirements. Cocaine intoxication may also result in an exaggerated hypertensive response to ephedrine and ketamine. In chronic users, depletion of neurotransmitters results in decreased need for anesthetic agents and decreased response to ephedrine [117].

In individuals who use cocaine, there is risk of compromised oxygenation and supply due to the vasoconstrictive properties and vasospasm associated with use. When intubating or placing adjuvant airways in cocaine use disorder patients, caution should be taken due to chronic intranasal use causing septal and soft palate destruction [124]. Chronic smoking or crack-cocaine can lead to pulmonary complications that may result in difficult oxygenation or ventilation [108].

Due to changes in circulating catecholamines, patients may become hypertensive or hypotensive intraoperatively and should be monitored closely for pressure changes and arrhythmias. It may be valuable to also obtain a platelet count in patients with cocaine use to manage cocaine-induced thrombocytopenia that takes place due to platelet activation from vasospasm or autoimmune response [28]. Discontinuation of cocaine may cause withdrawal symptoms of increased anxiety, psychomotor agitation, and tremors [108]. Some of the other adverse effects of cocaine use include anxiety, papillary dilation, asthma, pulmonary hemorrhage, angina, and myocardial infarction [28].

7.4 Amphetamines and methamphetamines

Acute intoxication and chronic use may lead to cardiac complications including arrhythmias, aortic dissection, acute coronary syndrome, and cardiomyopathy [108]. It is recommended to obtain an electrocardiogram in acute and chronic users.

Due to increased sympathetic stimulation during acute intoxication, anesthetic requirements may be increased. Chronic users will demonstrate decreased anesthetic requirements [117]. Chronic amphetamine/methamphetamine users may experience poor oral hygiene resulting in damaged and loose teeth. Caution should be taken as such poor oral hygiene may result in dislodged teeth during intubation [108]. Chronic intranasal use may result in septal destruction and caution should be taken in use of nasogastric tubes. Smoking route of use can lead to pulmonary complications of arteriole remodeling and pulmonary hypertension [108]. It is recommended to continue prescription amphetamines perioperatively to prevent hemodynamic instability, which may result from chronic stimulant use. Amphetamine withdrawal may result in decreased energy, sleep disturbance, changes in appetite, mood changes, notably dysphoria and anxiety, as well as the emergence of suicidal ideations (for more information about the mechanism of action refer to stimulants).

7.5 Marijuana

Marijuana has become increasingly accessibly in the United States with the legalization for medical and recreational use in multiple states. Marijuana contains cannabinoids and the active ingredient is tetrahydrocannabinol (THC). Inhalation effects of marijuana include bronchodilation in acute intoxication with possible airway obstruction in chronic use [108]. Cardiovascular effects of marijuana are dose dependent. At low doses, sympathetic stimulation results and at high dose sympathetic inhibition results [125]. Withdrawal from marijuana causes mild physiologic effects and may result in increased anxiety, increased appetite, irritability, and mood changes.

There is limited evidence regarding marijuana cessation prior to anticipated or elective surgery. If a patient utilizes marijuana *via* smoking or other inhalation methods, it would be beneficial to discontinue use at minimum of 72 hours prior to surgery with consideration of 4–8 weeks prior to surgery as is recommended in tobacco use due to the benefits on the pulmonary system.

7.6 Hallucinogens/lysergic acid diethylamide/phencyclidine

Acute intoxication with hallucinogenic substances typically manifests as hallucinations, tachycardia, hypertension, hyperthermia, and gastrointestinal symptoms. Patients using lysergic acid diethylamide (LSD) may experience mydriasis, tachycardia, tachypnea, fever, hyperglycemia with effects lasting from 6 to 10 hours after use [108].

Patients using phencyclidine (PCP) may present with nystagmus, tachycardia, hypertension, psychosis, agitation, and cerebral hemorrhage with effects lasting from 4 to 8 hours [108]. Avoid ketamine use in patients intoxicated with PCP as it is a derivative of the substance.

7.7 Inhalants

There are various substances including organic solvents and volatile agents used as inhalants. Toluene is one of the more commonly utilized inhalants and its acute intoxication may cause cardiac arrhythmias, bronchial irritation, acute respiratory distress syndrome, liver toxicity, pulmonary hypertension, methemoglobinemia, cerebral edema, and pulmonary edema [28]. Chronic use may lead to cerebellar degeneration and brain atrophy. General anesthesia may be the preferred option for patients acutely intoxicated with inhalants/solvents due to respiratory compromise and aspiration risk [28].

7.8 Opioids

Opioids continue to be an important pharmacologic agent in the management of certain types of pain, and it is important to acknowledge that this class of medications has significant potential for misuse. Natural and synthetic opioids bind mu receptors: u1, which plays a role in analgesia and u2, in respiratory depression. Acute intoxication causes sedation, reduced respiratory rate, hypoxia, and pupillary miosis. It also causes delayed gastric emptying time and increases aspiration risk [117]. Chronic use can cause constipation. Use *via* snorting may result in septal and soft palate destruction.

Tramadol, commonly used in chronic pain management, is linked to psychiatric symptoms including altered mood, hallucinations, confusion, sleep disturbance, and nightmares [8]. Notably, when Tramadol is combined with selective serotonin reuptake inhibitors (SSRIs) and tricyclic antidepressants (TCAs) in the risk of serotonin syndrome, it reduces the seizure threshold.

Opioid overdose causes respiratory depression and can be life threatening. Additionally, opioid intoxication and overdose may result in pulmonary edema [117]. Opiate overdose is most often reversed with the opioid antagonist, naloxone, which can be administered intranasally or intravenously in the pre-, intra-, and postoperative period. Repeated intravenous access for use may result in difficult access in the peri- and intraoperative period and should be considered in intravenous users [108].

Patients in recent or sustained opioid use disorder recovery may request induction agents other than fentanyl, in such cases ketamine may be a favored option. Patients in recovery may be utilizing medical assisted therapy to maintain sobriety and it is important to assess for such use including methadone, buprenorphine-naloxone combinations in sublingual form, naloxone in oral or injectable form, or buprenorphine in sublingual or injectable form. Patients on buprenorphine/naloxone combination medication should consider tapering prior to surgery to prevent the opioid antagonist from counteracting postoperative opioids for pain [117].

It is recommended to continue opioids perioperatively to avoid withdrawal and to decrease the need for scheduled additional pain medications in the perioperative setting. It is recommended to use a multimodal pain regimen in patients including but not limited to acetaminophen, non-steroidal anti-inflammatory drugs, gabapentin, regional anesthesia (including nerve blocks) where appropriate [108]. Opiate withdrawal onset varies based on amount used and type of opioid. For example, heroin withdrawal may begin in 6–18 hours, methadone withdrawal in 24–48 hours.

Opioid withdrawal may result in sympathetic hyperactivity, including tachycardia, hypertension, anxiety, insomnia, irritability, mydriasis, yawning, lacrimation, hyperreflexia, and muscle cramps. Rhinorrhea, piloerection, chills, myalgia, and arthralgia are common occurrences in opioid withdrawal. Gastrointestinal symptoms such as nausea, vomiting, and diarrhea may also occur. Supportive management is recommended, including hydration and electrolyte repletion. Clonidine is often used to help alleviate autonomic symptoms of opioid withdrawal [126].

7.9 Medication-assisted treatments (MATs)

MAT uses a combination of counseling, psychotherapy, and medications to assist patients with substance use disorders. Special care should be taken with patients who have a history of opioid use dependence as they are at high risk of relapse. In patients with this history, it may be beneficial to order a substance use disorder consult in addition to careful preoperative planning, which includes active patient participation in the weighing of the risks and benefits of different forms of pain management and frank discussion on the risk of relapse. Patients with a history of opioid abuse can benefit of becoming part of a MAT program as it has been shown to improve patient retention, increase abstinence, and decrease illicit opiate use [127–129]. There are many patients with opioid use dependence who are currently participating in MAT including methadone, suboxone, and naltrexone.

Methadone is a synthetic opioid that has been in use since 1972 [130]. It binds to the mu-opioid receptor and prevents opioid withdrawal for 24 hours or more. Methadone is available in several formulations, but it is advised to avoid switching formulations to decrease the chances of eliciting withdrawal symptoms. It can be continued at the outpatient dosage, which is notably not sufficient for pain management in the perioperative setting. If a patient is on methadone treatment, avoid using partial agonist opioids such as buprenorphine or butorphanol as this can also precipitate withdrawal symptoms.

Suboxone is a combination of buprenorphine and naloxone. It is used to treat opioid use disorder. Buprenorphine is a partial mu-receptor agonist and suppresses cravings and withdrawal symptoms while blocking the receptor against other opioids. Naloxone is a non-selective and competitive opioid receptor agonist. Per a review by Kohan *et al.* in *Regional Anesthesia Pain Medicine* in 2021, buprenorphine management in the perioperative period: educational review and recommendations from a multi-society expert panel, the most recently published recommendation is to continue buprenorphine throughout the perioperative period [131].

Naltrexone is an opioid antagonist that binds competitively to mu-receptors and therefore blocks endogenous and exogenous opioids. Thus, opioid intoxication and dependence is reduced, and increases patient abstinence. Since this medication inhibits analgesia, a “wash out” period is recommended. For injectable versions of naltrexone such as Vivitrol, it is recommended to wait 4 weeks from the last dosage prior to surgery. For oral naltrexone, a 72-hour washout prior to surgery is recommended [130].

For a general overview of side effects and recommendations, please refer to the Summary Table at the end of the chapter.

8. New psychotropic medications and considerations

This section contains some of the newer psychiatric medications that were recently approved by the FDA and released into the market. The new medications are of interest as there are limited data on potential drug-drug interactions with commonly used anesthetic agents. Regardless as they generally can cause various side effects, it is not unreasonable to speculate that the patients taking these medications would need to be monitored closely during procedures that require sedation, anesthesia, or analgesia.

8.1 Dexmedetomidine sublingual film (IGALMI™)

This formulation of alpha-2 adrenergic agonist received FDA approval in 2022 for acute treatment of agitation associated with Bipolar I or II Disorder or Schizophrenia [132]. Most common adverse effects reported from clinical trials include somnolence, dry mouth, hypotension, and dizziness [133]. There is a possible serious adverse effect such as orthostatic hypotension and QT prolongation. Since dexmedetomidine decreases sympathetic activity, hypotension and/or bradycardia can be pronounced in patients with hypovolemia, chronic hypertension, and patients who are elderly. Caution should be used if co-administered with other anesthetic agents.

8.2 Olanzapine and Samidorphan (LYBALVI®)

This combination of a second-generation antipsychotic and opioid antagonist was initially approved by FDA in 2021 for the treatment of schizophrenia, mania, or mixed episodes of Bipolar I Disorder as monotherapy or adjunct to lithium or valproate [134]. The medication is formulated to provide the efficacy of olanzapine and to mitigate the risk of olanzapine associated weight gain. Most common adverse effects reported during clinical trials were weight gain, somnolence, headaches, upper respiratory infections [135]. As with other antipsychotic medications, there is an increased risk for serious adverse reactions, such as neutropenia/agranulocytosis, lowering of seizure threshold, hypotension, and neuroleptic malignant syndrome [136]. Due to the opioid antagonist component, there is a risk of opioid intoxication if concurrent opioids are used to overcome the effect of antagonism. There is also a risk of precipitated withdrawal in those who are taking opioids. Thus, this medication is contraindicated in those using opioids and in those undergoing opioid withdrawal. Caution must be taken with regards to medication interactions, as CNS acting drugs such as anesthetics, sedatives, and hypnotics can potentiate the risk of orthostatic hypotension.

8.3 Lumateperone (Caplyta)

This is a new second-generation antipsychotic FDA approved for the treatment of schizophrenia in 2019 and Bipolar depression in 2022 [137]. It works as a presynaptic partial agonist and post-synaptic antagonist at D2 receptors and has high affinity for serotonin receptors [138]. Common side effects include fatigue, somnolence, sedation, constipation. Lumateperone shares serious side effects like other second-generation antipsychotics. Caution should be used when co-administering medications that affect CYP3A4: inhibitors require decrease in lumateperone dose and concomitant use of inducers should be avoided. Common agents that are CYP3A4 inducers are phenobarbital, primidone, fosphenytoin, and carbamazepine [139]. Like for other antipsychotics, vital signs should be monitored if anesthetic agents are administered.

9. Herbal supplements

Recent data show that more than 50% of U.S. adults aged 20 and use some form of dietary supplement. Its use was also found to increase with age, as 80.2% of U.S. adults 60 or older report using at least one form of dietary supplement [140]. Although concern has been raised by medical associations and physicians about the use of herbal remedies and supplements, most patients perceive herbal medicines as natural and safe products. As a result, many patients fail to disclose their current use of herbal remedies placing themselves in danger of potential side effects or even death.

Knowledge of herbal medicines is essential when the patient presents for a surgical procedure, elective or urgent, especially for the potential interactions with anesthetic agents and unexpected complications in the perioperative period. Herbs can cause hematologic, cardiovascular, and endocrine disturbances, hepatotoxicity, prolongation of anesthetic agents, and even organ transplant rejection. Even though the American Society of Anesthesiologists (ASA) advises that all herbal medicines and supplements must be stopped 2 weeks before surgery [141] anesthesiologists should be aware of the potential drug-drug interaction of the most common herbal remedies used by the psychiatric population and advise patients, as necessary.

9.1 St John's wort

Various herbal supplements have been linked to the treatment of depression. Generally, these should be discontinued at least 2 weeks prior to surgery but can vary with supplements. A commonly used supplement is St. John's Wort, which notably inhibits dopamine, norepinephrine, and serotonin and has the potential for serotonin syndrome [142]. St. John's Wort induces CYP3A4, which therefore reduces the efficacy of oral midazolam [14].

9.2 Ephedra Sinica

Ephedra sinica, also known as ephedra or ma-huang, is a central nervous system stimulant (CNS) that contains alkaloids ephedrine, methyephedrine, pseudoephedrine, and nor-pseudo-ephedrine. It works by stimulating α- and β-adrenergic receptors and increasing the release of norepinephrine from presynaptic neurons [143]. Due to its sympathomimetic effects, it is marketed for memory enhancement, weight loss, and asthma treatment. However, it is also used in the illegal manufacture of methamphetamine known as "Cloud 9" or "Herbal Ecstasy" [144]. A few side effects include hypertension, tachycardia, seizure, and stroke [145].

The effects of ephedra on anesthesia are well understood. Fatal arrhythmias associated with the simultaneous administration of ephedra and inhalation of the anesthetic agent halothane have been reported [146]. In addition to arrhythmias, if combined with other sympathomimetics it can also cause hyperthermia and hypertension [145]. Patients who have used this agent long term may benefit from direct-acting sympathomimetics as their endogenous catecholamine stores may be depleted, which increases the risk of intraoperative cardiovascular instability.

9.3 Ginkgo Biloba

Ginkgo biloba is a supplement commonly used to improve memory, mental alertness, treat intermittent claudication, and other circulatory disorders. The two main active medicinal groups of ginkgo are terpene lactones and ginkgo flavone [147]. The terpene lactones are known to inhibit the platelet-activating factor (PAF), which predisposes the patient to increased bleeding [148]. A case report described an event of spontaneous hyphemia with the combined use of ginkgo and high-dose aspirin [149]. In another case, a patient developed spontaneous bilateral subdural hematoma [150]. Caution is advised on patients with previous history of bleeding disorders or who are taking anticoagulant drugs (especially with non-steroidal anti-inflammatory drugs (NSAIDs), heparin, and warfarin) [147].

The reported medicinal components of ginkgo, terpenes, and flavones do not significantly inhibit the CYP450 enzymes, but other components of this herbal supplement do inhibit the CYP1A2 and CYP3A4 [151].

9.4 Ginseng

Ginseng is advertised for several things, especially as an energy booster and lowering blood glucose agent. It is also used as a stress-relieving and homeostatic product

[152]. Its pharmacological properties come from the ginsenosides that act as steroidal hormones. Ginseng interacts with coagulation cascade and inhibits platelet aggregation [153]. Due to its glucose blood lowering effects, it is sometimes used concomitantly with other glucose-lowering agents in patients with type II diabetes [154]. Therefore, serum blood glucose concentrations should be closely monitored in diabetic surgical patients taking ginseng. Additional precautions should also be exercised in patients receiving anticoagulants or blood thinners. Finally, during surgery, it may precipitate rapid heart rate and high blood pressure [155].

9.5 Valerian

Valerian is used to treat sleep disorders, anxiety, headaches, depression, irregular heartbeat, and tremors. Its active compounds are called sesquiterpenes. Valerian acts similar to St. John's Wort as it modulates the Gamma Aminobutyric Acid (GABA) neurotransmitter and has hypnotic and sedative properties. As a sedative, it can potentiate the effects of general anesthesia [156]. Therefore, it may make it harder to wake up after general anesthesia and can cause irregular heart rhythms [155]. Lastly, the abrupt discontinuation of this product can produce benzodiazepine withdrawal symptoms [156, 157].

9.6 Kava

Kava, a CNS depressant, is used for religious and medicinal purposes in the South Pacific Rim and is known to be beneficial in treating anxiety [158, 159]. Research suggests that the primary active ingredient (kavalactones) modulates GABA activity and inhibits dopamine and noradrenaline reuptake [160, 161]. Kava is also a muscle relaxant and, in toxic doses, can induce paralysis and reversible muscle weakness but no loss of consciousness. This supplement may decrease the dosage needed for relaxants during surgery and increase the potency of antiemetics, antipsychotics, and CNS depressants [162]. It can also cause liver damage [163].

10. Electroconvulsive treatment

Electroconvulsive therapy (ECT) is defined as the "induction of a series of generalized epileptic seizures for therapeutic purposes." ECT may be utilized as a first line treatment for severe depressive episodes, catatonia, schizoaffective psychosis, and neuroleptic malignant syndrome [164]. ECT is also utilized as a treatment for mania as well as depressive or psychotic symptoms due to organic disease and has been employed as a last resort treatment for epilepsy, dyskinesias, and Parkinson's disease [164]. The procedure is brief, with an expected seizure duration of 30 to 90 seconds and administered two to three times per week, 6 to 12 treatments in total per series [165]. **Table 3** shows a list of common anesthetics used during ECT.

The mechanism of action by which ECT achieves therapeutic results is unknown; however, studies have discovered that ECT affects neurotransmitter pathways in the brain (increasing GABA neurotransmission and increasing plasma levels of tryptophan as well as glutamate), affects the hypothalamic pituitary adrenal axis, and results in an increase in cerebral blood flow [164]. In patients suffering from psychotic depression, 90% will achieve remission from ECT treatment, with relief of symptoms occurring within 10 to 14 days [164].

Drug	Mechanism of action	Purpose of drug for ECT	Onset of action	Half life	Potential post-procedural side effects	Effect on seizure duration
Dexmetomidine	Highly selective a2 receptor agonist	Sedative	4–5 minutes	2–2.5 hours	Hypotension, bradycardia, arrhythmias	No effect
Etomidate	$GABA_A$ receptor modulator	Sedative	30–60 seconds	2–5 hours	Adrenal suppression, nausea, vomiting, clonus	Increase
Ketamine	NMDA receptor agonist	Sedative	1–2 minutes	2.5–3 hours	Secretions, disassociation, hypertension, tachycardia	Increase
Methohexital	$GABA_A$ receptor modulator	Sedative	30–60 seconds	3–6 hours	Fatigue, confusion, nausea, vomiting	No effect
Propofol	$GABA_A$ receptor modulator	Sedative	30–60 seconds	Initial: 40 minutes Terminal: 4–7 hours	Hypotension, myoclonus, QT prolongation	Decrease
Remifentanil	Opioid	Sedative	1–3 minutes	1–20 minutes	Hypotension, bradycardia, nausea, vomiting	No effect
Rocuronium	Depolarizing Neuromuscular Blocker	Paralytic	3–5 minutes	20–45 minutes	Respiratory complications, anaphylaxis	No effect
Succinylcholine	Non-depolarizing Neuromuscular Blocker	Paralytic	30–60 seconds	30–60 seconds	Residual paralysis, apnea, bradycardia, malignant hyperthermia	No effect

Table 3.
Common anesthetic agents utilized during ECT.

As the procedure is brief, ideal sedating agents and paralytics for ECT have a fast onset of action and a short distribution half-life [166]. It is important to note that the goal of an ECT session is to achieve adequate seizure duration (between 30 and 90 seconds) and anesthetic agents can influence seizure threshold and duration [166]. Ideally, the anesthetic agent should also be easy to administer and have minimal postoperative side effects [166].

In preparation for the procedure, it is equally important to recognize that psychiatric medications can also have an impact on seizure duration and require management strategies in the setting of ECT administration. Mood stabilizing agents including lithium, valproic acid, and carbamazepine may require dosing adjustments [165]. **Table 4** shows a list of psychiatric medications and their potential effects in the setting of ECT Administration.

There are no absolute contraindications for ECT administration; however, there are several relative contraindications that require careful consideration before performing the procedure [164]. Relative contraindications include increased intracranial pressure, intracranial bleeding, recent cerebral infarction or myocardial

Drug	Class	Potential complications	Recommendations
Lithium	Mood Stabilizer	• Delirium • Postictal confusion • Lithium toxicity • Increases seizure duration • Serotonin syndrome • Prolonged effects of neuromuscular blocking agents	• Consider substituting an atypical antipsychotic for lithium during ECT treatment course. • Recommend adjusting the dose to maintain a blood lithium level in the lowest therapeutic range. • Recommend utilizing reduced doses of neuromuscular blocking agents.
Valproic Acid	Mood Stabilizer	• Increases seizure threshold • Decrease seizure duration	• Consider reducing the dose of valproic acid during ECT treatment course. • Consider utilizing a sedative agent such as etomidate that increases seizure duration.
Carbamazepine	Mood Stabilizer	• Increases seizure threshold • Decreases seizure duration • Decreases efficacy of neuromuscular blocking agents	• Consider reducing the dose of carbamazepine during ECT treatment course. • Consider holding doses prior to ECT procedure (holding the nighttime dose prior to the procedure or holding the morning dose prior to the procedure). • Studies suggest succinylcholine and mivacurium are preferred paralytic agents for patients receiving carbamazepine.
Lamotrigine	Mood stabilizer	Theoretically increases seizure threshold.	No medication adjustments are necessary.
Gabapentin	Mood stabilizer	Theoretically increases seizure threshold.	No medication adjustments are necessary.
Topiramate	Mood stabilizer	Theoretically increases seizure threshold.	No medication adjustments are necessary.
Phenelzine, Tranylcypromine, Selegiline, Isocarboxazid	MAOI	Hypertensive crisis	• Recommend careful monitoring and avoidance of medications known to interact with MAOIs. • Consider switching patient to a reversible MAOI such as moclobemide.
Fluoxetine, Sertraline, Paroxetine, Escitalopram Citalopram	SSRI	Theoretically reduces seizure threshold.	• No medication adjustments are necessary. • Monitor for signs of serotonin syndrome.
Venlafaxine, Desvenlafaxine, Duloxetine	SNRI	Theoretically reduces seizure threshold.	No medication adjustments are necessary.

Drug	Class	Potential complications	Recommendations
Bupropion	NDRI	Theoretically increases seizure duration.	Consider reducing the dose of bupropion during ECT treatment.
Alprazolam, Clonazepam, Diazepam, Lorazepam, Midazolam, Temazepam	Benzodiazepines	• Increases seizure threshold • Decreases seizure duration	• Discontinue benzodiazepines or utilize sparingly during ECT treatment. • Long-acting benzodiazepines such as clonazepam should be discontinued days before ECT treatment.
Chlorpromazine, Loxapine, Haloperidol, Prochlorperazine, Perphenazine, Thiothixene	First-Generation Antipsychotics	Theoretically reduces seizure threshold.	• No medication adjustments are recommended • Monitor for anticholinergic and antiadrenergic side effects.
Clozapine	Second-Generation Antipsychotic	Clozapine reduces seizure threshold in a dose dependent manner.	Consider reducing the dose of clozapine during ECT treatment.
Methylphenidate	Stimulant	Theoretically increases seizure duration.	No medication adjustments are recommended.

Table 4.
Psychiatric medication management in the Setting of ECT administration.

infarction less than 3 months ago, intracerebral tumor, and vascular malformations [164]. Cardiac pathology (including coronary artery disease, unstable angina, cardiac arrythmias), orthopedic pathology (including severe osteoporosis), and respiratory pathology (including respiratory conditions such as severe COPD that would pose a life-threatening anesthesia risk as well as conditions that would predispose the patient to aspiration such as an esophageal hernia) are also relative contraindications [164].

11. Postoperative considerations for psychiatric patients

Several studies suggest that severe mental illness may suppress and dysregulate the immune system [167–169] and, thus, expose patients to higher risk of postoperative infection and mortality [167, 169]. Higher rates of postoperative infection have been reported for multiple surgeries including coronary bypass graft, hip surgery, total knee replacement, craniotomy, bariatric surgeries, and the implantation of ventricular assist devices [167, 170, 171]. Surgical procedures can also exacerbate cognitive impairment commonly associated with mental illness [8]. In addition, research has shown that depression and anxiety lower pain thresholds and that patients with these conditions prior to surgery have significantly higher postoperative pain and analgesic requirements. Depression and anxiety are also strong predictors of chronic surgical pain and are independent risk factors for postoperative delirium [8, 167].

Psychiatric patients undergoing surgery report a lack of mental health recognition, minimal discussion on the impact of surgery on mental health, a lack of specific mental health information prior to discharge, and inconsistent interaction with the mental health team. Surgeons report that they do not routinely ask their patients about their mental health status prior to surgery. Reasons cited by surgeons include a lack of time and fear of being inappropriate or disliked by patients. Surgeons also reported feeling less confident about managing patients with severe mental illness compared to medical comorbidities. In addition, patients may be fearful to discuss topics of mental health, as there continues to be a stigma toward mental illness in healthcare and studies suggest that this stigma may impact surgical decisions [172, 173].

Due to these concerns, several hospitals and insurance companies now require a surgical clearance assessment from a psychiatrist before patients can undergo major elective surgeries [167, 171, 174, 175]. For example, most patients that undergo bariatric surgery receive psychiatric clearance prior to the surgery. This psychiatric assessment helps determine if the patient is psychologically and emotionally prepared to undergo the procedure and helps identify if there are any issues that might impede a successful surgical outcome. The assessment also addresses whether the patient can make adequate lifestyle changes and if mental health support is needed following the surgery. Psychiatric evaluations have been shown to result in more favorable outcomes when mental health issues are treated prior to surgery [167, 171, 175].

Psychiatric evaluations should include a diagnostic interview, observation, and thorough review of medical records. Psychiatric evaluation should focus on history of major mental illnesses, substance use, cognitive skills, and capacity to make decisions, ability to adhere to treatment, coping skills, level of social support, and safety assessment including assessment for active suicidal or homicidal ideations [175, 176]. Patients with uncontrolled psychiatric illness and poor social support are at higher risk for surgical complications. Patients with active substance use are also at an increased risk for surgical complications and efforts should be made to connect these patients with drug and alcohol treatment prior to undergoing major elective procedures [176]. Surgery is a significant life event that can exacerbate mental illness [167, 173]. The patient should fully understand the surgical risks and benefits. A history of compliance with medical instructions, medications, and keeping appointments is also important. Patients should have established internal and external resources for coping with stress, depression, and anxiety.

Following major surgeries, there is often some loss of normal functioning and the need to modify lifestyle and depend on others for assistance. Disruption of the patient's normal routine, combined with loss of independence, can have a debilitating effect on mental health and exacerbate existing psychiatric conditions [167, 175]. There is growing awareness among surgeons that general anesthesia may be responsible for delirium, confusion, hallucinations, depression, mania, and psychotic behavior [167]. Therefore, patients and families should be educated on the early signs of worsening mental health and an action plan should be developed prior to discharge.

12. Discussion

Optimal perioperative outcomes require a multidisciplinary team to provide comprehensive and individualized care. Teamwork, interprofessional communication, and quality improvement efforts continue to play a vital role in the advancement of healthcare. It is important to consider protocols to screen patients for mental illness and facilitate communication between anesthesiologists and mental health professionals particularly when to prevent treatment errors, avoid higher treatment costs, and improve patient experiences. Moreover, efforts to increase communication such as electronic health records, TigerConnect, and TelmedIQ can be implemented in the hospital systems to ease the flow of information between providers and decrease the likelihood of sentinel events. In hospitals where access to these technologies is not possible, physician notes or letters can be given to the patient to share his/her personal health information across his/her health care providers.

As psychiatry continues to advance, it is expected to see new treatment methods and psychotropic medicines. One such new medicine is the novel recent FDA approved neurosteroid Zulresso® (brexanolone) injection for the treatment of post-partum depression. This medicine is administered as a continuous intravenous infusion, throughout 2.5 days, and is thought to work as a positive allosteric modulator of $GABA_A$ receptors [177]. Other common adverse effects are dizziness, vertigo, presyncope, and sedation [178]. Interactions with anesthetics or other sedatives have not been studied but caution is advised due to its mechanism of action.

Another promising new therapy is the use of propranolol for the reduction of post-traumatic stress disorder (PTSD) symptoms. In a randomized controlled trial, Bruner and colleagues found that patients taking propranolol had improved Clinician-Administered PTSD Scale (CAPS-5) scores compared to the placebo group [179]. Although these were exciting results, long-term follow-up studies and replication of this study are necessary to reach any conclusions.

The use of medical cannabis is growing in popularity across the U.S.A. but controlled studies in its efficacy and safety are lacking. An 8-week multicenter, double-blind randomized controlled trial on the use of cannabidiol (CBD) on patients with schizophrenia demonstrated that when compared to the placebo group, patients taking 1000-mg daily of CBD had decreased positive symptoms in the Positive and Negative Syndrome Scale (PANSS). Improvement in cognition was also documented and the treatment was well tolerated by the participants [180]. Although these results are promising the study had a small sample size, is pending replication, and to confirm these results a lasting phase-3 trial is necessary.

13. Conclusion

This chapter discusses the most common psychotropic medications, substances, and herbal supplements used by patients with psychiatric conditions. Anesthesiologists should exercise special caution to prevent discontinuation syndromes, withdrawal symptoms, or potentially lethal interactions with anesthetics. It is also essential to stay up to date with new drugs such as dexmedetomidine, olanzapine/samidorphan combination, and lumateperon for new data on anesthetic interactions. Lastly, anesthesiologists are encouraged to contact the patient's physician if questions about their psychotropic medications arise during the pre-operative examination (**Table 5**).

14. Summary table

Drug	Hold/continue	Interaction with anesthetics	Considerations
Antidepressants			
SSRI	Continue	Avoid serotonin crisis precipitants & methylene blue	Avoid pethidine, meperidine, tramadol, pentazocine, and dextromethorphan

Drug	Hold/continue	Interaction with anesthetics	Considerations
SNRI	Continue	Avoid serotonin crisis precipitants & methylene blue	Avoid pethidine, meperidine, tramadol, pentazocine, and dextromethorphan
MAOI	2-week Washout	Avoid indirect acting sympathomimetics (such as phenylephrine or ketamine), avoid serotonergic crisis precipitants such as meperidine or dextromethorphan	
TCA	Hold 2 days prior	Avoid sympathomimetics (ketamine, ephedrine, metaraminol, etc.)	May reduce seizure threshold and may augment anesthetic sedatives
Atypical Antidepressants (Mirtazapine, etc.)	Continue	Avoid serotonin crisis precipitants & methylene blue	
Ketamine	Continue		Potential decreased efficacy with lamotrigine
Anxiolytics			
Benzodiazepines	Continue		Avoid use with meperidine and tramadol
Buspirone	Continue		Avoid use with meperidine or tramadol
Hydroxyzine	Continue		Avoid anticholinergics
Mood stabilizer			
Lithium	Stop 72 hours prior	Prolongs depolarization and polarization phase of neuromuscular blockade by acting additively with depolarizing neuromuscular agents and synergistically with non-depolarizing neuromuscular agents.	Signs of toxicity: tremors, vomiting, confusion, diarrhea, increased deep tendon reflexes, hypotension, seizures. Obtain plasma lithium level if suspected toxicity
Valproic Acid	Continue	Can increase levels of highly protein bound anesthetics such as propofol.	Recommend preoperative screening for bleeding risk, as well as preoperative platelet count, bleeding time, PT, activated partial thromboplastin time, fibrinogen, and von Willebrand factor
Carbamazepine	Continue	Duration of effect of non-depolarizing aminosteroid neuromuscular blockers	Strong CYP450 Inducer, can decrease plasma concentration of many medications including

Drug	Hold/continue	Interaction with anesthetics	Considerations
		such as vecuronium can be shortened	cardiovascular drugs, such as amiodarone, β-blockers (metoprolol, propranolol), and calcium channel blockers (nifedipine, nimodipine, felodipine, and verapamil).
Lamotrigine	Continue	Can decrease Ketamine's dissociative effect	
Antipsychotics			
Antipsychotics	Continue	Avoid enflurane	Caution is advised with other seizure-threshold lowering drugs
Stimulants			
Amphetamines/Amphetamine-like substances	Continue	• Acute intoxication—anesthetic requirements increase • Chronic use—anesthetic requirements decrease	
Recreational drugs			
Tobacco	Stop at least 72 hours before elective surgery		
Alcohol	Stop 1–2 weeks prior to surgery	• Acute intoxication—anesthetic requirements decrease • Chronic use—anesthetic requirements increase	
Opioids	Continue prescription opioids for pain control as appropriate to avoid withdrawal		
Cocaine		• Acute intoxication—anesthetic requirements increase • Chronic use—anesthetic requirements decrease	• Acute intoxication—hypertension possible in response to ephedrine and ketamine • Chronic use—decreased response to ephedrine
Marijuana	Stop smoking use at least 72 hours prior to elective surgery		

Drug	Hold/continue	Interaction with anesthetics	Considerations
Inhalants			Acute intoxication—recommendation for general anesthesia due to respiratory compromise and aspiration risk
Medication assisted treatments (MATs)			
Methadone	Continue		Avoid buprenorphine or butorphanol, as it can precipitate withdrawal
Buprenorphine	Continue		Do not administer on patient on methadone
Naltrexone (oral)	Hold at least 72 hours prior to surgery	Inhibits anesthetics	
Naltrexone (Vivitrol)	Hold 4 weeks prior to surgery	Inhibits anesthetics	
New medications			
Dexmedetomidine Sublingual Film (IGALMI™)	Continue	Limited Data	Side effects can be similar to dexmedetomidine used intravenously
Olanzapine and Samidorphan (LYBALVI®)	Continue	Limited Data	Anesthetics, sedatives, and hypnotics can potentiate the risk of orthostatic hypotension.
Lumateperone (Caplyta)	Continue	Limited Data	Anesthetics, sedatives, and hypnotics can potentiate the risk of orthostatic hypotension.

Table 5.
Summary of recommendations.

Conflict of interest

The authors declare that the work for this book chapter was conducted in the absence of any commercial or financial relationships that could be considered a conflict of interest.

Author details

Maria Martinez-Baladejo[1], Franzes Anne Z. Liongson[1*], Dustin Wong[1], Christina Spoleti[1], Diyor Suyumov[1], Sanjay V. Menghani[2,3], Christopher McCarthy[1], Alec James Divito[1], Shani Varghese Daniel[1], Shilpa Salpekar[1], Rina Bhalodi[1], Maaz Siddiqui[1] and Christine Marchionni[1]

1 St. Luke's University Hospital Network (SLUHN), Bethlehem, PA, USA

2 University of Arizona College of Medicine – Tucson, Tucson, AZ, USA

3 Medical Scientist Training MD-PhD Program, University of Arizona College of Medicine – Tucson, Tucson, AZ, USA

*Address all correspondence to: franzes.liongson@sluhn.org

IntechOpen

© 2023 The Author(s). Licensee IntechOpen. This chapter is distributed under the terms of the Creative Commons Attribution License (http://creativecommons.org/licenses/by/3.0), which permits unrestricted use, distribution, and reproduction in any medium, provided the original work is properly cited.

References

[1] WHO. World mental health report: Transforming mental health for all - executive summary. In: WHO, editor. 2022. p. 1-28

[2] Dattani S, Ritchie H, Roser M. Mental Health - Our World in Data. Our World in Data. January 4, 2023 at 16:41 ed. Online2021

[3] Ruth Brauer BA, Blais JE, Chan EW, Chui CSL, Hayes JF, Man KKC, et al. Psychotropic medicine consumption in 65 countries and regions, 2008–19: A longitudinal study. Lancet. Psychiatry. 2021;**8**:1071-1082

[4] Moore TJ, Mattison DR. Adult utilization of psychiatric drugs and differences by sex, age, and race. JAMA Internal Medicine. 2017;**177**:274-275

[5] NIMH. Major Depression. 2022. Available from: https://www.nimh.nih.gov/health/statistics/major-depression.

[6] DSM5. Diagnostic and Statistical Manual of Mental Disorders. 5th ed. Washington D.C: American Psychiatric Association; 2013

[7] Malhi GS, Bell E, Morris G, Hamilton A. The delay in response to antidepressant therapy: A window of opportunity? The Australian and New Zealand Journal of Psychiatry. 2020;**54**(2): 127-129

[8] Attri JP, Bala N, Chatrath V. Psychiatric patient and anaesthesia. Indian Journal of Anaesthesia. 2012; **56**(1):8-13

[9] Preskorn SH. Clinically relevant pharmacology of selective serotonin reuptake inhibitors. An overview with emphasis on pharmacokinetics and effects on oxidative drug metabolism. Clinical Pharmacokinetics. 1997;**32**:1-21

[10] Raj KS, Williams N, DeBattista C. Mood Disorders (Depression & Mania). In: Papadakis MA, McPhee SJ, Rabow MW, editors. Current Medical Diagnosis & Treatment 2021. New York, NY: McGraw-Hill Education; 2021.

[11] Hillhouse TM, Porter JH. A brief history of the development of antidepressant drugs: From monoamines to glutamate. Experimental and Clinical Psychopharmacology. 2015;**23**(1):1-21

[12] Trindade E, Menon D, Topfer LA, Coloma C. Adverse effects associated with selective serotonin reuptake inhibitors and tricyclic antidepressants: A meta-analysis. CMAJ. 1998;**159**(10): 1245-1252

[13] Fanoe S, Kristensen D, Fink-Jensen A, Jensen HK, Toft E, Nielsen J, et al. Risk of arrhythmia induced by psychotropic medications: A proposal for clinical management. European Heart Journal. 2014;**35**(20):1306-1315

[14] Brentjens Tricia E, Warner David O. Pharmacology & Physiology in anesthetic practice, 4th Edition. Anesthesiology. Philadephia, PA: Lippincott Wililams and Wilkins; 2006;**105**(4):864

[15] Peck TE, Wong A, Norman E. Anaesthetic implications of psychoactive drugs. Continuing Education in Anaesthesia, Critical Care & Pain. 2010; **10**:177-181

[16] Polasek TM, Miners JO. Time-dependent inhibition of human drug metabolizing cytochromes P450 by tricyclic antidepressants. British Journal of Clinical Pharmacology. 2008;**65**(1):87-97

[17] Arlander E, Ekström G, Alm C, Carrillo JA, Bielenstein M, Böttiger Y, et al. Metabolism of ropivacaine in humans is mediated by CYP1A2 and to a minor extent by CYP3A4: An interaction study with fluvoxamine and ketoconazole as in vivo inhibitors. Clinical Pharmacology and Therapeutics. 1998;**64**(5):484-491

[18] Dean L, Kane M. Tramadol Therapy and CYP2D6 Genotype. In: Pratt VM, Scott SA, Pirmohamed M, Esquivel B, Kattman BL, Malheiro AJ, editors. Medical Genetics Summaries. Bethesda (MD): National Center for Biotechnology Information (US); 2012

[19] Inomata S, Nagashima A, Itagaki F, Homma M, Nishimura M, Osaka Y, et al. CYP2C19 genotype affects diazepam pharmacokinetics and emergence from general anesthesia. Clinical Pharmacology and Therapeutics. 2005; **78**(6):647-655

[20] Polasek TM, Elliot DJ, Somogyi AA, Gillam EM, Lewis BC, Miners JO. An evaluation of potential mechanism-based inactivation of human drug metabolizing cytochromes P450 by monoamine oxidase inhibitors, including isoniazid. British Journal of Clinical Pharmacology. 2006;**61**(5):570-584

[21] Chen CC, Lin CS, Ko YP, Hung YC, Lao HC, Hsu YW. Premedication with mirtazapine reduces preoperative anxiety and postoperative nausea and vomiting. Anesthesia and Analgesia. 2008;**106**(1): 109-113. table of contents

[22] Meyler's Side Effects of Drugs: The International Encyclopedia of Adverse Drug Reactions and Interactions (Fifteenth Edition). JK A, editor. 2006

[23] Shin JJ, Saadabadi A. Trazodone. Treasure Island (FL): StatPearls Publishing; 2022

[24] Heise CW, Skolnik AB, Raschke RA, Owen-Reece H, Graeme KA. Two cases of refractory cardiogenic shock secondary to bupropion successfully treated with Veno-arterial extracorporeal membrane oxygenation. Journal of Medical Toxicology. 2016; **12**(3):301-304

[25] Saraghi M, Golden LR, Hersh EV. Anesthetic considerations for patients on antidepressant therapy-part I. Anesthesia Progress. 2017;**64**(4):253-261

[26] Matveychuk D, Thomas RK, Swainson J, Khullar A, MacKay M-A, Baker GB, et al. Ketamine as an antidepressant: Overview of its mechanisms of action and potential predictive biomarkers. Therapeutic Advances in Psychopharmacology. 2020; **10**:2045125320916657

[27] Kim J, Farchione T, Potter A, Chen Q, Temple R. Esketamine for treatment-resistant depression - first FDA-approved antidepressant in a new class. The New England Journal of Medicine. 2019;**381**(1):1-4

[28] Hernandez M, Birnbach DJ, Van Zundert AA. Anesthetic management of the illicit-substance-using patient. Current Opinion in Anaesthesiology. 2005;**18**(3):315-324

[29] Peltoniemi MAST, Hagelberg NM, Reponen P, Turpeinen M, Laine K, Neuvonen PJ, et al. Exposure to oral S-ketamine is unaffected by itraconazole but greatly increased by ticlopidine. Clinical Pharmacology and Therapeutics. 2011;**90**(2):296-302

[30] Veraart JKE, Smith-Apeldoorn SY, Bakker IM, Visser BAE, Kamphuis J, Schoevers RA, et al. Pharmacodynamic interactions between ketamine and psychiatric medications used in the treatment of depression: A systematic

review. The International Journal of Neuropsychopharmacology. 2021; **24**(10):808-831

[31] Harbell MW, Dumitrascu C, Bettini L, Yu S, Thiele CM, Koyyalamudi V. Anesthetic considerations for patients on psychotropic drug therapies. Neurology International. 2021;**13**(4):640-658

[32] Howland RH. Potential adverse effects of discontinuing psychotropic drugs: Part 2: Antidepressant drugs. Journal of Psychosocial Nursing and Mental Health Services. 2010;**48**(7):9-12

[33] Foster AC, Kemp JA. Glutamate- and GABA-based CNS therapeutics. Current Opinion in Pharmacology. 2006;**6**(1): 7-17

[34] Griffin CE 3rd, KA, Bueno FR, Kaye AD. Benzodiazepine pharmacology and central nervous system-mediated effects. The Ochsner Journal. 2013;**13**: 214-223

[35] Kim JJ, Hibbs RE. Direct structural insights into GABA(A) receptor pharmacology. Trends in Biochemical Sciences. 2021;**46**(6):502-517

[36] Veselis Robert A, Reinsel Ruth A, Feshchenko Vladimir A, Wronski M. The comparative amnestic effects of midazolam, Propofol, thiopental, and fentanyl at Equisedative concentrations. Anesthesiology. 1997;**87**(4):749-764

[37] Linassi F, Obert DP, Maran E, Tellaroli P, Kreuzer M, Sanders RD, et al. Implicit memory and anesthesia: A systematic review and meta-analysis. Life (Basel). 2021;**11**(8):850

[38] Messina AG, Wang M, Ward MJ, Wilker CC, Smith BB, Vezina DP, et al. Anaesthetic interventions for prevention of awareness during surgery. Cochrane Database of Systematic Reviews. 2016; **10**(10):Cd007272

[39] Mijderwijk H, Vanb S, Duivenvoorden HJ, Stolker RJ. Effectiveness of benzodiazepine premedication on recovery in day-case surgery: A systematic review with meta-analysis. Minerva Anestesiologica. 2016; **82**(4):438-464

[40] Otani K. Cytochrome P450 3A4 and benzodiazepines. Seishin Shinkeigaku Zasshi. 2003;**105**(5):631-642

[41] Jones D, Story DA. Serotonin syndrome and the anaesthetist. Anaesthesia and Intensive Care. 2005; **33**(2):181-187

[42] Ungur AL, Neumann T, Borchers F, Spies C. Perioperative Management of Alcohol Withdrawal Syndrome. Visceral Medicine. 2020;**36**(3):160-166

[43] Kim SH, Fechner J. Remimazolam - current knowledge on a new benzodiazepine intravenous anesthetic agent. Korean Journal of Anesthesiology. 2022;**75**:307-315

[44] Hu Q, Liu X, Wen C, Li D, Lei X. Remimazolam: An updated review of a new sedative and Anaesthetic. Drug Design, Development and Therapy. 2022;**16**:3957-3974

[45] Wang M, Zhao X, Yin P, Bao X, Tang H, Kang X. Profile of Remimazolam in anesthesiology: A narrative review of clinical research Progress. Drug Design, Development and Therapy. 2022;**16**:3431-3444

[46] Mancuso CE, Tanzi MG, Gabay M. Paradoxical reactions to benzodiazepines: Literature review and treatment options. Pharmacotherapy. 2004;**24**(9):1177-1185

[47] Lee SJ, Sung TY. Emergence agitation: Current knowledge and unresolved questions. Korean Journal of Anesthesiology. 2020;**73**(6):471-485

[48] Fujisawa T, Miyata K, Nitta Y, Terui A, Ishikawa E, Hamaya E, et al. Cross-sectional study of propofol dose during intravenous sedation for dental surgery in patients with long-term oral benzodiazepine therapy: A secondary publication. Clinical and Experimental Dental Research. 2022;**8**:1124-1129

[49] Haybarger E, Young AS, Giovannitti JA Jr. Benzodiazepine allergy with anesthesia administration: A review of current literature. Anesthesia Progress. 2016;**63**(3):160-167

[50] Tai CY, Liu HY, Cata JP, Dai YX, Chen MH, Chen JT, et al. The association between general anesthesia and new postoperative uses of sedative-hypnotics: A Nationwide matched cohort study. Journal of Clinical Medicine. 2022; **11**(12):3360

[51] Wang L, Pan Y, Ye C, Guo L, Luo S, Dai S, et al. A network meta-analysis of the long- and short-term efficacy of sleep medicines in adults and older adults. Neuroscience and Biobehavioral Reviews. 2021;**131**:489-496

[52] Baandrup L, Ebdrup BH, Rasmussen J, Lindschou J, Gluud C, Glenthøj BY. Pharmacological interventions for benzodiazepine discontinuation in chronic benzodiazepine users. Cochrane Database of Systematic Reviews. 2018; **3**(3):Cd011481

[53] Hukins D, Macleod U, Boland JW. Identifying potentially inappropriate prescribing in older people with dementia: A systematic review. European Journal of Clinical Pharmacology. 2019;**75**(4):467-481

[54] Masudo C, Ogawa Y, Yamashita N, Mihara K. Association between elimination half-life of benzodiazepines and falls in the elderly: A meta-analysis of observational studies. Yakugaku Zasshi. 2019;**139**(1):113-122

[55] Bandelow B. Current and novel psychopharmacological drugs for anxiety disorders. In: Kim Y-K, editor. Anxiety Disorders: Rethinking and Understanding Recent Discoveries. Singapore: Springer Singapore; 2020. pp. 347-365

[56] Lenhardt R, Orhan-Sungur M, Komatsu R, Govinda R, Kasuya Y, Sessler DI, et al. Suppression of shivering during hypothermia using a novel drug combination in healthy volunteers. Anesthesiology. 2009;**111**(1):110-115

[57] Haberzettl R, Fink H, Bert B. Role of 5-HT(1A)- and 5-HT(2A) receptors for the murine model of the serotonin syndrome. Journal of Pharmacological and Toxicological Methods. 2014;**70**(2): 129-133

[58] Llorca PM, Spadone C, Sol O, Danniau A, Bougerol T, Corruble E, et al. Efficacy and safety of hydroxyzine in the treatment of generalized anxiety disorder: A 3-month double-blind study. The Journal of Clinical Psychiatry. 2002; **63**(11):1020-1027

[59] Aleo E, Picado AL, Abancens BJ, Soto Beauregard C, Tur Salamanca N, Esteban Polonios C, et al. Evaluation of the effect of hydroxyzine on preoperative anxiety and anesthetic adequacy in children: Double blind randomized clinical trial. BioMed Research International. 2021;**2021**: 7394042

[60] Bobo WV. The diagnosis and Management of Bipolar I and II disorders: Clinical practice update. Mayo

Clinic Proceedings. 2017;**92**(10): 1532-1551

[61] Chokhawala K, Lee S, Saadabadi A. Lithium. Treasure Island (FL): StatPearls; 2022

[62] Tondo L, Alda M, Bauer M, Bergink V, Grof P, Hajek T, et al. Clinical use of lithium salts: Guide for users and prescribers. International Journal of Bipolar Disorders. 2019;**7**(1):16

[63] Flood S, Bodenham A. Lithium: Mimicry, mania, and muscle relaxants. Continuing Education in Anaesthesia Critical Care & Pain. 2010;**10**(3):77-80

[64] Poels EMP, Bijma HH, Galbally M, Bergink V. Lithium during pregnancy and after delivery: A review. International Journal of Bipolar Disorders. 2018;**6**(1):26

[65] Kishimoto N, Yoshikawa H, Seo K. Potentiation of Rocuronium bromide by lithium carbonate: A case report. Anesthesia Progress. 2020;**67**(3):146-150

[66] Rahman M, Nguyen H. Valproic Acid. Treasure Island, (FL): StatPearls; 2022

[67] Abdallah C. Considerations in perioperative assessment of valproic acid coagulopathy. Journal of Anaesthesiology Clinical Pharmacology. 2014;**30**(1):7-9

[68] Kodama M, Higuchi H, Ishii-Maruhama M, Nakano M, Honda-Wakasugi Y, Maeda S, et al. Multi-drug therapy for epilepsy influenced bispectral index after a bolus propofol administration without affecting propofol's pharmacokinetics: A prospective cohort study. Scientific Reports. 2020;**10**(1):1578

[69] Ouchi K, Sugiyama K. Required propofol dose for anesthesia and time to emerge are affected by the use of antiepileptics: Prospective cohort study. BMC Anesthesiology. 2015;**15**:34

[70] Yang LQ, Yu WF, Cao YF, Gong B, Chang Q, Yang GS. Potential inhibition of cytochrome P450 3A4 by propofol in human primary hepatocytes. World Journal of Gastroenterology. 2003;**9**(9): 1959-1962

[71] Maan JS, Duong Tv H, Saadabadi A. Carbamazepine. Treasure Island (FL): StatPearls; 2022

[72] Andreasen AH, Brosen K, Damkier P. A comparative pharmacokinetic study in healthy volunteers of the effect of carbamazepine and oxcarbazepine on cyp3a4. Epilepsia. 2007;**48**(3):490-496

[73] Prabhavalkar KS, Poovanpallil NB, Bhatt LK. Management of bipolar depression with lamotrigine: An antiepileptic mood stabilizer. Frontiers in Pharmacology. 2015;**6**:242

[74] Verrotti A, Striano P, Iapadre G, Zagaroli L, Bonanni P, Coppola G, et al. The pharmacological management of Lennox-Gastaut syndrome and critical literature review. Seizure. 2018;**63**: 17-25

[75] Kornhall D, Nielsen EW. Failure of ketamine anesthesia in a patient with lamotrigine overdose. Case Reports in Critical Care. 2014;**2014**:916360

[76] Kessler RC, Birnbaum H, Demler O, Falloon IR, Gagnon E, Guyer M, et al. The prevalence and correlates of nonaffective psychosis in the National Comorbidity Survey Replication (NCS-R). Biological Psychiatry. 2005;**58**(8): 668-676

[77] Wu EQ, Shi L, Birnbaum H, Hudson T, Kessler R. Annual prevalence

of diagnosed schizophrenia in the USA: A claims data analysis approach. Psychological Medicine. 2006;**36**(11): 1535-1540

[78] Desai P, Lawson KA, Barner JC, Rascati KL. Estimating the direct and indirect costs for community-dwelling patients with schizophrenia. Journal of Pharmaceutical Health Services Research. 2013;**4**(4):187-194

[79] Arciniegas DB. Psychosis. Continuum (Minneap Minn). 2015;**21**(3 Behavioral Neurology and Neuropsychiatry):715-736

[80] Dorado P, Penas-Lledo EM, Llerena A. CYP2D6 polymorphism: Implications for antipsychotic drug response, schizophrenia and personality traits. Pharmacogenomics. 2007;**8**(11): 1597-1608

[81] Haddad PM, Anderson IM. Antipsychotic-related QTc prolongation, torsade de pointes and sudden death. Drugs. 2002;**62**(11):1649-1671

[82] Vieweg WV. New generation antipsychotic drugs and QTc interval prolongation. Primary Care Companion to the Journal of Clinical Psychiatry. 2003;**5**(5):205-215

[83] Miller DD. Atypical antipsychotics: Sleep, sedation, and efficacy. Prim Care Companion to the Journal of Clinical Psychiatry. 2004;**6**(Suppl. 2):3-7

[84] Kudoh A. Perioperative management for chronic schizophrenic patients. Anesthesia and Analgesia. 2005;**101**(6):1867-1872

[85] Brandt L, Bschor T, Henssler J, et al. Antipsychotic withdrawal symptoms: A systematic review and meta-analysis. Frontiers in Psychiatry. 2020;**11**:569912

[86] Horowitz M, Sameer J, Natesan S, et al. A method for tapering antipsychotic treatment that may minimize the risk of relapse. Schizophrenia Bulletin. 2021;**47**(4): 1116-1129

[87] Boulant JA. Role of the preoptic-anterior hypothalamus in thermoregulation and fever. Clinical Infectious Diseases. 2000;**31**(Suppl 5): S157-S161

[88] Henderson VWWG. Neuroleptic malignant syndrome: A pathogenetic role for dopamine receptor blockade? Neurology. 1981;**31**(2):132

[89] TI B. Neuroleptic Malignant Syndrome Medscape. 2020. Available from: https://emedicine.medscape.com/article/816018-overview

[90] Strawn JRKPJ. Caroff SN neuroleptic malignant syndrome. The American Journal of Psychiatry. 2007;**164**(6):870

[91] Chandran GJ, Mikler JR, Keegan DL. Neuroleptic malignant syndrome: Case report and discussion. CMAJ. 2003; **169**(5):439-442

[92] Caroff SNMS. Neuroleptic malignant syndrome. The Medical Clinics of North America. 1993;**77**(1):185

[93] Kogoj AVI. Olanzapine induced neuroleptic malignant syndrome–a case review. Human Psychopharmacology. 2003;**18**(4):301

[94] Desai DGK, Kumar R, Biswas A. Levosulpiride-induced neuroleptic malignant syndrome in rheumatoid arthritis. BML Case Reports. 2018;**2018**: bcr2018224679

[95] Jeffrey L. Neuroleptic malignant syndrome. The American Journal of Psychiatry. 1985;**142**(10):1137

[96] Mizuno YTH, Mizuta E, Kuno S. Malignant syndrome in Parkinson's disease: Concept and review of the literature. Parkinsonism & Related Disorders. 2003;**9**:S3-S9

[97] Onofrj M, Thomas A. Acute akinesia in Parkinson disease. Neurology. 2005; **64**(7):1162-1169

[98] Keck PE Jr. PHJ, Cohen BM, McElroy SL, Nierenberg AA risk factors for neuroleptic malignant syndrome. A case-control study. Archives of General Psychiatry. 1989;**46**(10):914

[99] Gurrera RJ. Is neuroleptic malignant syndrome a neurogenic form of malignant hyperthermia? Clinical Neuropharmacology. 2002;**25**(4):183

[100] Mason PJ, Morris VA, Balcezak TJ. Serotonin syndrome. Presentation of 2 cases and review of the literature. Medicine (Baltimore). 2000;**79**(4): 201-209

[101] Lazarus A. Neuroleptic malignant syndrome. Hospital & Community Psychiatry. 1989;**40**(12):1229-1230

[102] Couch GA, White MP, de Gray LE. Central nervous system stimulants: Basic pharmacology and relevance to anaesthesia and critical care. Anaesthesia & Intensive Care Medicine. 2020;**21**(10): 503-511

[103] Compton WM, Han B, Blanco C, Johnson K, Jones CM. Prevalence and correlates of prescription stimulant use, misuse, use disorders, and motivations for misuse among adults in the United States. The American Journal of Psychiatry. 2018;**175**(8):741-755

[104] Hashemian SM, Farhadi T. A review on modafinil: The characteristics, function, and use in critical care. Journal of Drug Assessment. 2020;**9**(1):82-86

[105] Administration SAaMHS. Results from the 2010 National Survey on Drug Use and Health: Summary of National Findings. In: Administration SAaMHS, editor. Administration SAaMHS, Rockville, MD, 2011.

[106] Campbell R, Young SP. Central nervous system stimulants: Basic pharmacology and relevance to anaesthesia and critical care. Anaesthesia & Intensive Care Medicine. 2018;**19**(1): 20-24

[107] Levine M, Brooks DE, Truitt CA, Wolk BJ, Boyer EW, Ruha AM. Toxicology in the ICU: Part 1: General overview and approach to treatment. Chest. 2011;**140**(3):795-806

[108] Moran S, Isa J, Steinemann S. Perioperative management in the patient with substance abuse. The Surgical Clinics of North America. 2015;**95**(2): 417-428

[109] Pachlopnik Schmid J, Lemoine R, Nehme N, Cormier-Daire V, Revy P, Debeurme F, et al. Polymerase ε1 mutation in a human syndrome with facial dysmorphism, immunodeficiency, livedo, and short stature ("FILS syndrome"). The Journal of Experimental Medicine. 2012;**209**(13): 2323-2330

[110] Kushikata T, Hirota K. Mechanisms of anesthetic emergence: Evidence for active reanimation. Current Anesthesiology Reports. 2014;**4**(1):49-56

[111] Kumar R. Approved and investigational uses of modafinil : An evidence-based review. Drugs. 2008; **68**(13):1803-1839

[112] Basurto Ona X, Osorio D, Bonfill CX. Drug therapy for treating post-dural puncture headache. Cochrane

Database of Systematic Reviews. 2015;**7**: CD007887

[113] Fischer SP, Schmiesing CA, Guta CG, Brock-Utne JG. General anesthesia and chronic amphetamine use: Should the drug be stopped preoperatively? Anesthesia and Analgesia. 2006;**103**(1):203-206 table of contents

[114] Der-Avakian A, Markou A. Withdrawal from chronic exposure to amphetamine, but not nicotine, leads to an immediate and enduring deficit in motivated behavior without affecting social interaction in rats. Behavioural Pharmacology. 2010;**21**(4):359-368

[115] Danielsson K, Lagström O, Ericson M, Söderpalm B, Adermark L. Subregion-specific effects on striatal neurotransmission and dopamine-signaling by acute and repeated amphetamine exposure. Neuropharmacology. 2021;**194**:108638

[116] Johnston RR, Way WL, Miller RD. Alteration of anesthetic requirement by amphetamine. Anesthesiology. 1972; **36**(4):357-363

[117] Zinboonyahgoon N, & Garfield, J Essential Clinical Anesthesia Review: Keywords, Questions and Answers for the Boards Cambridge: Cambridge University Press; 20215

[118] Steinhauer JRCJ. Spontaneous coronary artery dissection associated with cocaine use: A case report and brief review. Cardiovascular Pathology. 2001; **10**(3):141-145

[119] Fernandez-Sola JJA, Estruch R, et al. High alcohol intake as a risk and prognostic factor for community-acquired pneumonia. Archives of Internal Medicine. 1995;**155**(15): 1649-1654

[120] Newman R, Gallagher, MA, Gomez AE. Alcohol Withdrawal: StatPearls; 2021

[121] Liu Y, Xu Y, Li Q, Zhang L. Alcohol withdrawal management in patients undergoing head and neck reconstruction-a retrospective analysis. Frontiers of Oral and Maxillofacial Medicine. 2021;**3**:36

[122] Tønnesen H, Nielsen PR, Lauritzen JB, Møller AM. Smoking and alcohol intervention before surgery: Evidence for best practice. British Journal of Anaesthesia. 2009;**102**(3): 297-306

[123] Havakuk O, Rezkalla SH, Kloner RA. The cardiovascular effects of cocaine. Journal of the American College of Cardiology. 2017;**70**(1):101-113

[124] Birchenough SA, Borowitz K, Lin KY. Complete soft palate necrosis and velopharyngeal insufficiency resulting from intranasal inhalation of prescription narcotics and cocaine. The Journal of Craniofacial Surgery. 2007; **18**(6):1482-1485

[125] Ghuran A, Nolan J. Recreational drug misuse: Issues for the cardiologist. Heart. 2000;**83**(6):627-633

[126] SMH MR. Opioid Withdrawal. Treasure Island (FL): StatPearls Publishing; 2022

[127] Mattick RP, Breen C, Kimber J, Davoli M. Buprenorphine maintenance versus placebo or methadone maintenance for opioid dependence. Cochrane Database of Systematic Reviews. 2014;**2**:CD002207

[128] Krupitsky E, Nunes EV, Ling W, Illeperuma A, Gastfriend DR, Silverman BL. Injectable extended-release naltrexone for opioid

dependence: A double-blind, placebo-controlled, multicentre randomised trial. Lancet. 2011;**377**(9776):1506-1513

[129] Lee JD, Friedmann PD, Kinlock TW, Nunes EV, Boney TY, Hoskinson RA Jr, et al. Extended-release naltrexone to prevent opioid relapse in criminal justice offenders. The New England Journal of Medicine. 2016; **374**(13):1232-1242

[130] Ward ENQA, Wilens TE. Opioid use disorders: Perioperative Management of a Special Population. Anesthesia and Analgesia. 2018;**127**(2): 539-547

[131] Kohan L, Potru S, Barreveld AM, Sprintz M, Lane O, Aryal A, et al. Buprenorphine management in the perioperative period: Educational review and recommendations from a multisociety expert panel. Regional Anesthesia Pain Medicine. 2021;**46**(10): 840

[132] IGALMI™. Prescribing Information: BioXcel Therapeutics, Inc. 2022. Available from: https://www.accessdata.fda.gov/drugsatfda_docs/label/2022/215390s000lbl.pdf

[133] Preskorn SH, Zeller S, Citrome L, Finman J, Goldberg JF, Fava M, et al. Effect of sublingual Dexmedetomidine vs placebo on acute agitation associated with bipolar disorder: A randomized clinical trial. Journal of the American Medical Association. 2022;**327**(8): 727-736

[134] LYBALVI®. Prescribing Information.: Alkermes Pharma Ireland Limited; 2021 [Available from: https://www.accessdata.fda.gov/drugsatfda_docs/label/2021/213378s000lbl.pdf

[135] Kahn RS, Silverman BL, DiPetrillo L, Graham C, Jiang Y, Yin J, et al. A phase 3, multicenter study to assess the 1-year safety and tolerability of a combination of olanzapine and samidorphan in patients with schizophrenia: Results from the ENLIGHTEN-2 long-term extension. Schizophrenia Research. 2021;**232**:45-53

[136] Thomas K, Saadabadi A. Olanzapine. StatPearls. Treasure Island; (FL)2022

[137] CAPLYTA®. Prescribing Information: Intra-Cellular Therapies, Inc. 2021. Available from: https://www.accessdata.fda.gov/drugsatfda_docs/label/2021/209500s005s006lbl.pdf

[138] Maini K, Hollier JW, Gould H, Bollich V, John LaForge J, Cornett EM, et al. Lumateperone tosylate, A selective and concurrent modulator of serotonin, dopamine, and glutamate, in the treatment of schizophrenia. Health Psychology Research. 2021;**9**(1):24932

[139] Administration USFaD. Table of Substrates, Inhibitors and Inducers. 2022 [Available from: https://www.fda.gov/drugs/drug-interactions-labeling/drug-development-and-drug-interactions-table-substrates-inhibitors-and-inducers

[140] Mishra SSB, Gahche JJ, Potischman N. Dietary Supplement Use among Adults: United States, 2017–2018. Hyattsville, MD: National Center for Health Statistics; 2021

[141] Franco Ruiz SGMP. Dietary supplements and the anesthesiologist: Research results and the state of the art. Revista Colombiana de Anesthesiologia. 2014;**42**:90-99

[142] Malhi GSBE, Bassett D, Boyce P, Bryant R, Hazell P, Hopwood M, et al. Murray G the 2020 Royal Australian and new Zealand College of Psychiatrists clinical practice guidelines for mood

disorders. The Australian and New Zealand Journal of Psychiatry. 2021; **55**(1):7

[143] Tyler's Herbs of Choice: The Therapeutic Use of Phytomedicinals. In: Pharmaceutical Products Press; 3rd edition by Dennis V.C. Awang. Boca Raton, FL: CRC Press Taylor and Francis Group; 2009. pp. 103-104

[144] Wong ATS. Herbal medicines and anaesthesia. Continuing Education in Anaesthesia Critical Care & Pain. 2010; **11**(1):14-17

[145] Haller CABN. Adverse cardiovascular and central nervous system events associated with dietary supplements containing ephedra alkaloids. The New England Journal of Medicine. 2000;**343**(25):1833

[146] J G. PDR for Herbal Medicines. Montalve NJ: Medical Economic Company; 1998

[147] Biloba G. Natural Medicines. In: TRC Natural Remedies 2020. Denver CO: Therapeutic Research Center Healthcare; 2020

[148] Maerz S, Liu CH, Guo W, Zhu YZ. Anti-ischaemic effects of bilobalide on neonatal rat cardiomyocytes and the involvement of the platelet-activating factor receptor. Bioscience Reports. 2011;**31**(5):439-447

[149] Rosenblatt M, Mindel J. Spontaneous hyphema associated with ingestion of Ginkgo biloba extract. The New England Journal of Medicine. 1997; **336**(15):1108

[150] Rowin J, Lewis SL. Spontaneous bilateral subdural hematomas associated with chronic Ginkgo biloba ingestion. Neurology. 1996;**46**(6):1775-1776

[151] von Moltke LL, Weemhoff JL, Bedir E, Khan IA, Harmatz JS, Goldman P, et al. Inhibition of human cytochromes P450 by components of Ginkgo biloba. The Journal of Pharmacy and Pharmacology. 2004;**56**(8):1039-1044

[152] Brekhman II. New substances of plant origin which increase nonspecific resistance. Annual Review of Pharmacology. 1969;**9**:419-430

[153] Kimura YOH, Arichi S. Effect of various gingsengsaponin on 5-hydroxytryptamine release and aggregation in human platelets. The Journal of Pharmacy and Pharmacology. 1988;**40**:838-843

[154] Sotaniemi EAHE, Rautio A. Ginseng therpy in non-insulin-dependend diabetic patients. Diabetes Care. 1995;**18**:1373-1375

[155] Encyclopedia UoRMC-H. What to Know About Herbs and Surgery. Rochester, NY: University of Rochester Medical Center; 2022

[156] Ang-Lee MK, Moss J, Yuan CS. Herbal medicines and perioperative care. Journal of the American Medical Association. 2001;**286**(2):208-216

[157] Chaplin RLJ, Jedynak J, Johnson D, Heiter D, Shovelton L, Garrett N. The effects of valerian on the time course of emergence from general anesthesia in Sprague-Dawley rats. AANA Journal. 2007;**75**:431-435

[158] Witte S, Loew D, Gaus W. Meta-analysis of the efficacy of the acetonic kava-kava extract WS1490 in patients with non-psychotic anxiety disorders. Phytotherapy Research. 2005;**19**(3): 183-188

[159] Pittler MH, Ernst E. Kava extract for treating anxiety. Cochrane Database

of Systematic Reviews. 2003;**1**: CD003383

[160] Sarris J, LaPorte E, Schweitzer I. Kava: A comprehensive review of efficacy, safety, and psychopharmacology. The Australian and New Zealand Journal of Psychiatry. 2011;**45**(1):27-35

[161] Teschke R, Schwarzenboeck A, Hennermann KH. Kava hepatotoxicity: A clinical survey and critical analysis of 26 suspected cases. European Journal of Gastroenterology & Hepatology. 2008; **20**(12):1182-1193

[162] Lyons TR. Herbal medicines and possible anesthesia interaction. AANA Journal. 2002;**70**:47-51

[163] A D. Review of abnormal laboratory testresults and toxic effects due to use of herbal medicines. American Journal of Clinical Pathology. 2003;**120**(1):127-137

[164] Baghai TC, Möller HJ. Electroconvulsive therapy and its different indications. Dialogues in Clinical Neuroscience. 2008;**10**(1): 105-117

[165] Zolezzi M. Medication management during electroconvulsant therapy. Neuropsychiatric Disease and Treatment. 2016;**12**:931-939

[166] Lee K, Jenkins KD, Sparkle T. A narrative overview of current anesthetic drugs in electroconvulsive therapy. Life (Basel). 2021;**11**(9):981

[167] Ghoneim MM, O'Hara MW. Depression and postoperative complications: An overview. BMC Surgery. 2016;**16**:5

[168] Bufalino CHN, Aguglia E, Pariante CM. The role of immune genes in the association between depression and inflammation: A review of recent clinical studies. Brain, Behavior, and Immunity. 2012;**31**:31-47

[169] C V. Mental health and immunity (review). Experimental and Therapeutic Medicine. 2020;**20**(6):211

[170] Klement MR BA, Blizzard DJ, et al. Should We Think Twice About Psychiatric Disease in Total Hip Arthroplasty? 2016:221-6

[171] Vaishnav M, Gupta S, Vaishnav P. Psychiatric intervention pre- and post-bariatric surgery. Indian Journal of Psychiatry. 2022;**64**(Suppl. 2):S473-SS83

[172] McBride KESM, Steffens D, et al. Mental illness and surgery: Do we care? ANZ Journal of Surgery. 2019;**89**(6): 630-631

[173] McBride KE, Solomon MJ, Lambert T, O'Shannassy S, Yates C, Isbester J, et al. Surgical experience for patients with serious mental illness: A qualitative study. BMC Psychiatry. 2021; **21**(1):47

[174] McBride KE, Solomon MJ, Steffens D, Bannon PG, Glozier N. Mental illness and surgery: do we care? ANZ Journal of Surgery. 2019 Jun:**89**(6):630-631. DOI: 10.1111/ans.15248. PMID: 31179630

[175] Clay RA. How psychologists prepare patients for surgery. Monitor on Psychology. 2020;**51**(6):40

[176] G S. Pre-surgical psychiatric evaluation: 6 considerations. Current. Psychiatry. 2010;**9**(10):96

[177] ZULRESSO. Prescribing Information. Cambridge, MA: Sage Therapeutics, Inc; 6/2019

[178] Meltzer-Brody S, Colquhoun H, Riesenber R, et al. Brexanolone injection

in post-partum depression: Two multicentre, double-blind, randomised, placebo-controlled, phase 3 trials. The Lancet. 2018;**392**(10152):1058-1070

[179] Brunet A, Saumier D, Liu A, Streiner DL, Tremblay J, Pitman RK. Reduction of PTSD symptoms with pre-reactivation propranolol therapy: A randomized controlled trial. The American Journal of Psychiatry. 2018; **175**(5):427-433

[180] McGuire P, Robson P, Cubala WJ et al. Cannabidiol (CBD) as an adjunctive therapy in schizophrenia: A multicenter randomized controlled trial. The American Journal of Psychiatry. 2018;**173**(3):225-2321

Section 9

Trauma Medicine

Chapter 13

Anesthesiology for Trauma Medicine: Roles, Medications, Airway Management, and Multidisciplinary Team Coordination

Vanessa Reese, Wayne B. Bauerle, Anthony P. Allsbrook, Jennifer Hwang and Prabhdeep Hehar

Abstract

Given the complex nature of trauma, a highly organized, multidisciplinary approach is necessary to ensure the best possible outcomes. Anesthesia providers play a critical role in the management and effective treatment of trauma patients. This chapter will address both the multidisciplinary and multitiered management of trauma patients with a focus on the intersection of trauma staff and anesthesia in three phases: the initial evaluation (i.e., in the bay), intraoperative care, and postoperative care. Included is a brief discussion on more recent methodologies and newly incorporated technologies in the resuscitation of trauma patients.

Keywords: trauma, anesthesia, resuscitation, intraoperative care, postoperative care

1. Introduction

Multisystem trauma patients are medically complex largely due to the presence of shock. Therefore, their physiology significantly differs from those undergoing elective surgical procedures. Data has shown that emergent operative procedures demonstrate both increases in overall morbidity and mortality [1]. As perioperative partners, a collaboration between surgeons and anesthesia providers from the time of initial trauma response activation to immediate postoperative care is critical for improved patient outcomes. It is important to note that unlike other fields of surgery, trauma utilizes a well-established systematic approach to the initial management and stabilization of trauma patients.

The initial approach to trauma involves a rapid, systematic evaluation of the patient known as the primary and secondary surveys. Advanced Trauma Life Support (ATLS) is the most referenced approach that allows one to identify the most immediate threats to life through the ABCDEs of the primary survey [2]. The primary survey simplifies priorities. Any problems identified are promptly treated as they arise. This reduces the risk of not recognizing life-threatening injuries.

The primary survey progresses in sequential order from A to E as follows [2]:

Airway maintenance with cervical spine protection.
Breathing and ventilation.
Circulation with hemorrhage control.
Disability: neurologic status.
Exposure/**E**nvironmental control.

Objectives
In Bay

Primary Survey
• MTP for hemodynamic instability, active bleeding, transfusion in the trauma bay, or ABC score ≥ 2
• Continue primary and secondary survey
Reassess endpoints (if MTP initiated)
• Goals met: downgrade or stop MTP
    o Hemodynamically stable, anatomic control of hemorrhage, hemoglobin > 10g/dL, PT < 18 seconds, PTT < 35 seconds, PLT > 150 x 10^9, fibrinogen levels > 180 g/L
    o Imaging and further work up of identified injuries as needed
• Goals unmet: continue evaluation and resuscitation
    o Component specific resuscitation as needed
    o Operative intervention as indicated

Intra Op
Primary Survey • Continue or begin resuscitation efforts • Establish airway, peripheral and/or central access (if not already done), place arterial line if needed • Determine whether front of cervical collar can be removed (if present) Induction • In line RSI • Preventillate vs apneic intubation • Lung protective ventilation strategies Normothermia • Bair hugger
Post Op

Continue Resuscitation
• IV fluids to prevent AKI
• Reassess endpoints
    o TEG and ROTEM
    o Downgrade, discontinue, or adjust MTP based on endpoints
    o Electrolyte management: treat calcium, magnesium, and potassium derangements as needed
    o Correct acidosis
Normothermia
• Temperature management system
• Warm fluids
Tertiary Exam

Figure 1.
Stepwise approach to preoperative, perioperative, and postoperative phase of case. MTP = massive transfusion protocol, ABC score = Assessment of Blood Consumption score, RSI = rapid sequence intubation, AKI = acute kidney injury, TEG = thromboelastogram, ROTEM = rotational thromboelastometry. The figure above is an internal resource from the St Luke's University Hospital Network Trauma department.

A hard stop occurs at each section when an intervention needs to be performed. Utilizing a systematic approach is imperative in settings with limited resources. However, at major trauma centers, multiple injuries may be attended to simultaneously.

Adjuncts are utilized during or immediately following the primary survey. Examples of adjuncts include vital sign monitoring, insertion of a urinary catheter to monitor urine output, focused assessment with sonography for trauma (FAST), extended FAST (eFAST), X-rays, and bloodwork. The adjunctive data help guide resuscitative efforts and should be re-evaluated as needed to ensure appropriate resuscitation of the patient.

Once the primary survey is completed and the patient is demonstrating hemodynamic stability, the secondary survey may begin. The focus shifts to collecting a complete history and performing a thorough physical examination to ensure injuries have not been missed. Important questions to ask about the patient's history can be remembered using the mnemonic AMPLE: Allergies, Medications, Past illnesses/Pregnancy, Last meal, and Events/Environment related to the injury [2]. The head-to-toe physical exam should include a detailed neurological exam, and if indicated, the genitals and rectum should also be examined. Information regarding the mechanism of injury provides valuable insight into the types of injuries to expect and can help determine appropriate adjuncts to the secondary survey, including CT scans, additional X-rays, and other diagnostic imaging.

Overall, the medical approaches, diagnostic algorithms, and speed by which decisions are made in Trauma Medicine vary significantly in comparison to other medical fields. Unlike the Level I trauma patient that is transported to the emergency department, in the previous chapters, the majority of the patient populations were relatively hemodynamically stable, the patient's history and medical management were well documented, and the acuity of the medical care provided was performed in an elective manner.

In this chapter, we will provide a brief introduction to the epidemiology of unintentional injury in the United States and discuss clinical practice updates in the field of trauma medicine, with emphasis on certain medical management strategies provided by trauma anesthesiologists. After the introduction, we will discuss patient management in the trauma bay, along with appropriate intraoperative and postoperative care following major surgery (**Figure 1**). Finally, we will discuss future directions regarding the management of trauma patients from an anesthesiologist's perspective in conjunction with how the current landscape of trauma anesthesiology continues to evolve.

1.1 Epidemiology of Unintentional Injury

In the United States, the most common reasons for presentation to the emergency department are injury and poisoning [3]. Unintentional injury alone accounts for upward of 97.9 million ED visits [4]. The two age groups that tend to experience the worst outcomes from unintentional injury include those younger than 46 years of age and the geriatric population [5, 6]. Although young patients tend to experience significantly higher morbid levels of trauma, minor trauma experienced by the elderly portends significant morbidity and mortality due to their increased frailty [5]. In patients younger than 46 years of age, trauma is the leading cause of death [5].

In the United States, unintentional injuries were the fourth leading cause of death in the year 2020 following heart disease, cancer, and COVID-19 [7]. Unintentional injuries include unintentional poisoning/overdose, motor vehicle accidents (MVA), unintentional drowning, and unintentional falls [7]. From 1999 to 2006, the unintentional injury rate rose by 1.9%. From 2014 to 2017, the rate of unintentional injury rose even further, with an annual growth rate of 6.8% [8]. When comparing the rate of age-adjusted death due to unintentional injury in 2020 to 2019, there was a 16.8% increase, largely due to a rise in deaths due to unintentional poisoning/overdose [7, 9]. In 2020 alone, unintentional accidents accounted for 200,955 deaths in the United States [4].

Unintentional injury accounts not only for a substantial proportion of annual ED visits and deaths, but it is also considered a significant contributor to the cost burden placed on the United States healthcare system. In 2019, treatment of these unintentional injuries resulted in $4.2 trillion in costs, with $327 billion being directly related to medical care and the remaining difference being attributable to costs associated with days lost of work and quality of life [9].

Given that unintentional injury continues to grow at a steady rate and provided that this subgroup of patients accounts for a large proportion of ED visits, adequate and timely management of this patient population is essential, with the main goal being to provide scientifically sound and cost-efficient medical care. Trauma anesthesiologists provide a unique subset of skills in the multidisciplinary treatment of trauma patients, especially when considering that with many of these patients present in a hemodynamically unstable state, there is usually minimal time to prepare the patient for major operations, and the ability to act swiftly and efficiently within a truncated time period is essential to improved patient outcomes.

2. Methods

A literature search was performed using Google search keywords of "trauma anesthesia" and "anesthesia in trauma." The Advanced Trauma and Life Support (ATLS) literature and Trauma Quality Improvement Program (TQIP) literature were also searched for trauma anesthesia information. There were no de facto inclusion criteria and no specific time limitation or time frame to the articles; rather, the articles were included based on relevance or relation to anesthesia methods used for trauma patients.

3. Management in the Trauma Bay

3.1 Resuscitation of the Critically Ill Patient

Guidelines on trauma resuscitation have been implemented by several surgical societies in North America. In the United States, some of the more commonly followed guidelines have been published by the American College of Surgeons (ACS), the American Trauma Society (ATS), the American Association for the Surgery of Trauma (AAST), the Eastern Association for the Surgery of Trauma (EAST), and the Western Trauma Association (WTA) [10]. Resuscitation of a critically injured patient is essential as hemorrhage is the main cause of death within the "golden hour" on arrival at the trauma center. As defined in the guidelines provided by the ACS Trauma Quality Improvement Program (TQIP), massive transfusion protocol (MTP) is the supplementation of >10 units of red blood cells (RBCs) within 24 h [11]. In their guidelines, the ACS provides a set of criteria for initiating a MTP, the correct ratio of blood products to administer, and typical endpoints used to assess the adequacy of resuscitation efforts [11].

A MTP should be initiated if a critically ill trauma patient present in a persistent state of hemodynamic instability has active bleeding requiring a procedure, requires blood transfusion in the trauma bay, or has an Assessment of Blood Consumption

(ABC) score greater than 2 [11] (**Figure 2**). The ABC score was developed by Cotton et al. and is widely accepted due to its ease of use as no lab tests are required and accuracy, with a sensitivity ranging between 75% and 90% and a specificity range from 67% to 88% [12, 13]. This clinically validated scoring tool is endorsed by the ACS [11].

When initiating a MTP, resuscitation should begin with blood products over crystalloid or colloid solutions [11]. A rapid transfuser and blood warmer should be utilized to administer RBCs and plasma, and you should stay at least 1 blood cooler ahead of the current transfusion until the MTP has been terminated [11]. A blood warmer should not be used for products such as platelets and cryoprecipitate. The ideal ratio for blood product resuscitation is a 1:1 or 1:2 ratio of plasma to RBCs [11]. For every 6 units of blood given, supplement 1 unit of platelets [11]. The use of cryoprecipitate and/or fibrinogen during MTP varies widely by institution, and there are no specific guidelines for the administration of cryoprecipitate until laboratory studies and adjunctive testing such as thromboelastography (TEG) and rotational thromboelastometry (ROTEM) have been initiated [11].

When deciding on whether to stop the MTP, it is the role of the anesthesiologist in conjunction with the surgeon to decide if the resuscitation endpoints have been met. The assessment should include the physiological hemodynamic status and the anatomic control of the hemorrhage [11]. Endpoints to assess include hemoglobin >10 g/dL, prothrombin time < 18 seconds, partial thromboplastin time (aPTT) < 35 seconds, platelet count >150 × 10^9, and fibrinogen levels >180 g/L [11]. Based on the previously mentioned endpoints, MTP can be downgraded or completely stopped, and

Component	Score
Penetrating Mechanism	1
SBP ≤ 90	1
HR	1
Positive FAST	1
Score ≥ 2 is likely to require MTP	

Figure 2.
Components of the Assessment of Blood Consumption (ABC) score. Abbreviations: SBP = systolic blood pressure; HR = heart rate; FAST = focused abdominal sonogram for trauma; MTP = massive transfusion protocol. The figure presented above was created using data from the article by Cotton et al. [12].

more targeted blood component supplementation can be performed. MTP should also be withdrawn when it is determined that continued resuscitation would be futile [11].

3.2 Benefits of Massive Transfusion Protocols (MTP)

The use of MTPs in trauma centers has several benefits not only pertaining to patient outcomes but also in improving healthcare resource utilization and reducing healthcare costs. One of the most well-known trauma-based randomized clinical trials (RCTs) of the decade, the PROPPR trial, demonstrated that there was no difference in 24-h or 30-day mortality regardless of whether patients received a 1:1:1 or 1:1:2 ratio of plasma, platelets, and RBCs [14]. In general, the implementation of a MTP at major trauma centers is associated with a reduction in time to transfusion, a reduction in the volume of transfused blood products, and a reduction in overall mortality [15, 16]. In the retrospective cohort study conducted by O'Keeffe et al., the implementation of a MTP at a major trauma center resulted in the reduction of shipment times and a savings of $2270 per patient; however, there was no statistically significant difference in mortality [17]. Although MTPs provide several advantages, the type of blood product used for resuscitation, the protocol established by the institution, and the allocation of healthcare resources continue to be debated.

3.3 Crystalloids and Colloids

Besides blood component therapy and whole blood, crystalloids (normal saline, lactated Ringer's, and isolyte) and colloids (albumin, dextrans, and modified starches) can also be used for volume resuscitation. Crystalloid solutions differ from colloids in that they are composed of smaller molecules than that of colloids; crystalloids are less expensive, and they are easier to use [18]. Colloids are composed of either synthetic or natural molecules and are more likely to induce allergic reactions. The modified starches are no longer used as they can cause coagulopathy as well as acute kidney injury [19]. Benefits of colloids such as albumin are increased oxygen transportation, myocardial contractility, and cardiac output [19]. No survival benefit has been demonstrated for colloids as opposed to crystalloids, and given the cost, crystalloids are preferred. The current ATLS guidelines recommend the use of a 1-L bolus of crystalloid for the initial management of hypotension found during the primary survey [2]. Normal saline is the most used crystalloid solution partially due to its approval of use with blood transfusions; however, a noteworthy potential side effect of normal saline is hyperchloremic metabolic acidosis when large volumes are administered [20]. Lactated Ringer's solution is relatively contraindicated for blood transfusion because it contains calcium. The concern would be a reaction of the calcium with the citrate used to preserve the RBCs, leading to coagulation and clotting of the RBCs. Research has shown that there is no actual adverse effect of using lactated Ringer's solution during a blood transfusion [20]. Lacted Ringer's solution is also thought to promote the inflammatory response seen in shock and trauma states, increase bowel and liver apoptosis, and decrease serum calcium levels by sequestering calcium in the mitochondria [21]. Isolyte is a crystalloid solution with added acetate and gluconate as well as a lower chloride level. Its use is limited due to concerns for potential worsening organ failure as it has been shown to negatively impact peripheral vascular resistance and heart rate [20]. Crystalloids reduce oncotic pressure that can lead to pulmonary and peripheral edema; decreased tissue oxygen exchange, which delays wound healing; as well as exacerbated cell injury and dysfunction via worsening the extracellular calcium shifts seen in shock [21]. Although blood component therapy is the preferred solution for MTPs, colloid and crystalloid solutions may provide adequate volume resuscitation in certain patient populations. For example, normal saline is the preferred solution in patients with traumatic brain injury (TBI) [22]. On the other hand, it is best to avoid the use of colloids, such as albumin, in patients with TBI due to the concern for worsening cerebral pressure and the concomitant increase in mortality [22, 23]. Normal saline or lactated Ringer's are also the treatment of choice for post-traumatic acute kidney injury [20].

3.4 Thromboelastography (TEG) and Rotational Thromboelastometry (ROTEM)

There has been an increase in the number of United States trauma centers that have implemented TEG and ROTEM into their MTP protocols. They both assess clot formation, degradation, and strength but differ in the mechanics behind the rotational mechanism that generates various coagulation parameters. In TEG, the cylinder that contains the blood sample is what oscillates, and a pin that is suspended in the blood sample is stationary [24]. ROTEM utilizes mechanics opposite to TEG, with the blood sample cylinder being stationary and the pin oscillating [24]. The benefit of using TEG and ROTEM in the management of massive hemorrhage is that they rapidly and readily predict various coagulopathies within 15 min to help guide resuscitation efforts [25]. A sample TEG image is presented in **Figure 3** along with a description of the various parameters investigated and the recommended treatment based on the results for each parameter. Provided the numerous advantages of incorporating TEG and ROTEM into standard trauma management, more targeted resuscitation efforts can potentially improve morbidity and mortality (**Figure 4**) [25] . More recent studies have begun to investigate the use of guided resuscitation compared to the standard fixed ratio of platelets, packed RBCs, and plasma. Of the currently available studies regarding the use of TEG or ROTEM for guided resuscitation, the only available RCT, conducted by Gonzales et al., found that guided resuscitation with TEG improves survival while decreasing the number of units of plasma and platelets transfused [29].

3.5 Antifibrinolytics

In the process of hemostasis, a blood clot is formed when fibrinogen is converted to fibrin by thrombin-mediated proteolytic cleavage, with the end result being fibrils that mature to produce a clot that inhibits bleeding [30]. Typically, the clot is broken down by the protein plasminogen after it is converted into the active form, plasmin [31]. Antifibrinolytic agents, such as tranexamic acid (TXA) and amino caproic acid, are synthetic lysine derivatives that competitively inhibit the lysine binding sites on plasminogen, blocking the conversion of plasminogen to plasmin [32]. By doing so, these antifibrinolytic agents inhibit the proteolytic action of plasmin on the fibrin clot, thereby prolonging the life of the clot plug.

Aprotinin is an antifibrinolytic that is not currently available in the United States, and similar to TXA, it is a protease inhibitor. However, unlike TXA, aprotinin differs because it complexes with active serine residues on various proteases [33]. Aprotinin acts reversibly on trypsin, kallikrein, plasmin, and elastase [33]. Of all the available antifibrinolytics, aprotinin is the most potent pharmacological agent available. While this is the most potent agent available, it is seldom used secondary to its propensity to cause renal side effects [34].

Although the role of antifibrinolytics in trauma is not heavily established, more recent studies, such as the CRASH-2 study, have demonstrated that drugs like TXA

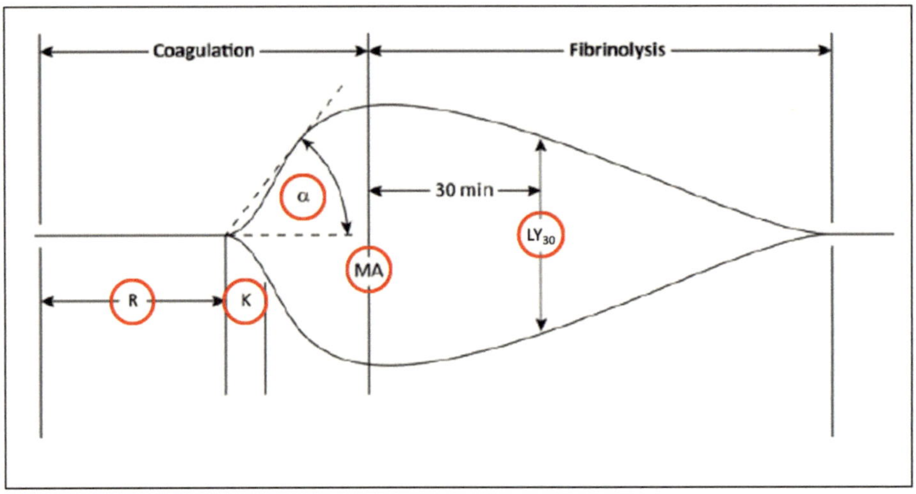

PARAMETER	DEFINITION	NORMAL RANGE	TREATMENT
R – Time	Time till clot initiation	4-8 min	When R-Time prolonged give **FFP**
K – Time	Time to reach 20 mm clot strength	1-3 min	When K-Time prolonged give **Cryo**
α – angle	Rate of clot formation	55-78 degrees	When α-angle decreased give **Cryo**
MA	When clot reaches its maximum strength	54-69 mm	When MA prolonged give **Platelets**
LY_{30}	Amplitude loss at 30 minutes	0-15%	When LY30 prolonged give **TXA**

Figure 3.
Sample image of TEG with the associated parameters and recommended treatment. R-time = reaction time, MA = max amplitude, FFP = fresh frozen plasma, LY30 = percentage lysis after 30 min of MA, Cryo = cryoprecipitate. The image presented above was extracted from the article by Pietri et al. and was slightly modified for simplification [26]. The normal ranges in the bottom portion of the figure were obtained from the article written by Cameron et al. [27]. The treatment approaches for each of the abnormal parameters presented in the bottom half of the figure were discussed in the article written by Johansson et al. [28].

may play a role in improving outcomes in bleeding trauma patients [35]. In their randomized control trial, more than 270 hospitals from over 40 countries were included, and the results of the study demonstrated that the application of TXA reduces all-cause mortality and the incidence of bleeding in patients experiencing traumatic injuries [35]. Current usage recommendations from TQIP indicate antifibrinolytic agents can be used empirically or in response to point of care testing showing increased fibrinolytic activity [11]. The TQIP guidelines for the dosing of TXA are more specific. Patients that are actively bleeding and present within 3 h of injury should be administered 1 g infused intravenously over a timeframe of 10 min, followed by another 1 g infusion over an 8 h period [11].

3.6 Vasopressors and Inotropes

Provided that the acidosis arm of the lethal triad is to some degree due to end-organ malperfusion, many consider the use of vasopressors in massive hemorrhage ill-advised [36]. The pathophysiology behind systemic vascular resistance is that in

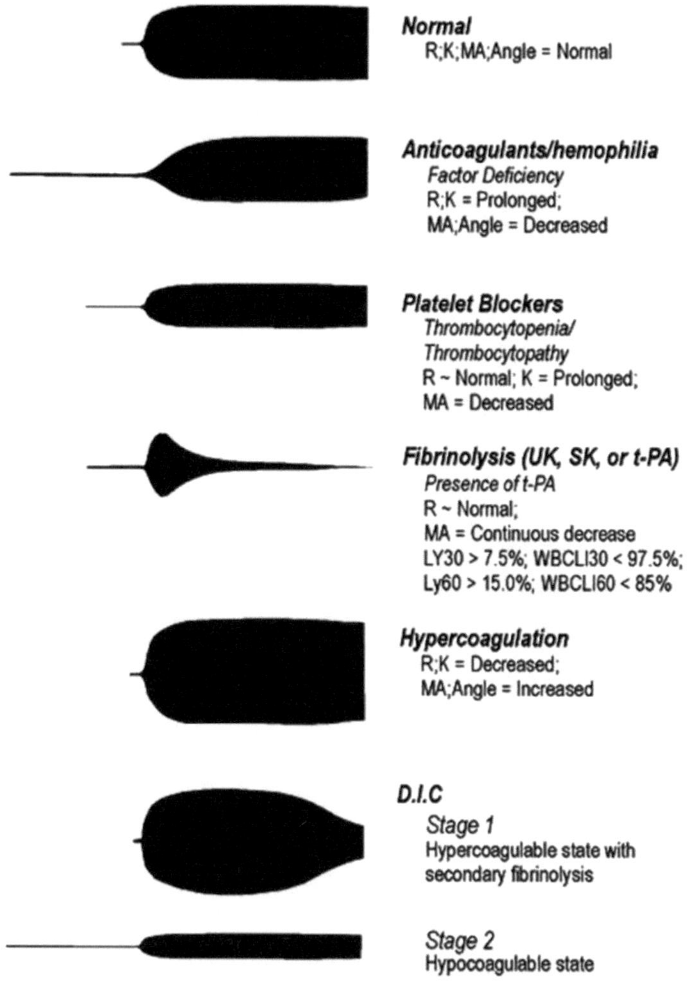

Figure 4.
Sample pathologic TEG waveforms. The image presented above was extracted from the article by Whiting and DiNardo [24].

the presence of massive intravascular volume loss, compensatory mechanisms induce vasoconstriction, and adding a vasopressor agent on top of the neuroendocrine response will only exacerbate end-organ malperfusion [36]. Of the vasopressor agents commercially available, the most commonly used vasopressors include norepinephrine, vasopressin, and phenylephrine (**Figure 5**). A common side effect of vasopressors is arrhythmia. They also can cause varying degrees of tissue necrosis in the setting of extravasation. Reflex bradycardia, decreased cardiac output, and ischemia (peripheral, mesenteric, renal, or myocardial) are associated with phenylephrine. Vasopressin can cause mesenteric ischemia, chest pain, coronary artery constriction or myocardial infarction, bronchial constriction, and hyponatremia [38]. In addition, norepinephrine use can also result in bradycardia and dysrhythmia.

More recently, controversy regarding the use of vasopressors in trauma has led to a valid argument that based on normal pathophysiological mechanisms alone, permissive hypotension would seem detrimental to the patient given the prolonged period of end-organ malperfusion. On the other hand, volume overload has been correlated with worse clinical outcomes, thereby providing a potential reason for vasopressors when the ideal middle ground is the ultimate goal for adequate perfusion [36]. An appropriate balance of volume replenishment and vascular resistance is essential to establishing homeostasis, and in select patients, vasopressors may be beneficial. In general, blood component therapy is the first line treatment for massive hemorrhage; however, in the presence of persistent hypovolemia and vasoplegic shock, vasopressors and inotropes may provide the necessary increase in vascular tone [39]. Larger prospective RCTs are currently being performed, and although vasopressors are typically frowned upon, patients with concomitant medical comorbidities such as cardiac dysfunction may benefit from inotropic agents like dobutamine, dopamine, and epinephrine that stimulate cardiac contractility [39]. Inotropes exhibit many of the same adverse effects that vasopressors do, namely, hypotension, dysrhythmias, myocardial infarction, and tachycardia. Additionally, the use of these agents can cause angina. Dopamine exhibits the most severe form of tissue necrosis (necrosis without extravasation and gangrene with extravasation) [38]. Epinephrine can cause anxiety, pulmonary edema, and tachycardia [38]. Vasopressors, inotropes, and leusitropes should be administered through a central venous access as prolonged delivery using peripheral IVs can exacerbate side effects.

Class	Agents	Mechanism	Uses
Vasopressors	Vasopressin Phenylephrine Norepinephrine	V1a, V1b, V2 α1 agonist α1, α2, β1, β2 agonist	Shock/hypotension
Inotropes	Epinephrine Dobutamine Dopamine	α1, α2, β1, β2 agonist α1, β1, β2 agonist α1, β1, β2, D agonist	Shock/hypotension
Leusitrope	Milronone	Phosphodiesterase inhibitor	Cardiac dysfunction
Experimental	Methylene Blue Esmolol Angiotensin II	Inhibits sGC, NO β1 > β2 antagonist AT-R1, AT-R2 agonist	Vasoplegia Shock Shock
Antifibrinolytics	Tranexamic Acid Amionocaproic Acid Aprotonin	Plasminogen lysine receptor inhibitor Serine protease inhibitor	Hemorrhage/coagulopathy
Electrolytes	Calcium Potassium Magnesium	N/A	MT associated electrolyte disturbances

Figure 5.
Adjunct pharmacologic agents used in trauma resuscitation. sGC = soluble guanylyl cyclase, NO = nitric oxide, AT-R1 = angiotensin receptor 1, AT-R2 = angiotensin receptor 2, CO = cardiac output, MT = massive transfusion, N/A = not applicable. The mechanism of action and uses of the agents in the figure were discussed in the article written by Levy et al [37].

3.7 Other pharmacological agents used in trauma

Along with vasopressors and inotropes, other pharmaceutical agents used during the management of massive hemorrhage and vasoplegia include hydrocortisone, leusitropic agents such as milrinone, and electrolyte replenishment. Hydrocortisone is beneficial for the management of hypotensive patients that have an impaired hypothalamic-pituitary-adrenal (HPA) axis. In cases where the endocrine function of the adrenal gland is in question, supplementation with hydrocortisone has been shown to reduce vasopressor requirements, although the outcomes following hydrocortisone administration are less clear [20]. Replenishment and monitoring of electrolytes is another important aspect of resuscitation efforts. Massive transfusion can lead to derangements in calcium, magnesium, and potassium [40]. Citrate that is incorporated into blood products for storage purposes can lead to calcium and magnesium chelation, eventually inducing hypocalcemia and hypomagnesemia, which can manifest as prolonged hypotension as well as a prolonged QT interval [20, 40]. This occurs with transfusion rates of >1 unit of RBCs/5 min or in patients with hepatic dysfunction [20]. Both hyperkalemia and hypokalemia can occur, with hyperkalemia being more common. Over time, the levels of potassium in stored RBCs increase, leading to hyperkalemia with massive transfusions. The mechanism of hypokalemia is multifactorial. Increased aldosterone and antidiuretic hormone release, chelation from citrate in stored RBCs, catecholamines, and activity of the RBC membrane ATPase pump all contribute to decreased potassium levels following a massive transfusion of blood products [20].

There are also experimental uses of agents like methylene blue, angiotensin II, or selective b-blockers such as esmolol [37]. While primarily used as a contrast agent, methylene blue (MB) has shown utility as an adjunctive treatment for severe vasoplegia in cardiac surgery and septic shock [41]. The mechanism of action involves direct inhibition of nitric oxide as well as the inhibition of soluble guanylyl cyclase (sGC), which is a peptide (classify) that increases cyclic guanosine monophosphate (c-GMP) [41, 42]. cGMP then causes relaxation of blood vessels. When given early in vasoplegia, MB helps increase mean arterial pressure (MAP) and improve cardiac function [41, 42]. Angiotensin II is another medication used in conjunction with vasopressors to treat septic shock. As demonstrated in the ATHOS studies, the use of angiotensin II leads to improvement in hypotension and catecholamine sparing [43, 44]. The use of esmolol has been shown on meta-analysis to improve survival, prevent myocardial depression by improving myocardial oxygen utilization, and decrease heart rate and troponin [45]. However, a recent pilot trial by Levy et al. has demonstrated that the use of esmolol within 6–12 h following vasopressor use results in increased risk of hypotension and diminished cardiac index [46].

Lastly, factor VIIa had been proposed as an additional therapeutic agent to help alleviate massive hemorrhage. Factor VIIa acts by binding to tissue factor that is exposed after endothelial damage, and by increasing the formation of thrombin, a fibrin clot is created [20]. Unfortunately, the use of Factor VIIa has not been shown to improve mortality and is not recommended for routine use in massive transfusion situations; however, more prospective RCTs are needed to definitively establish the role Factor VIIa may play in the future management of hemorrhagic trauma [20].

3.8 Current thinking on Massive Hemorrhage Resuscitation

More recently, traumatologists have circled back to the principle of whole blood resuscitation. Although whole blood resuscitation is used heavily in the military setting, significant barriers to more widespread adoption in the civilian setting are due to the portrayed risks of higher infections and immunological complications. Other drawbacks include a lack of clotting factors in whole blood, as well as increased potassium, hydrogen ions, and ammonia within whole blood.

Historically, whole blood was the principal resuscitation product during World War I, World War II, and the Korean War [47]. Although blood component therapy is now the most used method for civilian trauma resuscitation, there was a paucity of evidence to support the shift from whole blood to component therapy [47]. More recent data has suggested that whole blood transfusion provides civilian trauma patients with improved resuscitation status when compared to component therapies [47]. Whole blood requires significantly less volume versus component resuscitation (450–600 mL vs. 650 mL) and comes with a physiologic amount of platelets. The platelets in whole blood have a longer half-life than isolated platelets alone (21–35 days vs. 5 days), allowing for the expansion or preservation of platelet supplies. Whole blood is not recommended for use in rapid transfusers as the transfuser causes platelet destruction, though the decrease in platelets does not result in diminished platelet function or clot strength [47].

Individual components such as red blood cells, fresh frozen plasma, and cryoprecipitate are not without risk. Fresh frozen plasma has one of the highest risk profiles and can cause allergic reactions, transfusion-related acute lung injury (TRALI), fluid overload, and increased risk of infection.

Although the ability to collect low titer group O whole blood is much more difficult given that in certain regions of the United States, only 3% of the blood donor population meets the specified criteria, a more intuitive approach has been to test previously unrefutable medical principles [48]. Recent literature has suggested that the use of RhD-positive blood products results in a low risk of hemolytic disease of the newborn in females of childbearing age, a risk that is estimated to be only from 0.3% to 6.5% [48]. ABO incompatibility has also been further analyzed, and retrospective analyses have demonstrated no difference in mortality between those administered ABO-identical versus ABO-incompatible blood products [48]. By increasing the blood pool donor options, healthcare resources can become more accessible, and the likelihood of blood product shortages can be decreased.

3.9 Bridging the gap in modern resuscitation practices

Despite widespread support for whole blood resuscitation, there is still room for improvement in the current standards of care, including prehospital blood component administration and uniformity in MTPs.

Prehospital administration of plasma has been demonstrated to improve 30-day mortality in the PAMPer clinical trial, and post hoc analysis of the PAMPer and COMBAT clinical trials demonstrated a survival benefit with prehospital plasma administration when transport times exceeded 20 minutes [49, 50]. Even in light of strong evidence suggesting a benefit to prehospital administration of blood products, an analysis of the National Emergency Medical Services Information System (NEMSIS) 2019 dataset found that the use of prehospital blood transfusion for trauma resuscitation was extremely low [51].

Although the use of MTPs in trauma centers is the standard of care, the method for initiating the MTP and the actual format of the MTP vary between different institutions across the country. The ACS TQIP makes a note in their MTP guidelines that the creation of a MTP should "be developed by a multi-disciplinary committee" consisting of the blood bank, emergency medicine, anesthesia, and trauma services [11]. MTPs vary depending on the committees that form them, so there are discrepancies in their activation and constructs, leading to differences in patient outcomes. Etchill et al. found in their online survey conducted through the AAST that 7% of participants used a validated scoring system for MTP initiation, 9% consistently used TEG or ROTEM in their MTP, and the number of blood units readily available for use varied significantly among different institutions [52]. Given the major inconsistencies present in our healthcare system, there is a dire need for more uniform MTPs. However, despite these inconsistencies, the implementation of MTPs over the past decade has resulted in a reduction in mortality by 45%, a drop in median RBC units transfused from 12 to 4, and an increase in surviving patients being discharged back to their homes [53].

3.10 Operative vs. nonoperative management

The decision-making process in terms of operative or interventional management as opposed to nonoperative management of traumatic injuries is multifactorial and depends on the mechanism of injury, the structures that are injured, and the stability of the patient. Indications for prompt operative management include active bleeding/hemodynamic instability, aerodigestive injury, injury to major- or moderate-sized blood vessels, pericardial tamponade, positive FAST, blunt or penetrating abdominal trauma with peritonitis, expanding hematomas, and significant solid organ or internal injury that will require repair (i.e., grade V solid organ injuries or bowel perforations) [54]. Vascular injury such as partial or complete transection of blood vessels can occur from blunt or penetrating trauma via shearing or blast forces [55, 56]. Partial transection of blood vessels is more severe than complete transection being that a completely transected vessel is able contract and thus bleed less [56]. Intimal flaps with secondary thrombosis, pseudoaneurysms, and contusions can also occur.

Penetrating trauma involves kinetic energy and cavitation force leading to tissue injury and lacerations of solid or hollow organs as well as blood vessels. Blunt trauma (MVA, automobile vs. pedestrian accident, and falls from height) involves shearing, reactive forces in deceleration, rotational, and compressive forces. This tends to cause fractures, diffuse tissue injuries, compression and/or laceration of solid organs, perforation of hollow viscus organs, pneumothorax, and bronchial injury [55]. One of the most pertinent differences between blunt and penetrating trauma involves resuscitative thoracotomy. This procedure is not indicated in patients suffering from blunt trauma given the survival rate of 1% and the high incidence of significant neurologic morbidity in these survivors [54]. Patients with penetrating trauma to the chest causing cardiac injuries have a 35% survival rate provided they showed signs of life upon arrival to the emergency department or trauma bay [54].

4. Intraoperative care

4.1 General principles

After the decision has been made to proceed with operative intervention, there are a few general principles to consider from the anesthesiologist's perspective regarding the medical care of trauma patients. The patient must receive adequate resuscitation and maintenance fluids, the medical team must be able to accurately assess the patient for hemodynamic stability and physiological endpoints, and the anticipated supplies must be readily available as not to delay the troubleshooting of common complications.

Similar to the primary survey conducted at the beginning of the trauma patient's arrival, it is important to consider mechanical and pharmacological interventions for the airway, the pulmonary system, and the cardiovascular system.

For maintenance of the airway and pulmonary system, consider having the following supplies readily available: a laryngeal mask airway (LMA), various sized endotracheal tubes, Macintosh and Miller intubation blades, a videoscope, a bag valve mask, fiberoptic scopes, and oral and nasal airway systems.

For proper management of the cardiovascular system, utilize a rapid infuser and fluid warmer for resuscitation, consider placement of an arterial line and/or central line, ensure adequate peripheral access with two large-bore IVs (14G or 16G), consider the use of vasopressors, and place all necessary monitors (e.g., bispectral index monitor (BIM), pulse oximetry, a blood pressure cuff, 5 lead electrocardiogram (EKG), and core temperature monitor). Also, consider the maintenance of the patient's body temperature using a Bair hugger normothermia system and assess the operating room temperature in order to prevent hypothermia.

4.2 Current guidelines for intraoperative anesthesia care of trauma patients

Regarding intraoperative care, it is critical to be informed of the most recent literature pertaining to induction and maintenance goals, lung protective ventilation, and maintenance of normothermia.

The main goal of induction and maintenance is to maintain hemodynamic stability. If the patient is hemodynamically unstable, continue to resuscitate the patient preceding and during induction [57]. Adequate intravenous access is critical for timely resuscitation. If invasive access is needed, do not hesitate to proceed. It is best to ask the trauma team to maintain the patient's arms in an abducted position so that invasive access can be easily obtained without further delaying the surgery [57]. Given the time constraints, if possible, preoxygenate the patient with four vital capacity breaths prior to intubation. In certain scenarios, the patient may be obtunded. If so, proceed with apneic oxygenation [57]. When inducing, consideration should be given to the dose of the induction agent as trauma patients may require a much lower dose. Of the typical induction agents utilized, the most commonly used include ketamine, etomidate, and propofol [57].

Ketamine provides the ability to maintain systemic vascular resistance and spontaneous respirations; however, it is a cardiac depressant and should only be given at a dose of 1 mg/kg [57]. This makes ketamine an ideal choice for patients who have difficult airways. Dissociative delirium and increased secretions are well-known side effects. Etomidate is also used to maintain hemodynamic stability but can cause myoclonus, adrenal suppression, and postoperative nausea and vomiting [57]. Typical dosing is from 0.2 to 0.3 mg/kg. Propofol, although preferred by many due to its fast onset, has a significantly higher risk of decreasing systemic vascular resistance. Therefore, many anesthesiologists administer a vasopressor concomitantly in order to counteract the decrease in systemic vascular resistance [57]. A multicenter retrospective trial published by Leede et al. in 2021 showed no significant difference in systolic blood pressure for rapid sequence induction between these three agents [58]. Baekgaard et al. conducted a systematic review of the literature and found that there were no differences in transfusion or 30-day mortality rates between the ketamine, etomidate, and propofol [59]. As such, no specific recommendation can be made regarding the use of one of these agents over the other.

Aspiration is a significant risk to consider when inducing trauma patients as we often have to assume that they do not fall within the nil per os guidelines. Patient may be obtunded, may have received opioids that delay gastric emptying, and may have eaten recently. When performing rapid sequence intubation, it is advised to administer succinylcholine 1 mg/kg or rocuronium 1.2 mg/kg [57]. The onset of both previously mentioned pharmaceuticals is comparable, although rocuronium has a longer duration of action. Potential side effects of succinylcholine include myalgias, increased intraocular pressure, increased intracranial pressure, and hyperkalemia [57]. Succinylcholine should be avoided in patients with spinal cord or burn-related injuries and prolonged immobilization and pediatric patients [57].

Special consideration must be given to patients who present in a C-collar [57]. Due to the potential for injury, first establish if the front portion of the collar can be removed. The trauma team should be positioned so that one team member stabilizes the shoulders, another holds the patient's head, and the trauma anesthesiologist performs the intubation [57]. When deciding the intubation method with which to proceed, randomized control trials demonstrated no difference in C-spine manipulation when direct laryngoscopy or videoscope was performed [60].

When ventilating the patient, it is best to incorporate lung protective ventilation strategies to reduce iatrogenically induced pulmonary injury [61]. Tidal volumes should be set to 6–8 ml/kg, with positive end-expiratory pressure (PEEP) initially set to 5 and titrated accordingly based on individual patient characteristics [61, 62]. In general, patient characteristics that portend the greatest risk to postoperative pulmonary complications include age greater than 50 years old, body mass index greater than 40 kg/m^2, American Society of Anesthesiology (ASA) grade greater than 2, obstructive sleep apnea, preoperative anemia, preoperative hypoxemia, emergency or urgent surgery, ventilation duration exceeding 2 h, and intraoperative factors such as hemodynamic impairment and low oxyhemoglobin saturation [61].

Normothermia is an important physiologic parameter to maintain. If the patient becomes hypothermic, which is defined as a core body temperature of less than 35°C, the hypothermia cascades into a state of coagulopathy and metabolic acidosis. This lethal triad prolongs hemorrhage in surgically uncontrolled bleeding, preventing tissue regeneration and physiologic recovery [63]. Hypothermia can be classified even further into mild (32–35°C), moderate (28–32°C), and severe (<28°C) stages [63]. Hypothermia is a well-known predictor of worse outcomes in trauma and TBI patients and is associated with higher rates of mortality, greater blood transfusion requirements, and prolonged stays in both the hospital and ICU [64]. In order to proactively prevent hypothermia, strategies to maintain normothermia include keeping the operating room temperature elevated and utilizing an underbody, upper body, and lower body Bair hugger to heat the air immediately encompassing the body of the patient [65].

4.3 What is awareness, and how is it prevented?

In the realm of Anesthesia, awareness is the explicit recall of sensory events during the procedure. Patients undergoing obstetric procedures, cardiac surgery, or major trauma surgery are at an increased risk of intraoperative awareness. In cardiac surgery, the incidence varies between 1.1 and 1.5%, whereas in major trauma cases, the incidence may range from 11 to 43%. Three factors that contribute to the increased occurrence of intraoperative awareness are light use of anesthesia, resistance to anesthetics, and inadequate delivery of the anesthetic secondary to a machine malfunction or misuse of the anesthetic machinery. Light anesthesia is considered to be the most likely culprit of intraoperative awareness. Given the dose of the anesthetic is limited in trauma surgery due to the higher likelihood of hemodynamic instability with higher doses, the purposeful light anesthesia predisposes trauma patients to an increased likelihood of experiencing intraoperative awareness.

Fortunately, several preventative measures can be taken preoperatively and intraoperatively to reduce the likelihood of awareness. Consideration should be given regarding the use of a premedication drug such as benzodiazepines or scopolamine [66]. The use of amnestic drugs should be given stronger consideration if the patient will be given light anesthesia for a valid reason, such as a hemodynamically unstable trauma patient undergoing major surgery [66]. It is best to avoid muscle paralysis so that voluntary responses can still be observed [66]. Provide a volatile agent with a minimum alveolar concentration (MAC) of 0.6 or more, and utilize a combination of agents, such as opioids and nitric oxide, to aid induction of unconsciousness, noting that the use of opioids or nitrous oxide alone is not enough to produce unconsciousness. Knowing that machine misuse and malfunction is one of the three main causes of intraoperative awareness, continuously check the anesthesia machinery [66]. If there is ample time, it is ideal to talk to the patient about auditory options to block operative noises, such as the use of earphones [66]. Lastly, it is important to make the operative team aware of the phenomena, as a better understanding of the phenomena can allow the team to make the necessary changes to preoperative preparation and intraoperative management of the anesthetic settings [66]. Currently, bispectral index monitoring (BIS) is utilized to measure the patient's anesthetic depth. The consciousness level of the patient is measured by interpreting electroencephalographic signals, with the data converted into a score and a value between 40 and 60 being the current standard to prevent awareness [67]. There remains much controversy in the reliability of the BIS monitor; however, at this time, this is the only technology available in the United States that can aid in monitoring awareness.

4.4 Damage Control Surgery

When a trauma patient undergoes operative intervention to control massive hemorrhage, it is essential to establish the nature of the procedure and whether the end goal of the index procedure is to definitively correct traumatic injuries or to stabilize the patient so that a definitive operation can take place at a later date. The latter is referred to as damage control surgery (DCS), which is the approach utilized to control hemorrhage, control or reduce contamination, and re-establish physiologic homeostasis [20].

During damage control surgery, specifically for intrabdominal trauma or bleeding, a laparotomy to stop bleeding and control peritoneal contamination is performed. A staged repair then follows the initial laparotomy once adequate ICU resuscitation has been achieved. As the patient undergoes operative intervention, blood component therapy and resuscitation are aggressively provided. Originally an approach only utilized by military medicine, DCS is now becoming more heavily utilized in the civilian population [20].

It is important to acknowledge that unlike typical resuscitation efforts, DCS focuses on preventing the exacerbation of the lethal triad: hypercoagulability, hypothermia, and acidosis [20]. The DCS approach implements blood component resuscitation earlier and more aggressively, utilizes hypotensive resuscitation, and corrects for coagulopathy during the initial resuscitation measures [68].

Hypotensive resuscitation, also referred to as permissive hypotension, is unlike standard large-volume resuscitation in that a lesser volume of fluid and blood product is used so that the patient is maintained at below-normal blood pressure during the operative intervention [68]. By maintaining a mean arterial pressure (MAP) of 50 mmHg, as done in permissive hypotension, rather than a MAP of 65 mmHg, permissive hypotension has been shown to decrease postoperative coagulopathy and death [69]. Interestingly, among the randomized control trials that have investigated hypotensive resuscitation, outcomes following hypotensive resuscitation were not worse than the standard resuscitation measures [68]. Although mortality did not significantly differ in 4 of the 5 more well-known randomized control trials, the RCT conducted by Bickell et al. found that patients given hypotensive resuscitation had improved survival rates (70% vs. 62%, p = 0.04) [68, 70]. The exception to permissive hypotension in DCS are patients with neurologic trauma such as traumatic brain injury or spinal cord injury. Recommendations are to maintain a MAP of 65 mmHg or a systolic blood pressure of 90–100 mmHg to maintain adequate cerebral perfusion pressure ranging from 60 to 70 mmHg [68, 71].

Although patients that undergo DCS are at an increased risk of morbidity, it is still commonly performed despite a paucity of evidence to support its widespread use. In the systematic review conducted by Roberts et al., a total of 39 studies were included in their review, and overall, only 10 of the 59 indications for DCS had strong evidence for validity [72]. Given that the indications for DCS are less well-established, it is critical to develop a more uniform indication system. Future directions include establishing a more definitive scoring system such as the DECIDE score that was developed by Urushibata et al. using the Japan Trauma Data Bank. However, the sensitivity and specificity of their scoring system were only 64.8% and 70.0%, respectively [73]. More granular, prospectively validated scoring systems for civilian trauma could provide the solution to improve mortality while predisposing fewer patients to severe morbidity.

4.5 Considerations for postoperative care

After completing the index trauma procedure, several considerations must be given as to where the patient will be transferred and whether the patient is at high risk for unplanned admission to the ICU if transferred from the postanesthesia care unit to the floor. Part of the decision will be established before the index procedure is completed, as in the case of damage control surgery where the patient will be transported to the ICU for further resuscitation, electrolyte management, acidosis correction, and assessment of coagulopathy. In other cases, the patient's index procedure may be definitive, and ICU care is unnecessary. Transfer to the ICU still requires significant anesthesia involvement, particularly with intubated patients. There are no specific recommendations regarding propofol versus dexmedetomidine or benzodiazepines with narcotic titrations. Rather, sedation for these patients should be individualized based on their clinical pathology and condition [71]. Benzodiazepines, while possessing a stable hemodynamic profile, should be used with significant caution in the elderly and in patients with renal failure [74]. There is also a risk of ICU delirium with prolonged use of benzodiazepines. Propofol's vasodilatory affects seen with larger doses can be poorly tolerated by unstable patients [74]. Dexmedetomidine is a versatile medication as it can be used for sedation in intubated patients as well as analgesia in non-intubated patients. However, dexmedetomidine can cause hypotension, bradycardia, and heart block (if overdosed).

Within the ICU, resuscitation efforts become more goal-directed. ROTEM or TEG is used to monitor and guide the hematologic resuscitation, while laboratory studies guide electrolyte repletion and treatment of acid-base derangements. Once hemorrhage has been definitively addressed via surgery or interventional procedure, permissive hypotension can be discontinued. There is no absolute MAP or SBP goal, but resuscitation goals are aimed at a return to a more normotensive state to facilitate organ perfusion. Crystalloid use in the postoperative phase is predominantly focused on decreasing the incidence of post-traumatic acute kidney injury (AKI). Fluids are titrated to produce a urine output of 1–2 mL/kg/h [20]. A tertiary examination of the patient should also be completed in the postoperative period to assess for any missed injuries.

A concrete understanding of the patient's risk factors for unplanned ICU admission is essential to provide adequate care and anticipate potential barriers to timely medical management and discharge. In the systematic review conducted by Onwochei et al., independent risk factors for unplanned ICU admission included age, anemia, ASA physical status, body mass index (BMI), comorbidity burden, emergency surgery, high-risk surgery, male sex, obstructive sleep apnea, increased blood loss, and operative duration [75]. Out of the previously described risk factors, the most common in the United States included age, body mass index, comorbidity extent, and emergency surgery [75]. In conjunction with the previously mentioned risk factors, it is important to have a multidisciplinary discussion, and healthcare resource allocation should be taken into account when deciding on the most feasible medical ward for the patient's postoperative medical care.

5. Discussion

The future of trauma resuscitation involves technologies and methods geared toward better addressing the supply of blood products and novel methods of controlling hemorrhage. Resuscitative endovascular balloon occlusion of the aorta (REBOA, seen in **Figure 6**) has highly specific indications as a temporizing measure to control bleeding from non-compressible torso injuries (disruption of the axial torso vessels, solid organ injuries, pulmonary parenchymal injuries, and so on) as well as hemorrhage below the diaphragm [77]. The thoracoabdominal aorta is accessed via femoral catheterization, and a balloon is inflated in aortic zone 1 (the origin of the left subclavian artery to the celiac artery) or aortic zone 3 (from the lowest renal artery to the aortic bifurcation) depending on the injuries present. Zone 2 is from the celiac trunk to the lowest renal artery. Occlusion at this zone has no current indications and is technically challenging to achieve in an emergent situation as it requires contrast to accurately delineate the anatomy. This technique can be used for a maximum of 30–90 min depending on the injury zone; however, REBOA can only be attempted if there is capability to provide definitive care at the facility that performs the REBOA [78, 79]. It is contraindicated in major thoracic hemorrhage and pericardial tamponade, both of which are better addressed via resuscitative thoracotomy. Adverse effects of REBOA include spinal cord injury, increased mortality with >30 min use in zone 1, aortoiliac injury, balloon rupture, and ischemia reperfusion injuries (acute kidney injury and multisystem organ failure). There are also complications that can occur at the level of access such as femoral artery dissection, pseudoaneurysm, or hematoma [78].

Advances in lyophilization (freeze drying) techniques now allow for the destruction of pathogens such as hepatitis and HIV and have led to a resurgence in the development and use of lyophilized blood components [80]. Spray-dried plasma has been shown to be both safe and efficacious and is available in ABO universal forms [81]. Currently, these products are being used in South Africa and Europe with some prehospital use in Europe as well. Formulation and development are underway for the United States. The shelf-life ranges from 15 months to 2 years (as opposed to 12 months for FFP), and there is one formulation that can be stored at room temperature [81]. Reconstitution of the products occurs in minutes, making these products a viable solution for current blood product supply issues. Lyophilized platelets have a short duration of action and circulation (4–6 h) with only partial functionality in comparison to pooled platelets. Further progress is also necessary in terms of developing a working model of freeze-dried RBCs. Existing formulations sustain significant functional impairment of the cells in addition to substantial RBC death during reconstitution [81, 82]. Cryopreservation of RBCs requires −80°C freezers with a preparation and washing time of approximately 1.5 h, making this method impractical for use in trauma situations [82].

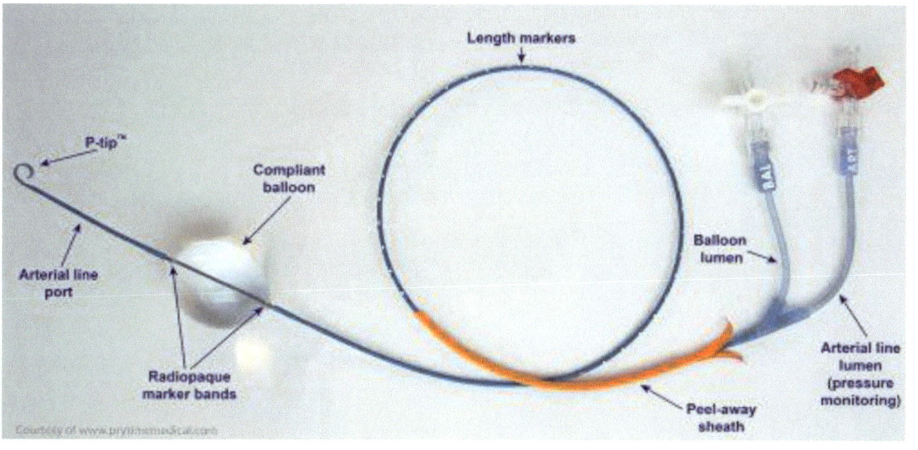

Figure 6.
REBOA catheter. The image presented above was extracted from the article by McGonigal [76].

Another methodology under ongoing investigation is the use of induced hypothermia for body and neurologic preservation, also called emergency preservation and resuscitation (EPR) [80]. Hypothermia to 10°C is rapidly induced via resuscitative thoracotomy and maintained for 60 min. A nonrandomized clinical trial of EPR called the EPR-CAT trial is underway with a scheduled conclusion in December of 2023 [83]. There is also the possibility of prehospital induction of hypothermia with portable equipment [80].

6. Conclusion

As one of the leading causes of emergency department visits and death in the United States, trauma is a field that is high-acuity and requires multidisciplinary teamwork. Although guidelines are constantly changing, the general principles of the primary and secondary surveys remain widely accepted for initial evaluation of the patient's injuries. It is during these initial assessments that decisions regarding adequate resuscitative interventions and need for operative intervention are made. Trauma patients needing emergent operative intervention tend to be in critical condition, so the anesthesia provider's expertise in areas such as resuscitation, intubation, induction, and awareness is crucial in making immediate decisions. Anesthesia providers also have a role in formulating standardized trauma-related protocols that can result in a widespread improvement in patient outcomes. Ultimately, the focus of every trauma activation is the patient outcome, which hinges on the preparation and contribution from each specialty in the trauma team. Anesthesia providers have an integral role, particularly in operative trauma cases, and staying updated in current trauma activation guidelines is imperative to appropriately resuscitate trauma patients and maintain hemodynamic stability in the operating room.

Author details

Vanessa Reese[1*], Wayne B. Bauerle[2], Anthony P. Allsbrook[2], Jennifer Hwang[2], and Prabhdeep Hehar[3]

1 Department of Research and Innovation, St. Luke's University Health Network, Bethlehem, USA

2 Department of Surgery, St. Luke's University Health Network, Bethlehem, USA

3 Department of Anesthesia, St. Luke's University Health Network, Bethlehem, USA

*Address all correspondence to: vanessa.reese@sluhn.org

IntechOpen

© 2023 The Author(s). Licensee IntechOpen. This chapter is distributed under the terms of the Creative Commons Attribution License (http://creativecommons.org/licenses/by/3.0), which permits unrestricted use, distribution, and reproduction in any medium, provided the original work is properly cited.

References

[1] McCunn M, Dutton RP, Dagal A, Varon AJ, Kaslow O, Kucik CJ, et al. Trauma, critical care, and emergency care Anesthesiology: A new paradigm for the "acute care" anesthesiologist? Anesthesia & Analgesia. 2015;**121**(6):1668-1673

[2] Rotondo MF et al. Advanced trauma life support (ATLS®): The ninth edition. Journal of Trauma and Acute Care Surgery. 2013;**74**(5):1363-1366

[3] Weiss AJ (IBM Watson Health), Jiang HJ (AHRQ). Most Frequent Reasons for Emergency Department Visits, 2018. HCUP Statistical Brief #286. December 2021. Agency for Healthcare Research and Quality, Rockville, MD. Available from: http://www.hcup-us.ahrq.gov/reports/statbriefs/sb286-ED-Frequent-Conditions-2018.pdf" www.hcup-us.ahrq.gov/reports/statbriefs/sb286-ED-Frequent-Conditions-2018.pdf

[4] Cairns C, Kang K, Santo L. National Hospital Ambulatory Medical Care Survey: Emergency department summary tables. 2018. Available from: https://www.cdc.gov/nchs/data/nhamcs/web_tables/2018_ed_web_tables-508.pdf

[5] Choi J, Carlos G, Nassar AK, Knowlton LM, Spain DA. The impact of trauma systems on patient outcomes. Current Problems in Surgery. 2021;**58**(1):100849

[6] Rhee P, Joseph B, Pandit V, Aziz H, Vercruysse G, Kulvatunyou N, et al. Increasing trauma deaths in the United States. Annals of Surgery. 2014;**260**(1):13-21

[7] Murphy SL, Kockanek KD, Xu J, Arias E. Mortality in the United States, 2020. 2021 (No. 427)

[8] Olaisen RH, Rossen LM, Warner M, Anderson RN. Unintentional injury death rates in rural and urban areas: United States, 1999-2017. Centers for Disease Control and Prevention. 2019;**343**:1-8

[9] Peterson C, Miller GF, Barnett SBL, Florence C. Economic cost of injury—United States, 2019. Morbidity and Mortality Weekly Report. 2021;**70**(48):1655-1659

[10] Ball CG, Grondin SC, Schieman C, Feliciano DV, Dixon E, Kirkpatrick AW, et al. Trauma surgery associations and societies: Which organizations match your goals? Journal of Trauma Management & Outcomes. 2014;**8**:6

[11] Trauma CO. ACS TQIP Massive Transfusion in Trauma Guidelines. 2014

[12] Cotton BA, Dossett LA, Haut ER, Shafi S, Nunez TC, Au BK, et al. Multicenter validation of a simplified score to predict massive transfusion in trauma. The Journal of Trauma. 2010;**69**(Suppl. 1):S33-S39. DOI:10.1097/TA.0b013e3181e42411

[13] Nunez TC, Voskresensky IV, Dossett LA, Shinall R, Dutton WD, Cotton BA. Early prediction of massive transfusion in trauma: Simple as ABC (assessment of blood consumption)? The Journal of Trauma. 2009;**66**(2):346-352. DOI:10.1097/TA.0b013e3181961c35

[14] Holcomb JB, Tilley BC, Baraniuk S, Fox EE, Wade CE, Podbielski JM, et al. Transfusion of plasma, platelets, and red blood cells in a 1:1:1 vs a 1:1:2 ratio and mortality in patients with severe trauma: The PROPPR randomized clinical trial. Journal of the American Medical Association. 2015;**313**(5):471-482

[15] Lim G, Harper-Kirksey K, Parekh R, Manini AF. Efficacy of a massive transfusion protocol for hemorrhagic trauma resuscitation. The American Journal of Emergency Medicine. 2018;**36**(7):1178-1181

[16] Consunji R, Elseed A, El-Menyar A, Sathian B, Rizoli S, Al-Thani H, et al. The effect of massive transfusion protocol implementation on the survival of trauma patients: A systematic review and meta-analysis. Blood Transfusion. 2020;**18**(6):434-445

[17] O'Keeffe T, Refaai M, Tchorz K, Forestner JE, Sarode R. A massive transfusion protocol to decrease blood component use and costs. Archives of Surgery. 2008;**143**(7):686-691

[18] Lewis SR, Pritchard MW, Evans DJ, Butler AR, Alderson P, Smith AF, et al. Colloids versus crystalloids for fluid resuscitation in critically ill people. Cochrane Database of Systematic Reviews. 2018;**8**(8):Cd000567

[19] Choi PT-L, Yip G, Quinonez LG, Cook DJ. Crystalloids vs. colloids in fluid resuscitation: A systematic review. Critical Care Medicine. 1999;**27**(1):200-210

[20] Tobin JM, Varon AJ. Update in trauma anesthesiology: Perioperative resuscitation management. Anesthesia & Analgesia. 2012;**115**(6):1326-1333

[21] Institute of Medicine (US). Committee on fluid resuscitation for Combat casualties. In: Pope A, French G, Longnecker DE, editors. Fluid Resuscitation: State of the Science for Treating Combat Casualties and Civilian Injuries. Washington, DC: National Academies Press (US); 1999

[22] Saline or albumin for fluid resuscitation in patients with traumatic brain injury. New England Journal of Medicine. 2007;**357**(9):874-884

[23] Gantner D, Moore EM, Cooper DJ. Intravenous fluids in traumatic brain injury: What's the solution? Current Opinion in Critical Care. 2014;**20**(4):385-389

[24] Whiting D, DiNardo JA. TEG and ROTEM: Technology and clinical applications. American Journal of Hematology. 2014;**89**(2):228-232

[25] Brill JB, Brenner M, Duchesne J, Roberts D, Ferrada P, Horer T, et al. The role of TEG and ROTEM in damage control resuscitation. Shock. 2021;**56**(1s):52-61

[26] De Pietri L, Ragusa F, Deleuterio A, Begliomini B, Serra V. Reduced transfusion during OLT by POC coagulation management and TEG functional fibrinogen: A retrospective observational study. Transplantation direct. 2015;**2**(1):e49. DOI:10.1097/TXD.0000000000000559

[27] Taylor JR, Cotton BA. Coagulation Issues and the Trauma Patient. Current Surgical Therapy. Elsevier. 2020:1251-1259

[28] Johansson PI, Stensballe J, Oliveri R, Wade CE, Ostrowski SR, Holcomb JB. How I treat patients with massive hemorrhage. Blood. 2014;**124**(20):3052-3058. DOI:10.1182/blood-2014-05-575340. Epub 2014 Oct 7

[29] Gonzalez E, Moore EE, Moore HB, Chapman MP, Chin TL, Ghasabyan A, et al. Goal-directed hemostatic resuscitation of trauma-induced coagulopathy: A pragmatic randomized clinical trial comparing a viscoelastic assay to conventional coagulation assays. Annals of Surgery. 2016;**263**(6):1051-1059

[30] Pieters M, Wolberg AS. Fibrinogen and fibrin: An illustrated review. Research and Practice in Thrombosis and Haemostasis. 2019;**3**(2):161-172

[31] Minors DS. Haemostasis, blood platelets and coagulation. Anaesthesia & Intensive Care Medicine. 2007;**8**(5):214-216

[32] Reed MR, Woolley LT. Uses of tranexamic acid. Continuing Education in Anaesthesia Critical Care & Pain. 2014;**15**(1):32-37

[33] Davis R, Whittington R. Aprotinin. A review of its pharmacology and therapeutic efficacy in reducing blood loss associated with cardiac surgery. Drugs. 1995;**49**(6):954-983

[34] Pusateri AE, Weiskopf RB, Vikhyat B, Butler F, Cestero RF, et al. Tranexamic acid and trauma: Current status and knowledge gaps with recommended research priorities. Shock. 2013;**39**(2):121-126

[35] CRASH-2 trial Collaborators, Shakur H, Roberts I, et al. Effects of tranexamic acid on death, vascular occlusive events, and blood transfusion in trauma patients with significant haemorrhage (CRASH-2): A randomised, placebo-controlled trial. The Lancet. 2010;**376**(9734):23-32

[36] Richards JE, Harris T, Dünser MW, Bouzat P, Gauss T. Vasopressors in trauma: A never event? Anesthesia & Analgesia. 2021;**133**(1):68-79

[37] Levy B, Fritz C, Tahon E, et al. Vasoplegia treatments: The past, the present, and the future. Critical Care. 2018;**22**:52

[38] VanValkinburgh D, Kerndt CC, Hashmi MF. Inotropes and Vasopressors, StatPearls [Internet]. Treasure Island (FL): StatPearls Publishing; 2022

[39] Gupta B, Garg N, Ramachandran R. Vasopressors: Do they have any role in hemorrhagic shock? Journal of Anaesthesiology Clinical Pharmacology. 2017;**33**(1):3-8

[40] Hayter MA, Pavenski K, Baker J. Massive transfusion in the trauma patient: Continuing professional development. Canadian Journal of Anesthesia/Journal Canadien d'Anesthésie. 2012;**59**:1130-1145. DOI:10.1007/s12630-012-9795-4

[41] Booth AT, Melmer PD, Tribble B, Mehaffey JH, Tribble C. Methylene blue for vasoplegic syndrome. The Heart Surgery Forum. 2017;**20**(5):E234-E238. DOI:10.1532/hsf.1806

[42] Kofler O, Simbeck M, Tomasi R, Hinske LC, Klotz LV, Uhle F, et al. Early use of methylene blue in vasoplegic syndrome: A 10-year propensity score-matched cohort study. Journal of Clinical Medicine. 2022;**11**(4):1121. DOI:10.3390/jcm11041121

[43] Khanna A, English SW, Wang XS, Ham K, Tumlin J, Szerlip H, et al. Angiotensin II for the treatment of vasodilatory shock. The New England Journal of Medicine. 2017;**377**(5):419-430. DOI:10.1056/NEJMoa1704154

[44] Bellomo R, Forni LG, Busse LW, McCurdy MT, Ham KR, Boldt DW, et al. Renin and survival in patients Given angiotensin II for catecholamine-resistant vasodilatory shock. A clinical trial. American Journal of Respiratory and Critical Care Medicine. 2020;**202**(9):1253-1261. DOI:10.1164/rccm.201911-2172OC

[45] Li P, Wu Q, Tang Y, Zhou Z, Feng F. The influence of esmolol on septic shock and sepsis: A meta-analysis of randomized controlled studies. The American Journal of Emergency Medicine. 2018;**36**(3):470-474. DOI:10.1016/j.ajem.2017.11.013

[46] Levy B, Fritz C, Piona C, et al. Hemodynamic and anti-inflammatory effects of early esmolol use in

hyperkinetic septic shock: A pilot study. Critical Care. 2021;**25**:21. DOI:10.1186/s13054-020-03445-w

[47] McCoy CC, Brenner M, Duchesne J, Roberts D, Ferrada P, Horer T, et al. Back to the future: Whole blood resuscitation of the severely injured trauma patient. Shock. 2021;**56**(1s):9-15

[48] Yazer MH. The evolution of blood product use in trauma resuscitation: Change has come. Transfusion Medicine and Hemotherapy. 2021;**48**(6):377-380

[49] Sperry JL, Guyette FX, Brown JB, Yazer MH, Triulzi DJ, Early-Young BJ, et al. Prehospital plasma during air medical transport in trauma patients at risk for Hemorrhagic shock. New England Journal of Medicine. 2018;**379**(4):315-326

[50] Pusateri AE, Moore EE, Moore HB, Le TD, Guyette FX, Chapman MP, et al. Association of Prehospital Plasma Transfusion with Survival in trauma patients with Hemorrhagic shock when transport times are longer than 20 minutes: A post hoc analysis of the PAMPer and COMBAT clinical trials. JAMA. Surgery. 2020;**155**(2):e195085

[51] Hashmi ZG, Chehab M, Nathens AB, Joseph B, Bank EA, Jansen JO, et al. Whole truths but half the blood: Addressing the gap between the evidence and practice of pre-hospital and in-hospital blood product use for trauma resuscitation. Transfusion. 2021;**61**(S1):S348-SS53

[52] Etchill E, Sperry J, Zuckerbraun B, Alarcon L, Brown J, Schuster K, et al. The confusion continues: Results from an American Association for the Surgery of Trauma survey on massive transfusion practices among United States trauma centers. Transfusion. 2016;**56**(10):2478-2486

[53] Cole E, Weaver A, Gall L, West A, Nevin D, Tallach R, et al. A decade of damage control resuscitation: New transfusion practice, new survivors, new directions. Annals of Surgery. 2021;**273**(6):1215-1220

[54] Townsend CM et al. Sabiston Textbook of Surgery: Management of Acute Trauma. Vol. 20E. New York, NY: Elsevier; 2017. pp. 408-448

[55] Feliciano DV, Mattox KL, Moore EE. Trauma. 7th ed. New York: McGraw-Hill; 2013. pp. 2-17, 632-640

[56] Wani ML, Ahangar AG, Ganie FA, Wani SN, Wani NU. Vascular injuries: Trends in management. Trauma Monthly. 2012;**17**(2):266-269. DOI:10.5812/traumamon.6238. Epub 2012 Jul 31

[57] Tobin JM, Barras WP, Bree S, Williams N, McFarland C, Park C, et al. Anesthesia for trauma patients. Military Medicine. 2018;**183**(suppl_2):32-35

[58] Leede E, Kempema J, Wilson C, Rios T, Alejandro J, Cook A, et al. A multicenter investigation of the hemodynamic effects of induction agents for trauma rapid sequence intubation. Journal of Trauma and Acute Care Surgery. 2021;**90**(6):1009-1013. DOI:10.1097/TA.0000000000003132

[59] Baekgaard JS, Eskesen TG, Sillesen M, Rasmussen LS, Steinmetz J. Ketamine as a rapid sequence induction agent in the trauma population: A systematic review. Anesthesia & Analgesia. 2019;**128**(3):504-510. DOI:10.1213/ANE.0000000000003568

[60] Robitaille A, Williams SR, Tremblay MH, Guilbert F, Thériault M, Drolet P. Cervical spine motion during tracheal intubation with manual in-line stabilization: Direct laryngoscopy versus GlideScope videolaryngoscopy. Anesthesia and Analgesia. 2008;**106**(3):935-941, table of contents

[61] Young CC, Harris EM, Vacchiano C, Bodnar S, Bukowy B, Elliott RRD, et al. Lung-protective ventilation for the surgical patient: International expert panel-based consensus recommendations. British Journal of Anaesthesia. 2019;**123**(6):898-913

[62] Coppola S, Froio S, Chiumello D. Protective lung ventilation during general anesthesia: Is there any evidence? Critical Care. 2014;**18**(2):210

[63] Dyer M, Neal MD. Defining the lethal triad. In: Pape H-C, Peitzman AB, Rotondo MF, Giannoudis PV, editors. Damage Control Management in the Polytrauma Patient. Cham: Springer International Publishing; 2017. pp. 41-53

[64] Rösli D, Schnüriger B, Candinas D, Haltmeier T. The impact of accidental hypothermia on mortality in trauma patients overall and patients with traumatic brain injury specifically: A systematic review and meta-analysis. World Journal of Surgery. 2020;**44**(12):4106-4117

[65] Peng RY, Bongard FS. Hypothermia in trauma patients. Journal of the American College of Surgeons. 1999;**188**(6):685-696

[66] Ghoneim MM, Weiskopf RB. Awareness during Anesthesia. Anesthesiology. 2000;**92**(2):597

[67] Phongchiewboon A, Bunchungmongkol N. Bispectral index for improving anaesthetic delivery and postoperative recovery. Cochrane database of Systematic Reviews. 2014;**17**(4):1-80

[68] Carrick MM, Leonard J, Slone DS, Mains CW, Bar-Or D. Hypotensive resuscitation among trauma patients. BioMed Research International. 2016;**2016**:8901938

[69] Morrison CA, Carrick MM, Norman MA, Scott BG, Welsh FJ, Tsai P, et al. Hypotensive resuscitation strategy reduces transfusion requirements and severe postoperative coagulopathy in trauma patients with hemorrhagic shock: Preliminary results of a randomized controlled trial. Journal of Trauma and Acute Care Surgery. 2011;**70**(3):652-663

[70] Bickell WH, Wall MJ Jr, Pepe PE, Martin RR, Ginger VF, Allen MK, et al. Immediate versus delayed fluid resuscitation for hypotensive patients with penetrating torso injuries. New England Journal of Medicine. 1994;**331**(17):1105-1109

[71] Sugeir S, Grunstein I, Tobin JM. Damage control anesthesia. In: Duchesne J, Inaba K, Khan M, editors. Damage Control in Trauma Care. Cham: Springer; 2018. DOI:10.1007/978-3-319-72607-6_16

[72] Roberts DJ, Bobrovitz N, Zygun DA, Kirkpatrick AW, Ball CG, Faris PD, et al. Evidence for use of damage control surgery and damage control interventions in civilian trauma patients: A systematic review. World Journal of Emergency Surgery. 2021;**16**(1):10

[73] Urushibata N, Murata K, Otomo Y. Decision-making criteria for damage control surgery in Japan. Scientific Reports. 2019;**9**(1):14895

[74] Louro J, Varon AJ. Essentials of Trauma Anesthesia. United Kingdom: Cambridge University Press; 2017

[75] Onwochei DN, Fabes J, Walker D, Kumar G, Moonesinghe SR. Critical care after major surgery: A systematic review of risk factors for unplanned admission. Anaesthesia. 2020;**75**(S1):e62-e74

[76] McGongal M. Available from: https://thetraumapro.com/2021/01/22/

reboa-a-comparison-of-the-hardware-from-two-companies/

[77] Moore LJ, Brenner M, Kozar, Rosemary A, Jason P, Wade CE, et al. Implementation of resuscitative endovascular balloon occlusion of the aorta as an alternative to resuscitative thoracotomy for noncompressible truncal hemorrhage. Journal of Trauma and Acute Care Surgery. 2015;**79**(4):523-532. DOI:10.1097/TA.0000000000000809

[78] Bulger EM, Perina DG, Qasim Z, et al. Clinical use of resuscitative endovascular balloon occlusion of the aorta (REBOA) in civilian trauma systems in the USA, 2019: A joint statement from the American College of Surgeons Committee on Trauma, the American College of Emergency Physicians, the National Association of Emergency Medical Services Physicians and the National Association of Emergency Medical Technicians. Trauma Surgery and Acute Care Open. 2019;**4**:e000376

[79] Thrailkill MA, Gladin KH, Thorpe CR, et al. Resuscitative endovascular balloon occlusion of the aorta (REBOA): Update and insights into current practices and future directions for research and implementation. Scandinavian Journal of Trauma, Resuscitation and Emergency Medicine. 2021;**29**:8. DOI:10.1186/s13049-020-00807-9

[80] Alam HB, Velmahos GC. New trends in resuscitation. Current Problems in Surgery. 2011;**48**(8):531-564. DOI:10.1067/j.cpsurg.2011.04.002

[81] Pusateri AE, Given MB, Schreiber MA, Spinella PC, Pati S, Kozar RA, et al. Dried plasma: State of the science and recent developments. Transfusion. 2016;**56**:S128-S139. DOI:10.1111/trf.13580

[82] Arav A, Natan D. Freeze drying (lyophilization) of red blood cells. The Journal of Trauma: Injury, Infection, and Critical Care. 2011;**70**(5):S61-S64. DOI:10.1097/TA.0b013e31821a6083

[83] Available from: https://clinicaltrials.gov/ct2/show/NCT01042015

Section 10

Geriatric Medicine

Chapter 14

The New Trend, Geriatric Surgery: Considerations in Geriatric Surgery

Ellen McHugh

Abstract

Current demographic trends reveal we are experiencing an aging population. Life expectancy has extended, individuals are living longer, and electing to have surgery in their older age. Often older patients are more medically complex when compared to their younger counterparts, this places them at a higher risk for developing a complication after surgery. In addition, older patients may have a poor tolerance to anesthesia making their surgical care challenging. Complications after surgery can lead to longer hospital stays, readmissions back into the hospital, and can disrupt the patients' quality of life. Presurgery screening and identification of any modifiable health concerns are the keys to prevention of bad outcomes after surgery. Surgeons, anesthesiologists, and the surgical team must be aware of the unique needs of the aging population to understand specific measures that can be taken to keep patients safe. Information that was presented in this chapter was obtained from clinical experience and an extensive literature search. A literature search was performed using search engines such as EBSCOhost, MEDLINE with Full Text, CINAHL Complete, Health Business Elite, Cochrane Database of Systematic Reviews, Cochrane Clinical Answers, E-journals, Google search engine, and Full-text Finder.

Keywords: aging population, senior, older age, elderly, geriatrics, geriatric surgery, anesthesia and elderly, anesthesia in the older adult, postoperative complications, comprehensive geriatric assessment, presurgery screening, optimization

1. Introduction: What is geriatric surgery?

Current demographic trends reveal we are experiencing an aging population. Life expectancy has extended, individuals are living longer, and electing to have surgery in their older age. The United States (U.S.) census data reveals every day 10,000 Americans turn age 65 years [1, 2]. This is expected to continue for the next thirty years, which will double the U.S. population of older adults from now 46 million to 90 million in the year 2050 [2]. When it is all said and done, senior citizens will make up 75% of the surgical workload [2].

A *senior* is defined as a person who is age 65 years or older [3]. In medicine, the term *senior citizen* describes an individual who has reached the milestone of age 65 years [3]. Geriatrics rather is a term used to describe the health condition of an individual, specifically an older individual, who has begun to experience age-related changes that are making them more vulnerable to life stressors [3, 4].

IntechOpen

As we age our bodies change, we begin to slow down, lose muscle mass, lose our senses, react differently to medications, and we may have chronic illnesses that start to take a toll on our bodies [3, 4]. The aging process, which tends to include an increased number of illnesses, malnutrition, difficulties in communication, difficulties in comprehension, and psychological and social alterations, can complicate the surgical process and serve as a precursor to poor outcomes after surgery [4]. Please refer to **Table 1** for a summary of the *Physiological Decline Seen in Older Adults*. More than half of older adults who are 70 years of age or older, suffer from one chronic disease, and 30% of this same population suffer from two or more chronic diseases [4]. This can make the surgical care of older adults challenging and places them at a higher risk for developing a complication after surgery. In addition, older adults may have a poor tolerance to anesthesia making their surgery very risky.

Body system	Physiological decline in body function
Cognitive	• Cognitive decline/impairment • Memory loss • Depression • Increase risk of acute delirium • Onset of dementia
Head, eyes, ears, nose, and throat (HEENT)	• Decrease or loss of sensory functions (loss of taste and smell, hearing loss, vision loss such as cataracts, glaucoma, macular degeneration, and impairment in swallowing) • Disruption of oral health (dry mouth, gum disease, and oral cancer) • Impairment of mouth cavity/teeth (missing or broken teeth, poorly fitting dentures, and sore gums) • Thinning hair, hair loss, and brittle nails • Dysphagia
Cardiac	• Atherosclerosis • Increase in cardiac disease • Decreased cardiac output
Pulmonary	• Decline in pulmonary capacity • Time of onset of chronic obstructive pulmonary disease (COPD)
Gastrointestinal	• Decrease in gastric mobility • Decrease in metabolism • Decrease in absorption of medications • Increase risk of malnutrition • Constipation
Genitourinary/ anorectal	• Renal insufficiency, decrease in Glomar infiltration rate affecting elimination of wastes production • Incontinence • Increase in urinary tract infections (UTI)
Musculoskeletal	• Demineralization of bones, bone loss • Onset of osteoporosis, increase in pain • Increase risk of injuries and falls

Body system	Physiological decline in body function
Integumentary	• Skin atrophy • Decrease in skin temperature • Easy bruising
Psychiatric/ behavioral	• Onset of anxiety/depression • Onset of chronic pain • Decline in mental health • Onset of dementia

Table 1.
Physiological decline seen in older adults [1–7].

Complications after surgery can lead to longer hospital stays, readmissions back into the hospital, and can disrupt the quality of life. Major complications seen after geriatric surgery include acute delirium, Small-Bowel Obstructions (SBO), Pulmonary Embolism (PE), and Urinary Retention (UR) leading to an Acute Kidney Injury (AKI). Delirium, an acute change in mental status, is the most common complication seen and occurs in 14–50% of older hospitalized adults with associated mortality ranging from 25% to 33% [4, 5]. Delirium is one of the main causes of hospital falls and has been linked to functional decline, increased hospital cost per day, longer hospital stays, restraint use, and increased mortality rates [5–7].

Just like there are doctors for our children (pediatricians) and doctors for our hearts (cardiologists), we have doctors for older age, known as geriatricians. A geriatrician is trained to recognize the unique needs of older adults and treat these conditions [3].

When you bring the two specialties together, geriatrics and surgery, you have a subspecialty of surgery that incorporates the unique needs of older adults into their surgical care [3]. No longer is the surgical care solely focused on the patient's body part to be operated on ("knee surgery" or "abdominal surgery"). Geriatric surgery is looking at the patient as a whole person, everything that is going on simultaneously, not just the body part that is being operated on. Unfortunately, a surgeon may not have the time or expertise to investigate and treat the patient's entire health history. That is one of the benefits of having a geriatric surgery program in place where a team of healthcare professionals can work together to meet the specific needs of the older surgical patient.

1.1 Story Time: (real patient encounter/true story experienced by author Ellen McHugh)

I will never forget one of my first patients. She was an 85-year-old female undergoing a hip replacement. She had lost her husband the previous year and was actively dealing with sadness and grief. She was having severe hip pain that was slowing her down. She elected to undergo a hip replacement to help decrease her pain and improve her quality of life. When she came into the surgery center, I can remember my first assessment of her, she is weak. She stepped on the scale and said, "I knew that was coming." She had lost a significant amount of weight. She was not surprised. She explained that she was no longer cooking because it was too painful for her to stand. Prior, her husband was her motivation to push through the pain and cook. Now that he was gone, she lost all motivation and did not need to eat. My second assessment of her was that she was very weak and frail, I was afraid this surgery would harm her. Yet, surgery was essential to improving her quality of life. I remember saying, we need to make some changes and get you in shape before this surgery! That is when she looked up at me and said, "will you please help me get started." I replied "Yes, absolutely!" Geriatric surgery is compassion! Having compassion and patience for the unique needs that the older adult brings to the table, including their chronic conditions, age-related conditions, and social needs while preparing them for surgery.

2. What is the comprehensive geriatric assessment (CGA)

We can expect to see more and more surgeries being performed in the elderly population, especially as older adults elect to have surgery to help improve and maintain a better quality of life. With geriatric surgery on the rise, every institution should have a surgical program in place that is designed to meet the needs of the older surgical patient. Having geriatric surgery program in place gives the surgical team an opportunity to meet the patient before surgery, perform comprehensive health screenings, and spend an adequate amount of time with the patient to really get to know them. This allows healthcare providers to identify any areas of health concern. In return they can put interventions in place to improve these areas of concern before surgery. With the end goal of getting the patient in their best health prior to their operation will lead to better outcomes and an improved quality of life.

Currently recommended for the older adult is a comprehensive health assessment, better known as, the comprehensive geriatric assessment (CGA). CGA can be described as a multidisciplinary diagnostic process that evaluates medical, functional, psychological, social capabilities, frailty status, and various geriatric syndromes [8, 9]. An easier way to sum up basis of the CGA is simply say, performing health screenings from head to toe. Performing a CGA can be useful in identifying patient health deficits that may not be assessed on a standard History and Physical (H&P) [9]. In addition, the CGA uses a multidisciplinary approach where healthcare providers work together to coordinate care and communicate for the patients. As a result, the surgical experience becomes less complicated and less confusing for the patient. Presurgery screening and identification of any modifiable health concerns are the key to prevention of bad outcomes after surgery. CGA can lead to early recognition of problems that can be modified presurgery to assist in preventing bad outcomes after surgery.

It is important to note that the CGA is an extremely timely process and is unrealistic to be completed by the surgeon alone. This CGA should include input from the surgeon, anesthesiologist, and geriatric nurse specialist. Other specialties that may be called into the assessment and treatment are nurses, dietitians, social work case managers, pharmacists, and or physical/occupational therapists. The American College of Surgeon's (ACS) National Surgical Quality Improvement Program (NAQIP) and the American Geriatrics Society (AGS) published guidelines that identify the core domains to be assessed in the CGA, which include: cognitive function, depression screening, nutritional assessment, functional mobility and falls, frailty, polypharmacy, cardiac and pulmonary assessments, comorbidities, geriatric syndromes (urinary incontinence, dental needs, visual, and hearing impairment), and patient's health goals [8–11].

A review of the literature found a meta-analysis of 29 trials, which showed that hospitalized older adults who received the care of a CGA team were more likely to be alive and in their homes 12 months after surgery and hospitalization [12]. Kim et al. [10] identified supporting data concluding that older adult patients are more likely to survive surgery and return to their home if they receive a CGA during their surgical care. This is very appealing to older adults who are unsure about moving forward with surgery, due to their fear of the unknown or possible unfavorable outcomes after surgery. A geriatric surgery program can help alleviate anxiety and fear that older adults may have surrounding surgery in their older age. Thus, making the whole surgical experience better for them.

Xue et al. [9] reviewed a few studies that found the health information identified on the CGA directly predicts postoperative complications in patients.

A meta-analysis study in gastrointestinal cancer patients identified that the CGA is effective in identifying patients with multiple comorbidities, polypharmacy, and ADL dependency; all syndromes that are directly associated with development of major postoperative complications [9]. When healthcare providers can identify high risk patients, interventions can be put into place to help decrease the chance of these bad outcomes from occurring. Decreasing bad outcomes after surgery favorably affects length of stay and readmissions back into the hospital. Harari et al. [13] revealed that the use of presurgery proactive care bundles (PCB) in older patients undergoing surgery (compared to patients who received standard care) significantly lower rates of postoperative complications such as pneumonia (20% VS. 4%), delirium (19% VS. 6%), and pressure ulcers (19% VS. 4%). Cohen et al. [14] determined that health data collected in the presurgery assessment phase, such as a low Braden scale score (<18); was associated with a significantly higher risk of developing 30-day complications, longer length of stay (LOS) and were more likely discharged to a nursing home versus home.

If a CGA is unable to be completed, research implies at the least; comorbidity, polypharmacy, and functional status should routinely assess for all geriatric patients undergoing surgery due to the high predictability of postoperative complications [9]. Review of a meta-analysis conducted by Kim et al. [10] showed that patients who completed the CGA showed a benefit on short term mortality, reduced complications, reduced readmissions, improved cognitive function, and improve physical function after surgery. Available studies proved that the CGA reduces post-op delirium and improves surgery outcomes in patients with hip fractures, possibly due to the multi-component interventions it uses [11].

There is so much evidence pointing to the benefits of utilizing the CGA. Performing a CGA also provides a time to discuss some of those uncomfortable topics that may have been rushed and/or overlooked at the initial decision to have surgery. Topics such as the patient's expected life span, the benefits and risk associated with surgery, the patient's overall health goals, and any unfavorable outcomes that may affect the patient's quality of life after surgery [4]. See **Appendix 1** for a visual diagram of the CGA workflow available at St. Luke's Hospital in Bethlehem Pennsylvania. The next section of this chapter will review each of the categories of the assessments used in the CGA.

3. Preoperative geriatric assessment tools (POGAT)

3.1 POGAT: mini-cognitive assessment (MCA)

In the general adult surgical population, the incidence of postop delirium was found to be (2.5–4.5%), which increased to (12–23%) in patients who were 60 years and older [11]. Understanding acute delirium and being able to recognize symptoms postoperatively will help keep patients safe and prevent further complications from developing. Studies reported a higher incidence of postoperative delirium in patients undergoing cardiovascular surgery at (15.3–23.4%), and hip fracture surgery (16.9%) [11]. Noting that cardiac and major lower joint surgeries are two of the most common surgeries performed in the elderly.

Mental cognitive impairment (MCI) and/or mental decline has become a rather general term that is used to describe a variety of conditions that affects an individual's mental state. Often it is used to describe any condition that interferes with brain function like; difficulty remembering things, difficulty learning new things, repeating the same stories over, asking the same questions over, the inability to make life decisions, etc. Most of the time, individuals with MCI can still function safely in everyday life. It may be seen that the term MCI is frequently miss used when trying to describe an acute delirium and/or chronic dementia. Knowing the differences between the three conditions, MCI, delirium, and dementia, will help healthcare providers understand their patients better and allow them to provide individualized care, specific to the patient's needs. As we see more and more surgeries being performed in the elderly, which is the number one population that these conditions affect, it becomes essential to understand these terms.

Delirium is an acute condition, the onset is abrupt, and can last hours to days. During that time span, the patient's mentation may wax and wean, showing improvements in mental cognition at times and then becoming worse again, especially, during the evening hours. Symptoms of delirium may be mild (impaired orientation and alertness) to severe (hallucinations and illusions). Delirium is reversible and most often resolves when the underlying cause is treated. Some causes of delirium may be electrolyte imbalance after surgery, infections, and the use of new medications. Patients with delirium cannot safely function alone [12].

There is a large amount of evidence that suggest postoperative delirium is directly associated with an increase mortality rate, and it is significantly linked to cognitive decline, and can lead to onset and/or development of dementia [11]. Specific to surgery, emergence delirium occurs during or immediately after emergence from general anesthesia and usually resolves within minutes or hours, and postoperative delirium mainly occurs 24–72 hours after surgery and resolves within hours to days [11].

Dementia is a long term, chronic, and disease process. Onset is gradual, and one's mental cognition will continue to slowly decline over months to years. Dementia is irreversible, but one may be able to slow down the progression with sustained treatment. Some risk factors include advanced age, head injury, atrophy of brain cells. Patients cannot safely function alone (19).

All these conditions increase with older age, and impaired cognition may go unrecognized in up to 81% of affected patient's [13]. The importance of presurgery cognitive screening is becoming more and more evident as (1) cognitive disorders are seen frequently in the elderly population and (2) research shows patients with MCI are at the highest risk for poor outcomes after surgery, such as longer hospital stays, higher hospital cost, increase chance of admission to an institution for rehab, and altered quality of life [4]. Recognition of any these cognitive concerns before surgery is essential as cognitive decline and/or postop delirium can persist for months or years and have a detrimental impact on the patient's quality of life, long-term survival, and increases the risk of developing dementia [11].

The use of at least one of the several cognitive assessment tools available should be considered during the perioperative stage when caring for an elderly patient. This can help alert healthcare providers to patients who are at a higher risk for developing a delirium after surgery. More importantly, this will provide the surgery team a clear baseline picture of the patient's mental status, which can be used for comparison after surgery if changes in cognition have been suspected.

Let us look at some of the tools that can be used in the cognitive assessment. Cognitive function can be assessed by direct interaction, and observation of the patient, concerns raised by family and friends, and self-reported by patient [13]. Cognitive assessment should be performed during the history taking both before and after surgery. Obtaining a baseline mental status is key in assisting suspected postoperative changes.

A more detailed assessment, like the mini-cognitive assessment (MCA) is a three-word recall and clock drawing activity that improves detection of MCI or dementia from 59% to 83% [13]. This assessment does not diagnose dementia, but alerts healthcare providers to those patients who may be at a higher risk for developing a delirium after surgery. Most favored due to its easy to use and time efficiency.

Other cognitive screening tools: such as, the Mini-mental state examination (MMSE), Confusion Assessment Method (CAM), digital span test (DST), and the Montreal Cognitive Assessment (MoCA) have all been validated assessments and easily incorporated into the perioperative environment [11, 13–15]. Please refer to **Table 2** for a summary of the cognitive assessments screening tools available to healthcare providers. Concerns identified on any of the screens should lead to a more detailed comprehensive evaluation that can be done by primary care doctor or a geriatric specialist.

Cognitive screens	Details	Summary of results
• Mini-Cognitive Assessment (MCA)	Clock drawing activity and 3-word recall. Patient is given three words to remember and then instructed to draw a clock. Patient is instructed to draw a time on the clock and then word recall is done.	Assessments are made to determine if patient can place the numbers correctly on the face of a clock (attention to position of 12, 3, 6, 9) and identify the specific time announced. After clock drawing patients are asked to recall three words. Points are accumulated for a score (1–5). • 0–2 suspect cognitive impairment • 3–5 no concerns
• Mini-Mental State Examination (MMSE)	Provider administers questionnaire. Includes questions and activities in the domains of orientation, registration, attention and calculation, recall, language, and copying.	Questions are used to assess cognitive function. Points are accumulated for a score (0–30). • 0–17 severe cognitive impairment • 18–23 mild cognitive impairment • 24–30 no cognitive impairment
• Confusion Assessment Method (CAM)	Provider completes 2-part assessment form after interviewing patient. Domains assessed are acute onset of confusion, inattention, disorganized thinking, and altered level of consciousness.	If all items in part one is YES and one item in part two: diagnosis of delirium expected
• Digital Span Test (DST)	Verbal test to exam short term memory. Provider has patient repeat back a series of numbers, up to a group of five.	Repeating sequence of numbers (two trails each series). Scoring is pass or fail.
• Montreal Cognitive Assessment (MoCA)	Provider administered questionnaire. Includes questions in activities in the domains of short-term memory, visual abilities, command functions, attention span, language, reasoning, and orientation.	Points are accumulating for score (1–26) • 0–16 impairment • 16–25 mild to moderate impairment • 26–30 no impairment

Table 2.
Cognitive assessment screening tools [11, 13–15].

Patients who are identified as being high risk of developing delirium after surgery should have both nonpharmacological and pharmacological recommendations in place. During surgery preparation in the perioperative stage, patients should be encouraged to remain on a healthy diet and continue oral hydration, (until diet restrictions for surgery start, NPO), encourage daily exercise, avoid toxins (drugs and alcohol), and stay socially active. Emphasis should include ways to stay mentally active through reading, playing games, and doing puzzles. A meta-analysis of 11 studies, showed that an exercise program, when routinely completed, greatly improved global cognition (believed to be related the aerobic component) and is something that can be incorporated into a patient at home surgery preparation plan [13]. A thorough medication review should be done assessing for any medication that may flag immediate geriatric concerns. Assessment for polypharmacy, medication redundancy, and medication safety are essential. Identification of any medications that can increase the risk of delirium, such as benzodiazepines and anticholinergics, should be noted, and consideration should be taken to decide if these medications should be stopped and/or decreased prior to surgery [11]. Recommendations such as the use of a geriatric pain protocol (the use of pain medications at a lower dose and slowly titrating up while monitoring for any changes in the patient's mental status) after surgery should be made. During the intraoperative phase interventions such those noted on the **Table 7** Geriatric ERAS should be put into place. Lastly, an inpatient consult to the facilities inpatient geriatrics team should be placed so the patient could be seen after surgery, at the bedside, to ensure standards of geriatric care being delivered. This team of experts makes sure that patients are participating in activities of daily life (ADL). For example, if the surgeon has cleared the patient to get up, that they are getting Out Of Bed (OOB) and moving, if the patient is cleared to eat that they are getting adequate nutrition. The geriatric team is also specialized in recognizing signs that point to changes in mental status.

3.2 POGAT: depression screening

Depression can be defined as feelings of sadness, hopelessness, and or despair that are occurring every day, for two or more weeks. Research reveals that depression has been directly linked to longer recovery times after surgery, which can lead to a longer hospital stay [9, 13]. Longer hospital stays may lead to deconditioning, weakening, and an increased risk of developing a postsurgical complication. Development of postoperative complications creates overall higher hospital costs for the patient and the institution. All these things are not safe for the patient and not ideal for the institution, thus making presurgery depression screening more and more important.

This is a topic that is rarely discussed, if at all. After most surgeries, there may be a period of physical limitations and restrictions. One may need help with basic activities of life (ADL) like going to the bathroom, bathing, and getting dressed. There may be restrictions set in place after surgery like not driving a car for a few weeks. Patients will need to rely on family and friends for help. This can create a lot of stress.

Patients have described feelings of anxiety, depression, and fear. There is a fear of the unknown. They fear things like; will I wake up from anesthesia, will I fully recover, who will take care of me after surgery? Even down to who will take care of my dog while I am hospitalized? These are all-natural human responses to stress and are preoperative psychological burdens that patients endure and may complicate the surgical experience [9]. This can be referred to as a situational depression, having these feelings related to the situation at hand. Often the patient will have surgery, start recovery, and day-by-day these feelings will begin to fade and eventually subside.

The real concern is patients who have an underlining chronic depression. These are the patients that may find it difficult to process the feelings surrounding surgery. Depression has been linked to longer recovery times, which then leads to longer hospital stays [9]. In the elderly specifically, depression was directly associated with pain and frailty, giving them a 3-fold risk of developing a delirium after surgery [9, 13]. Patients with MCI alone, are at a higher risk for being depressed due to the loss of independence [9]. Depression can lead to significant weight loss, decline in functional status, increase risk of suicide, overall increase in mortality, and increased use of healthcare services, all of which can complicate the surgical process [13].

Depression may present itself in different forms such as lethargy, weight loss, cognitive impairment, functional decline, and failure to thrive [13]. The standard history and physical conducted prior to surgery may miss the identification of depression. Specific prescreening for depression will allow healthcare providers to obtain a baseline picture of the patient's mental health, which will give a better understanding of any specific needs they may have throughout the entire surgical process. Interventions can be put into place to help monitor and prevent bad outcomes.

Screening for depression can be done with a brief 2-item screen, known as the patient health questionnaire-2. A positive result score of two on this simple screen should be followed by the patient health questionnaire-9, which is a more detailed assessment and has been validated as a reliable measure of depression severity and older adults [13]. Geriatric Depression Scale (GDS) is another screening tool that can be used for screening. Please see **Table 3** for a summary of depression tools. A retrospective study of patients greater than 75 years of age with colorectal cancer revealed that the GDS was an independent factor of postoperative delirium [9]. Another study that evaluated patients who were 75 years and older, diagnosed with thoracic cancer, showed that the use of GDS was able to predict the incidence of major complications [9].

Interventions in the presurgery phase may be as simple as having the patient speak with someone about their fears and concerns related to surgery. Offering support groups or access to online communities of patients who suffer from the same diagnosis process have shown to be very helpful. Specifically, in patients who are undergoing abdominal

Depression screens	Details	Summary of results
Patient health questionnaire -2 (PHQ-2)	Two-item questionnaires self-reported or administered by provider, if fails patient advances to the PHQ-9	• Score 0–1, stop • Score two or more, advanced to further screening via PHQ-9
Patient health questionnaire – 9 (PHQ-9)	Nine-item questionnaire self-reported or administered by provider	Score • 1–4 minimal depression • 5–9 mild depression • 10–14 moderate depression • 20–27 severe depression
Geriatric Depression Scale (GDS)	30-item questionnaire Self or assisted Yes or no format	Scores • 0–9 normal • 10–19 mild depressive • 20–30 severe depressive

Table 3.
Depression screening tools [9, 13].

surgery that results in creation of a colostomy bag. These patients benefit tremendously from meeting with a community of patients who have undergone the same procedure. Example: *living life after colostomy*. Online communities and blogs are terrific options as they can be attended from the comfort of patient's own home. Patients have expressed feelings of fear and thoughts that their life is over now having to have a colostomy bag attached to them. Not to mention feelings of isolation and embarrassment. Patients who have attended these support groups have come back expressing much relief and calmness after speaking with other patients who went through the same procedure and now are living a normal life.

When concerns arise about the depression screening, healthcare providers always want to identify if this is a new depression or chronic depression. Any new depression should be assessed in further detail and a referral placed to the appropriate provider and/or resources the patient may need. If it is a chronic depression, make sure the family physician is aware and patient is on appropriate treatment. Evaluation of all the medications they are taking to make sure the dose is appropriate and/or assessment of any medication changes they may need throughout the surgical phases. Some patients may benefit from starting a selective serotonin reuptake inhibitors (SSRI) during their surgical phase.

After surgery, it is important to continue to monitor the patient's mental status and mood. This will allow for quick interventions if needed. This will also allow for assessment of potential development of postoperative delirium. A thorough medication review should be conducted and determine if patient would need further readjustments of any medications. Last, an inpatient consult with the institution's psychology team may want to be considered.

3.3 POGAT: nutritional assessment

The World Health Organization (WHO) defines malnutrition as having deficiencies, either a lack of, an excess of, or an imbalance in patient's intake of energy, vitamins, minerals, and other nutrients [16]. Malnutrition can be used to describe two conditions, both undernutrition and/or overnutrition "overweight" [16]. Undernutrition is a state of deficit where there is lack of nourishment from poor diet intake and/or poor access to healthy foods. Overnutrition is too much, as in overweight, and excess of caloric- energy intake. Overnutrition can lead to an overweight state, increasing a patient's weight and Body Mass Index (BMI), which contributes to poor health and an increased the risk of diabetes, heart disease, stroke, and cancer [16]. Elderly patients are at risk for overnutrition and becoming overweight due to their sedentary lifestyle as they get older. Patients who are overweight should be considered for weight management programs to help improve their health and quality of life. Especially patients who are electing to have a major lower joint replacement as the extra weight can place stress on the new replacement and lead to higher rates of dislocation.

Unexpected weight loss and undernutrition are also very common in older age, especially the geriatric cancer population. A review of a study conducted by Tatum et al. [13], revealed among older adults receiving home care after surgery, 12% were malnourished and 51% were at risk for malnourishment [13]. Significantly increasing their chance of poor wound healing and surgical site infections (SSI). Malnutrition can be caused by physical, psychological, or social changes associated with aging, leading to decreased resistance to infection, immune function, and quality of life [17].

As we age, our bodies change and we begin to lose our senses, which causes a decrease or loss in appetite. Other conditions that can cause malnutrition in the elderly are medication use, decrease in exercise, difficulty swallowing, poor dentition, poorly fitting dentures, and difficulty digesting certain types of food [18]. Studies also show that malnutrition was directly related to an increase in the length of stay, an increase in the risk of readmission back into the hospital, and an increase in the over mortality of patients [18]. Preoperative nutrition screening is recommended and can help improve care of surgical patients, unfortunately, it is commonly overlooked.

Knowing the nutritional status of our patients is key to providing better care. More and more research showS just how important understanding nutrition is, however, it is still often underlooked at. Serum albumin less than 3.5 have been shown to be predictor of mortality and postoperative pulmonary complications (PPC) [4]. Malnutrition has been related to poor wound healing, increased risks of surgical site infection, and precursor to frailty. Nutritional screening should be done prior to the operation. If deficits are identified, patient-specific plans should be put in place to optimize the patient, for example, implementation of protein supplements should be considered prior to surgery, and education on the appropriate diet should be provided to patient.

Nutritional screening should be conducted prior to surgery. A simple question: such as, have you had any unintentional weight loss? A yes to this question should trigger a more thorough nutritional exam to be completed. Assessment of the patient's BMI and any BMI result of less than (<18), should trigger a more detailed nutritional assessment. In addition, there are several different patient health questionnaires that can be used to screen for malnutrition.

The Mini-Nutritional Assessment (MNA) form looks at different domains such as has the patient had any unintentional weight loss, whether there has been a decrease in food intake and why, have they had any psychological stress in the last year, and assessment of the patient's BMI. Answers to these questions are linked to points, points are accumulated and used to determine the risk of malnutrition.

Some more nutrition screening tools that can be incorporated into the presurgery screening process include the Geriatric Nutritional Risk Index (GNRI), Subjective Global Assessment, and the Malnutrition Screening Tool. See **Table 4** for a breakdown summary of nutritional screening tools available. The GNRI evaluates the patient's albumin level, in comparison to their present body weight, and ideal body weight. The GNRI has been used to help predict the risk of nutrition-related morbidity and mortality in elderly patients [17]. The GNRI was defined as a crucial independent prognosis for both overall survival and disease-specific survival [17].

One prospective study reviewed by Xue et al. [9] found that patients who were identified as malnourished *via* SGA were at a higher risk for postoperative morbidity [9].

Patients who are identified as at risk for malnutrition or malnourished, should follow the institutions' nutrition protocol or be enrolled in the nutrition program. If there are none in place, providers can refer patients to their family doctor for a complete nutritional assessment and any possible blood work they may need (prealbumin, albumin). The presurgery assessment phase is a great time to complete a thorough nutritional assessment. After the assessment, time should be set aside with the patient to review the findings. During this time, the provider can review the best diet type for the patient. Labs, prealbumin, and albumin levels can be obtained. Patients should be educated on how many grams of protein a day they should be

Nutrition screens	Details	Summary of results
Mini Nutritional Assessment (MNA)	Six-item questionnaire helps determine if patients are well-nourished, at risk for malnutrition, or malnourished	Points are assigned to each answer • 0–7 pts. malnourished • 8–11 at risk for malnutrition • 12–14 normal nutritional status
Malnutrition Screening Tool (MST)	3-step questionnaire used more in acute care and inpatient setting	Points are assigned to each answer • 0–1 pts. not at risk • 2 - < at risk
Geriatric Nutritional Risk Index (GNRI)	Predicts the risk of complications and mortality linked to malnutrition.	• Very severe GNRI <73 • Severe GNRI 73–82 • Moderate GNRI 82–92 • Mild GNRI 92–98 • Norm >98
Subjective Global Assessment (SGA)	**Gold standard** Used often in long-term care.	Clinical assessment: Assessment includes history of recent intake, weight changes, GI symptoms, and clinical evaluation.

Table 4.
Nutrition screening tools [9, 17].

consuming. A simple calculation can be done. It is recommended that healthy adults should consume 0.4 grams of protein for every pound of weight [16, 18]. Grams of protein a day should be increased from the patient's baseline during all phases of surgery to help build strength and promote tissue repair. Examples of different ways in which a patient can achieve their goal should be explored and taught to patient. Several weeks before surgery is an ideal time to begin protein supplements for ampule time to make improvements. Placing a consult to the institution's nutrition team to see the patient after surgery, at the bedside. For maximal benefits Protein supplements should begin 30 days before the operation to significantly decrease the chance of poor wound healing and surgical site infections. A medication review should be conducted. The American Geriatrics Society (AGS) recommends providers review the medication list and discontinue any medications that contribute to weight loss and diminished appetite [13]. Lastly, providing a list of appealing peeling foods, ensuring social support, and offering feeding assistance when patients are identified as at risk for malnutrition [13].

Nutritional assessments often get overlooked as they are not considered urgent matters like those of the heart and lungs. Not mandatory, but highly recommended in all presurgery assessments, at the least, nutritional screening should be a must in major abdominal surgeries. This is extremely important as weight loss can be expected with many abdominal surgeries, especially, when there is a bowel prep involved, surgery, inpatient hospital stay, and diet restrictions. Nutrition is key, the better your nutrition is before surgery the better your body will heal after surgery, which could mean shorter recovery times.

3.4 Storytime (Real patient encounter/true story experienced by author Ellen McHugh)

My mother had a very difficult time healing after her foot surgery. Not only was it painful, but the surgical wound was positioned right where the inner edge of her shoe lay, hence, impairing her walking. The wound was not healing and within weeks the wound grew bigger and was infected. This required multiple trips to the wound care center, which had taken time from both of our days and disrupted her quality of life. Not to mention, it required multiple resources from the hospital supplies and increased cost for all involved. I often question to this day, if she would have benefited from a nutritional evaluation prior to her surgery. (Later, a low albumin and protein level revealed itself on random blood work she had done). I often think about if we could have worked on improving her nutrition prior to her operation, could we have possibly prevented this outcome? Ultimately adding to a better quality of life (less pain, less anxiety, less burden of wound care, and no extra trips to the hospital). In addition, saving extra costs for everyone involved. Improving your nutrition may be one of the easier tasks to achieve in your health, something so simple that was overlooked. The better your nutrition is before surgery, the better your body will recover after surgery!

3.5 POGAT: cardiac and pulmonary assessments

Aside from postoperative delirium, cardiac and respiratory complications are the most common adverse events in elderly patients when recovering from surgery [19]. These events are seen more frequently in the advanced age, >80 years of age population [19]. Cardiac and respiratory complications can lead to an admission to the Intensive Care Unit (ICU), and admissions to ICU can lead to increased risk of death, all of which are not safe for the patient and not ideal for the institution [19]. The standard cardiac and pulmonary assessments are recommended to be included in the CGA. The patient's heart health should be evaluated prior to surgery to make sure their heart is strong enough to undergo anesthesia and have the operation. During completion of the H&P, any past and present heart conditions can be identified. The surgery team should be aware of any cardiac history and if the patient follows up with a cardiologist. Information should be collected on when the patient saw their cardiologist last and what were the recommendations at the end of the visit. Were those recommendations followed? Simple yes or no questions, such as, does the patient have chest pain (CP) or a new shortness of breath (SOB) in the last few months should be included in the assessment. Screening through a more detailed questionnaire such as a risk and triage, patient questionnaire to obtain a metabolic equivalent of task (METS) score is recommended. Any METS score less than four should be further investigated. Last, has the patient had any recent cardiac testing done like an electrocardiogram (ECG) or echocardiogram (ECHO). A complete review of those tests should be done and determine if any further cardiac testing is needed before moving forward. This is a time in which the healthcare team can discuss the patient's cardiac risk of having surgery.

Aging reduces the capacity of all pulmonary functions due to a decline in thoracic elasticity and weakening of respiratory muscles [4]. All underlying pulmonary diseases should be optimized prior to surgery. Again, the H&P is a good time to collect this information. Chronic obstructive pulmonary disease (COPD) is a frequent condition seen in the elderly and is a recognized risk factor for postop complications [4]. If the patient has a diagnosis of COPD, the patient should be assessed to ensure their breathing is stable and COPD is optimized. Questions to ask: are you compliant with your daily inhalers? when is the last time you used your rescue inhaler? and does your COPD affect your everyday life? If the patient is following up with a pulmonologist, information should be collected on when was their last visit and what were the recommendations made at that visit.

Active smokers who are interested in quitting smoking before the operation should be offered tobacco therapy. Tobacco therapy, the use of nicotine replacement therapy should be started as soon as possible. Ideal timing is 30 days prior to surgery, minimum is 2 weeks prior to surgery. Arrangements should be made to continue tobacco therapy treatment on admission for surgery.

The aging process reduces the capacity of lung functions from weakened respiratory muscles over time, and you may see a decrease in the protective reflexes such as coughing and swallowing leading to an increased chance of postoperative aspiration pneumonia [4]. During the CGA visit, lung exercises can be taught. Incentive spirometer can be taught. Deep breathing and cough exercises can be taught so the patient can begin their lung exercises immediately to help reduce risk of postoperative pneumonia.

3.6 POGAT: functional mobility

As our bodies age, our functional status (FS) and mobility begin to decline. Functional mobility can be described as a person's ability to move independently and safety in their environment [4]. FS can be defined as the number of behaviors that are needed to maintain daily activities, including social and cognitive function, it determines the patient's ability to actively mobilize and attend to basic activities of daily life (BADL) and instrumental activities of daily life (IDAL) by themselves [4]. Without good mobility, a person is at risk for further deconditioning, weakening of their body, and FS decline. Older age goes hand and hand with FS decline and can be seen in almost every frail patient. There is more and more evidence suggesting that impaired FS status is associated with poor postoperative outcomes [4, 9, 20] and unfortunately, most anesthesiologists and surgeons do not measure physical needs in the preop phase [4]. It is recommended that patients undergo presurgery screening and assessment of functional mobility and their ability to perform BADLs and IADLs. Information about the patient's ability to form BADLs/IADLs should be documented prior to surgery. This should include the patient's ability to bathe, dress, ambulate, budget the checkbook, their nutritional status, and their social needs [4, 9]. ADL dependency and deficiencies in performing ADLs are shown to be a direct predictor of 30-day postoperative complications [4, 9, 11, 20]. In addition, patients with an ADLs deficiency may not have enough physiological reserve to endure and rehabilitate from major surgery and this should be discussed with the patient and their family before the decision is made [9]. During FS screening, assessment of home safety and fall risk should also be included. Knowing the patient's fall risk is huge as it is detrimental to the geriatric population. Falls have also been related to 30-day mortality in patients who are 85 years of age and older [20, 21]. Falls can lead to further complications and impair the quality of life in the older adult population. More and more research shows that when we can accurately identify older patients who are at risk for falling, we can then implement interventions that reduce the rates of injurious falls, and/or detrimental outcomes [21]. Identification of any physical needs presurgery can give the team time to implement presurgery treatment with the goals of improving physical limitations prior to surgery.

There are different screenings and assessment tools that can be used to evaluate one's functional status. Please refer to **Table 5**, for a summary of FS assessment tools. The easiest way to assess one functional mobility is by direct observation. This can be done by the provider by watching the patient walk throughout the office visit and

Functional status screens	Details	Summary of results
Direct provider observation	Provider observes patient ambulate	Assessments made: • Steady or unsteady • Fast or slow
Fall screening	Simple yes or no question. Have you fallen in the last 6 months?	Answer of yes indicates high risk of falling again
Time Up to Go (TUG)	Timed physical activity test. Provider observes patient stand from chair, ambulate 10 feet, turn around, walk back, and sit down.	More than 15 seconds to complete this activity indicates high risk of falls
Barthel scale: Basic Activities of Daily Life (B-ADL)	Ambulating, transferring, dressing, eating, drinking, personal hygiene, and taking medication	Each activity is a point: Abilities maintain for each group • 5–6 independence • 3–4 intermediate dependence • 1–2 total dependence
Barthel scale: Instrumental activities of daily life (IDAL)	Driving, preparing meals, doing housework, shopping, managing finances, managing medication, and using telephone	Each activity is a point: Abilities maintain for each group • 5–6 independence • 3–4 intermediate dependence • 1–2 total dependence

Table 5.
Functional status screening tools [4, 10, 13].

paying attention to their ability to get up and down from chair to chair and move. Assessments should be made on how fast or slow their gait is. How steady or unsteady their gait is. Reduced gait speed has been associated with increased falls and reduced survival rates [13]. One activity that can be used to test the patient's functional mobility is the Time Up to Go (TUG). This activity requires a nurse to observe a patient getting up from a chair, walking straight for 10 ft, then turning around, walking back, and sitting back down [4, 13]. The activity should be timed. Studies suggest that patients who take longer to do the TUG (>15 seconds) are at a higher risk for falls [10]. A standardized assessment tool, such as the Barthel scale for ADLs, which gathers information on the patient's ability to perform everyday activities may be used. Fall risk can be assessed with a single screening question; have you fallen in the past 6 months? [13]. A positive answer to falling is associated with a 2.8 times higher likelihood of falling again within the next year, which is extremely important to note in elderly's having major lower joint surgeries [13].

Identifying FS decline and high fall risk can allow healthcare providers to implement interventions that can maximize independence and safety [13]. Patients who are identified as having an impaired FS and/or high fall risk should be taught bilateral upper extremity and bilateral lower extremity exercises for muscle strengthening and balance coordination. Generic exercises can be taught at the time of the presurgery assessment. An exercise routine should be developed for the patient that fits into their life and accommodates their physical needs. For example, if the patient is currently walking 1000 steps a day, set a goal to increase to 2000 steps a day. Wieland and Ferrucci [21] investigated the effectiveness of patient's using a wearable activity tracker device to monitor and improve patient's functional status prior to surgery [21]. They completed a systematic review of 26 studies with a total of 2767 participants that showed those who wore the device had increased their physical activity by almost 27% over their baseline [21].

Patients who are at high risk for falling should be taught exercises that can be done sitting or lying down. For severe FS decline, it may be beneficial for the patient to see a physical therapist or occupational therapist prior to the operation to address impairments [9]. Education on fall prevention should be provided to the patient. Home safety should be included. Emphasis on ways to prevent falls after your operation should be discussed. Including an FS evaluation in the anesthesia consult provides useful information about the surgical risk and can help develop a patient's specific plan for postoperative care [4].

This is also a good time to document any functional sensory impairments the patient may have. Other assessments that are rarely taken into consideration are assessing the patient's vision and hearing. Evaluation of the patient's vision, hearing, smell, and tactile abilities should all be documented in the presurgical phase. This can help determine a patient's baseline which can be used as a comparison if there are any changes suspected after surgery. Hearing loss is often unrecognized by patients and affects more than 80% of adults older than 80 years of age [13]. Moderate to severe hearing loss is associated with a 3–4-fold higher incidence of dementia [13]. Hearing loss can also be mistaken for depression. Urinary incontinence can impair in patient's quality of life and should also be documented [13].

3.7 POGAT: frailty

Understanding a patient's physical needs and frailty status is key in providing best care and can make a huge impact on recovery after surgery and improve surgical outcomes. Identifying if your patient is frail, pre-frail, or at risk for frailty is important because there is so much evidence to show that frail patients typically do not do well after surgery. Frailty is directly associated with major complications in the 30-day postoperative phase [4, 8, 9]. In fact, frail patients have a 4-times higher risk of developing 30-day postoperative major complications [9]. Patients who are frail are at a higher risk for developing complications after surgery leading to longer recovery times, physical deconditioning, discharge to nursing facilities, and even death. Frail patients are at a higher risk for developing cardiac and pulmonary complications that can lead to ICU stays, in addition, frailty is a direct risk factor for postoperative delirium [4]. Regarding surgery, frailty has been shown to be an independent risk factor for length of stay, postop complications, morbidity, and mortality [8]. All these complications will create chaos in the surgical experience and can disrupt the patient's quality of life.

Let us start by defining frailty. Frailty can be defined as a medical syndrome with numerous causes and contributing factors that are characterized by diminished strength, decreased endurance, and reduced physiological function that increases an individual's vulnerability to developing increased dependency and/or death [22–24]. Other studies defined frailty as a distinct clinical syndrome meeting three or more or five criteria, including weakness, slowness, low-level physical activity, self-reported exhaustion, and unintentional weight loss [8, 22]. Several factors that contribute to frailty are advanced chronological age, poor mechanical performance, decrease in level of energy, decreased metabolism, weakness, slowness, exhaustion, low activity, and weight loss [22]. Frailty is common health problem recognized among the older adult and has been shown to increase the risk of moderate to severe adverse outcomes, including longer recovery times, falls, delirium, higher readmission rates, and even death [20, 22]. Assessing for frailty in the older patient is crucial, as it has been a direct indicator of those patients who may do well versus those patients who may not do well after surgery [21]. Screening patients in the presurgery phase can help identify high-risk patients. Once patients are identified, the surgical team can put individualized care plans in place to help optimize them before their surgery and prevent these bad outcomes.

Refer to **Table 6** for a summary of frailty screening tools. The gold standard of measuring frailty is using the CGA, frailty can easily be defined by confirmative deficits identified in the comprehensive geriatric assessment [20, 21]. Concerns for frailty can be identified on almost all the assessments that are performed during the CGA (through a single assessment and/or combination). There are multiple other tools that have been used to identify states of frailty. The use of a hand-held device, known as a hand dynamometer, measures a patient's grip strength (in lbs. or kg) and has been used to identify patients who are prefrail, or frail. Patient has three trials of squeezing the hand dynamometer. Scores are average. Assessments in the form of

Frailty screens	Details	Summary of results
Comprehensive Geriatric Assessment (CGA)	**Gold standard:** Assessment domains: cognitive, depression, nutrition, functional status, frailty, polypharmacy, and patient's health goals	Can be a positive score on one of domain or a combination of domains
Hand dynamometer	Three trial physical assessment. Patient squeezes a handheld device three times. Strength of grip measured in pounds or kilograms	Number is calculated from average of three scores. Scores are compared on the B&L engineering grip strength norm chart: designed for ages 6–19 and adults 20 to 75+. Patient will fall in out of range for their age group.
Clinical Frail Scale (CFS)	Clinical judgment. Physician assigned scores to categories	Score • 1- very fit • 2- well • 3- well with treated comorbid diseases • 4- vulnerable • 5- mildly frail • 6- moderately frail • 7- severely frail
Frailty index	Evaluates the presence of health deficits: Morbidity, symptoms, disabilities, and diseases.	Provider assessment
Frail scale	Self-reported. five domains: Fatigue, resistance, ambulation, illness, or weight loss.	Score (# deficits present) • 0-no frailty • 1–2-pre-frail • 3 or more frail
Frailty phenotype	Checklist of five criteria: weight loss, weakness, self-reported exhaustion, slowness, and low activity questionnaire.	Score (# criteria present) • 0- not frail • 1–2- pre-frail • >3 - frail

Table 6.
Frailty screening tools [4, 8, 9, 20, 21].

patient questionaries include the Clinical Frailty Scale (CFS), freed criteria, frailty index, and the frail scale. The questionnaires that are available look into different domains such as comorbidities, social factors, psychological conditions, functional decline, and cognitive decline answers are incorporated into an index with a higher number of conditions indicating a higher level of frailty [22]. The TUGT, summarized in **Table 5**, is a physical assessment that is used for functional screening, and can also be an indicator of frailty and a predictor of falls.

Frailty is a common problem among older adults. Frailty increases the risk of adverse outcomes, falls, hospitalization, and death [22]. Identifying patients who are frail is key, however, emphasis needs to be placed on treatment and management to make a real difference [8]. Patients who are pre-frail, frail, or at risk for frailty should be evaluated and considered for prehabilitation (prehab) prior to their surgery. Most are familiar with the term rehabilitation (rehab), which is therapy after surgery, prehab refers to therapy before surgery to improve the patient's state of health. The goal is to increase their stamina and endurance. Prehab may consist of a variety of interventions, but most commonly include physical therapy (PT) and nutrition supplementation. PT for muscle strengthening and balance coordination and nutrition supplements to get the patient stronger and help tissue repair after surgery. Additional types of interventions included in prehab are vitamin D therapy, reduction of polypharmacy, multicomponent-focused interventions, and individually tailored geriatric care models [8, 22]. Vitamin D has been shown to help reduce falls, hip fractures, and overall mortality [8]. For best results, these interventions should be put into place at least 3–6 months prior to their operation [22].

Understanding frailty is important, when assessed correctly it can help us alert the patients who will not do well after surgery. The important takeaway is to identify frail syndromes and implement individual tailored geriatric interventions that can lead to continuous care and emphasize interventions that focus on improving clinical outcomes of the older adult [10]. With the goal of restoring a patient's preexisting reserves to bring them to a better state of health, one that can withstand surgical stress and maintain baseline functions postoperatively [23]. This is especially important as frailty has been directly related to adverse health outcomes, unplanned repeated hospitalizations, extended hospital stays, and high patient mortality [10], all things that are not safe for our patients and not ideal for the institution.

3.8 POGAT: polypharmacy

Changes in the pharmacodynamics and pharmacokinetics induced by aging make this population very sensitive to medications, especially those medications administered in the pre and intraoperative phases of surgery [4]. In the geriatric population, there is an increased incidence of unexpected reactions to medications, anesthesia, and surgery, making it extremely important to understand your patient's full medication history [4]. A thorough medication review should be done at the time of the CGA. This is critical as many elderly patients describe some confusion around their medication use, specifically, on what the medications are used for and how to take them correctly. It is very common to see misuse, underuse, and abuse of medications in this population [4]. Most older patients are on several medications and it may be hard for them to keep track. It was reported that geriatric patients are great consumers of medications (four drugs a day for ages 65–80 years, 4.5 drugs a day for ages >80 years) [9]. Providers should conduct a thorough medication review looking for polypharmacy, medication redundancy, and medication safety. Polypharmacy is a term used to describe the use of multiple medications; polypharmacy is defined as the use of >5 drugs a day [9]. Polypharmacy was found to be a direct predictive factor of 30-day postoperative major complications [9].

During the review, the provider should be assessing effectiveness of each medication with the goal of discontinuing or substituting medications that could potentially cause unsuitable side effects in the geriatric patient [9, 13]. Some medications may need to be reduced and/or placed on hold during the different surgery phases. Medications that are sensitive to the geriatric population and should be used cautiously are anticholinergic drugs such as (antiemetics, bronchodilators, antiarrhythmias, antihypertensive, anti-Parkinson's), which have been shown to disrupt cognitive function [4, 11]. Inappropriate drugs that act on the central nervous system such as benzodiazepines have been shown to increase the risk of falls, confusion, and cognitive deterioration [4, 9, 11].

The Beers, STOPP (screening tool for older person prescriptions), and START (screening tool to alert doctors to right treatment) criteria are helpful resources to utilize during the medication review. The Beers, STOPP, and START criteria lists potentially inappropriate medications, medications to avoid, medication combinations that may lead to harmful interactions in older adults, and dose adjustments for patients with chronic kidney disease (CKD) [13].

Education should be provided to the patient on each medication, including the use, dose, frequency, side effects, and interactions. Providers should assess the patient's ability to understand this information by having the patient recite the medication instructions by to them. If cognitive impairment is expected, information should be given to the patient's main caregiver. Providers should ensure that patients are able to adhere to the daily medication routine. Any medications that can be taken as a single daily dose should be prescribed that way to reduce the need for frequent dosing. Strategies to improve medication adherence include identifying a main caregiver to assist patient, recommending the use of pill boxes and daily organized medication blister packs, once-a-day medication instead of more frequent administration, and offering direct patient education with the pharmacist [13].

3.9 POGAT: substance abuse

If there are any concerns for substance abuse, substance abuse screening can be conducted at the time of the CGA. Standard tools such as the CAGE questionnaire (cutting down, annoyance, guilty, eye-opener) and alcohol screening are most used. Any abnormal finding on the screenings should alert healthcare providers to push for further investigation and treatment. Patients can be offered outpatient therapy and inpatient rehab depending on severity of their needs. Consideration of starting preop vitamins such as folic acid and thiamine may be beneficial. All findings should be documented and communicated with the surgical team. Assessments of potential withdrawal concerns should be made and implementation of Ethanol (ETOH) withdrawal monitoring protocols should be set in place as needed.

3.10 POGAT: caregiver needs

During the CGA, a main caregiver for the patient should be identified. Complete documentation in the health records on caregiver name and contact information. If the patient is without a caregiver, time should be spent with the patient to help determine who could help them. For example, discussing with the patient if they have family, friends, or neighbors that would be willing to help throughout the surgery process.

3.11 POGAT: patient health goals

When performing the CGA, time should be set aside to review the patient's overall health goals. Healthcare providers should present questions to the patient such as: What is important to you? What are your goals for after surgery? What is one thing that you cannot live without? Healthcare providers should explore these topics with the patient and review all options available to them, including surgical and nonsurgical treatment plans. Once identified, the patient's health goals should be documented in their health record and incorporated into their surgery plan of care. Evaluation of goals can be made throughout all phases of surgery and even used to remind the patient of the intended outcome after surgery.

Discussions should include what the patient's quality of life looks like with and without surgery. Although almost all surgical procedures enhance the quality of life, the balance between the expected benefits and the risk of adverse events (such as cognitive disorders, infections, or other medical complications) should be explored [4, 24]. In the advanced age adult, surgery should be considered when the disease process produces continued discomfort, unmanageable pain, disability, economical loss, and interference with a normal routine of life [25]. However, evaluating the surgical risks must be balanced against the expected beneficial results, the current enjoyment of life, and life expectancy with and without surgery, as unfavorable outcomes are a key issue [4, 25].

4. Enhanced Recovery After Surgery (ERAS)

Enhanced Recovery After Surgery (ERAS) protocols are one-way healthcare institutions can ensure that a thorough surgical plan has been developed, implemented, and carried out. ERAS protocols are designed to assign specific care measures to be delivered to patients at each phase of their surgical experience to help reduce and/or eliminate stressors on the body caused by surgery. ERAS protocols aim to produce better outcomes for patients after surgery. ERAS refers to condition-specific care pathways that use a multidisciplinary team approach, which begins in the preoperative phase, to effectively reduce the perioperative stress response, which then reduces the incidence of infectious complications, and chronic complications after surgery and achieves the goal of rapid rehabilitation [26]. ERAS protocols are available for many surgical conditions (colorectal, orthopedics, vascular, etc.) and universal guidelines recommend that a total of 20 elements of care, be divided into the perioperative, intraoperative, and postoperative phases of surgery [27]. The way in which an institution plans to deliver the different phases of the ERAS protocol may vary from place to place. Most intuitions assign each phase of care to be delivered (pre, intra, and post) to the appropriate units, which the patient will visit throughout the surgical experience.

Paduraru et al. [27] found that elderly patients who followed an ERAS protocol had fewer postoperative complications and a shorter hospital stay when compared to patients who received conventional care [27]. After the review of 18 independent studies, Paduraru et al. [27] concluded that ERAS can safely be applied to the elderly patients, both in emergency and elective surgery, to reduce post-op complications, shorten duration of hospital stay, and reduce readmissions [27]. Yu et al. [19] reviewed a study that utilized "care bundles" to closely follow patient's medical conditions and provide recovery care. Results showed patients who received care bundles, compared to patients who received conventional care, had a shorter duration of intubation, shorter length in PACU stay, and less adverse events such as respiratory tract, cardiovascular complications, and postoperative pain agitation were discovered during recovery [19].

ERAS protocols can serve as a great guide for pharmacological considerations in the geriatric population. Reference should be made to consider *2019 AGS BEERS Criteria Update Expert Panel* [28, 29]. Special attention should be placed on minimizing and/or avoiding the use of the medication class benzodiazepines. Some medications to avoid include: diphenhydramine, meperidine, metoclopramide, and pancuronium. Induction dosing of propofol should be decreased between 20% and 60% in the geriatric population (consider an initial dosing of 1 mg/kg) [28, 29]. If a provider chooses to use inhalation agents consider with MAC levels decrease with age decade over 40) [28, 29]. Drug distribution is altered with normal aging due to a decrease in total body water and increase in adipose tissue resulting in a smaller volume of distribution and increased plasma concentration of water-soluble medications. There is an increased volume of distribution with possible delay in the onset of action and accumulation of more lipid-soluble drugs such as fentanyl. Phase I metabolism through the liver is also impacted by normal aging secondary to decreased enzymatic activity and number of hepatocytes resulting in an increased half-life for several medications. Creatinine clearance may decrease up to 40% by age 80 and analgesic doses should be adjusted accordingly [28, 29]. Regional anesthesia should be prioritized in the orthopedic trauma patient, with strict consideration of avoiding hypotension.

With the aging population and growing number of geriatric surgeries seen, encouraging the use of a geriatric ERAS pathway is essential and has been shown to improve the surgical outcomes of older adults. Please refer to **Table** 7, for an example of a *geriatric enhanced recovery after surgery protocol.*

Preadmission testing phase (PAT):	• Discuss personal goals and treatment preferences • Provide realistic expectations of postoperative functional decline, loss of independence, and skilled care burden • Identify advance directive and a designated health care proxy • Discuss resuscitation wishes • One-on-one teaching (surgery type, smoking cessation, ETOH cessation) • Provide references to preoperative education and counseling • Chlorhexidine skin cleansing twice in 24 hrs prior to surgery • Consider performing a comprehensive geriatric Assessment or minimal cognitive and physical assessment • NPO guidelines: No solids after midnight except medication, with clear liquids, if ordered use of carbohydrate drink prior to surgery
Preoperative management:	• Chlorhexidine skin cleansing repeated inhouse • Fingerstick blood glucose check • Evaluation for VTE prophylaxis: both mechanical and pharmacological • Preoperative warming device (Bair Hugger) to keep temperature > 35C. • Consider regional anesthetic or neuraxial use for case type, perform in preoperative setting • Consider oral premedication: Acetaminophen, Gabapentin, Celebrex • Scopolamine transdermal patch for motion sickness, PONV prophylaxis • Perform a cognitive assessment test to document a baseline (if not already performed in PAT process)

Intra-operative management:	• Maintain MAP >70 mmHg, heart rate within 20% of baseline • Minimize or avoid narcotics; consider total IV anesthesia (TIVA) • Hyperglycemia control, goal for blood glucose level: < 180 mg/dL • IV antibiotics within 1 hour before skin incision, redose as per pharmacy guidelines • Maintain normothermia (>96.5 degrees Fahrenheit) • Goal hemoglobin levels: > 10 Hb? • Maintain euvolemia • Identify glomerular filtration rate (GFR) to determine risk for AKI, if high risk • Lung protective ventilation • PONV prophylaxis > 2 antiemetics (dexamethasone, ondansetron) • Consider nonopioid pain management regimen • Full reversal of neuromuscular blockade is required • Consider postoperative ventilation if neuromuscular blockade is questionable
Postoperative management:	• Blood glucose check • Analgesia as needed, minimize narcotics • Initiate epidural infusion if appropriate • Initiate clear liquids if cleared by surgery • Consider postoperative delirium screening tool prior to discharge from PACU • Diet: advance as tolerated • IV fluids: discontinue as soon as tolerating oral hydration • Continue hyperglycemia screening as protocol dictates • Consider bowel regimen if appropriate • Continue antibiotics at surgeon's direction • Continue VTE prophylaxis • Continue multimodal postoperative pain regimen • Begin ambulation as soon as possible with surgeries direction after evaluation of her fall risk • Discontinue Foley catheter as soon as possible • Begin postoperative education • Aggressive pulmonary rehab (incentives spirometry) • Begin postoperative physical/occupational/speech therapy as needed. • Daily evaluation • Delirium/cognitive impairment • Postoperative acute pain • Pulmonary complications • Fall risk • Nutrition • UTI prevention • Functional decline • Pressure ulcers • Daily family communication

Table 7.
Geriatric enhanced recovery after surgery (ERAS) protocol [1–7, 19, 25–27, 30–32].

DOI: http://dx.doi.org/10.5772/intechopen.111527

5. Anesthesia in the older adult

Surgical procedures have numerous benefits, including saving and prolonging life, providing continuous physical comfort, relieving pain, and can serve for functional and social usefulness [25]. These are all attractive benefits to the older adult, especially those who are looking to improve and maintain a good quality of life. That is why more and more adults are electing to have surgery in their older age and geriatric surgery is becoming the new trend. Unfortunately, we cannot ignore that surgical procedures and the anesthesia required can cause stress on all organs in the body and can disrupt hemostasis. Older adults with reduced physical reserve may not be able to tolerate the stress of surgery and/or the use of the anesthetics that are required. Changes in pharmacodynamics and pharmacokinetics induced by the aging process can make elderly patients very sensitive to medications, especially those administered in the pre and intraoperative phases of surgery [4]. Studies show that older adults are at an increased risk of adverse events even after induction of anesthesia alone, and a presedation assessment should be conducted to ensure that the patient is indeed a candidate for moderate sedation and analgesia (MSA) [30, 31]. The preoperative phase is the best time to conduct a presedation assessment. The sooner a patient's needs are identified the more time healthcare providers will have to intervene. Older adults undergoing surgery should have the standard history and physical (H&P) completed, in addition, an assessment for frailty, functional status, and cognitive impairment should now be included [30]. This is supported by the Association of Peri-Operative Registered Nurses (AORN) and the American Society of Anesthesiologists (ASA) and has made perioperative anesthesia management a challenge [30].

Perioperative anesthesia management is a challenge in the geriatric population; hence, the anesthetic plan should always be individualized to each patient's needs and then cautiously administered [31]. One way to accomplish this is to extend the anesthesia consult to incorporate additional assessments that are specific to the geriatric population. Two known risk factors seen in older patients that directly increase the patient's surgery risk include functional decline and multiple comorbidities [4]. Elderly patients with comorbid diseases like diabetes, and/or hypertension have been shown to lead to higher complication rates after surgery and significantly increase the length of stay and hospital costs [4]. These patients have an increased incidence of unexpected reactions to medications and anesthesia, particularly developing an acute delirium [4]. Geriatric screening tools used to assess cognition, frailty, and functional status should be incorporated into the assessment and the findings should be used to develop a plan of care that will choose the safest anesthetic regimen, keep patients safe, and produce the best outcomes after surgery. For example, patients who are identified with cognitive decline should be evaluated to see if they would be a good candidate for an epidural or nerve block with their surgery to reduce the number of sedatives they would need. In all geriatric patients, especially those with cognitive decline, the use of a geriatric pain protocol should be implemented. A consult with the institution's inpatient geriatric team can be ordered so the patient can be evaluated after surgery, at the bedside, and ensure best geriatric care is being delivered. Patients who are identified as prefrail, frail, and/or who have impaired functional status should be considered for prehabilitation (prehab) prior to their surgery.

Once the patient assessment is completed, providers should educate patients on the different types of anesthetics available to them and allow them to participate in the decision-making process. Studies revealed that when anesthesiologists provided preoperative education and followed plans of care specific to a patient's individual needs, patients reported less anxiety and showed better cooperation in the postoperative period [26].

The discussion should always start with the surgeon when the surgery is determined beneficial and then be reinforced by the anesthesiologist and other members of the surgical team. Once the patient assessment is obtained, information gathered should be used to determine if they are a good candidate for the use of a nerve block or an epidural with their surgery. Consideration of the risks and benefits of the use of nerve blocks, epidurals, and/or IV sedation with and/or without general anesthesia should all be reviewed with the patient in the presurgery phase. Research shows extreme benefits of using nerve blocks in the elderly population, as they have been beneficial in providing postoperative analgesia, and lessened the amount of reported postoperative nausea, vomiting, and sedation [32]. The use of nerve blocks and/or epidurals with surgery has been shown to offer better postop pain control [32]. This is beneficial as increased amounts of pain after surgery are associated with the development of postop complications such as pneumonia and deep vein thrombosis [32]. Numerous studies have shown that when measures are taken to minimize the side effects of anesthesia, opioids patients have reported improved satisfaction and acceleration in their recovery [32].

Presurgery	• Identification of health needs through CGA • Cardiac and pulmonary assessments • Assessment of chronic diseases and any organ reserve decline • Development of surgery care plans to improve surgery outcomes • Planning for choice of anesthesia • Discussion of utility of surgery • Identification of patient's wishes for resuscitation • Identification of health goals
Intraoperative	• Anesthesia mode-least invasive • Pharmacology-geriatric dosing • Continuous monitoring—avoiding ischemic complications • Volume management: blood pressure fluctuations • Transfusion management • Lung ventilation and protection • Prevention of hypothermia • Prevention of skin breakdown
Postoperative	• Assess for cognitive impairment • Assess for deconditioning and body system • Analgesia management-geriatric dosing • Respiratory distress–postop pneumonia • Urinary retention, acute kidney injury • Functional decline, physical deconditioning • Higher morbidity or mortality rates • Loss of independence failure to thrive

Table 8.
Anesthetic considerations in the geriatric patient [1–7, 24, 25, 30–32].

A study conducted by Li et al. [32], demonstrated a significant decrease in delayed postoperative mobility, improved surgical results, and faster rehabilitation in patients who had received nerve block anesthesia [32]. During their presurgery screening, they should be evaluated to see if they are a good candidate for a nerve block or epidural with their surgery to help manage postop pain and decrease opioid use. Choices should be based on avoiding deep anesthesia, cerebral oxygen desaturation, and avoiding intraoperative hypothermia, all measures that can directly cause postoperative delirium [11].

For the most part, presedation assessment is standardized and only captures a small portion of the necessary information, especially, about functional status and frailty [4]. The unique needs of the older adult should be taken into consideration. Please refer to **Table 8** for a breakdown of *anesthetic considerations in the geriatric patient*. Surgical procedures and anesthetic drugs disrupt the hemostasis of the human body, so it is important that both surgeon and the anesthesiologist consider the preexisting physical conditions and comorbidities of this fragile population to ensure the safest outcomes after surgery [4].

6. Conclusions

The number of older patients who are medically complex with significant past medical histories, and who are electing to undergo surgery, will continue to grow over the years. Comprehensive health screening can be a lengthy job, but it is worth it and proves to be very meaningful. Presurgery identification of any of these issues is key to the prevention of bad outcomes. Through this extensive screening, we have the potential to improve our patient's overall health, which will lead to a safer surgical experience and better postoperative outcomes. With better surgery outcomes we can reduce length of stay, and overall morbidity and mortality. Presurgery preparation just makes sense. Ideally, the presurgical assessment team should include, at the least, a geriatric specialist, the surgeon, and anesthesia. Mid-level providers such as advanced practice nurses are most appropriate to accommodate leading this team and serving as a patient advocate.

If you prepare for anything in life, most likely you will do better. If a student studies and prepares for the examination, most likely they will do better. If an athlete trains and practices before the big game, most likely they will do better. When you prepare for surgery you can only hope to do better. Research supports that presurgery identification of medically complex patients or functionally debilitated patients can assist in reducing preventable adverse outcomes [4]. Many studies revealed that using a comprehensive geriatric assessment conducted by interdisciplinary team has shown large improvements in the outcomes of elderly surgical patients, including an increased survival rate, improved physical function, and decreased nursing home place placement [21].

Conflict of interest

The authors declare no conflict of interest.

Videos

Talk With Your Doctor - Surgical Optimization | St. Luke's Talk with your Doctor | wfmz.com

Appendix

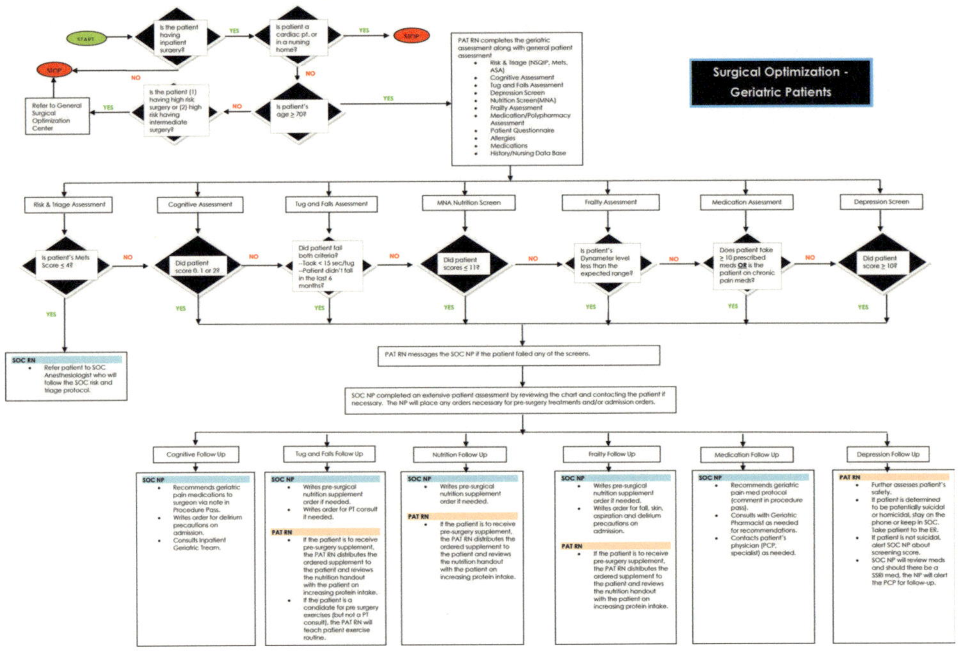

Appendix 1.
Compressive geriatric assessment (CGA) workflow diagram.

Author details

Ellen McHugh
St. Luke's University Health Network, Bethlehem, Pennsylvania, USA

*Address all correspondence to: ellen.mchugh@sluhn.org

IntechOpen

© 2023 The Author(s). Licensee IntechOpen. This chapter is distributed under the terms of the Creative Commons Attribution License (http://creativecommons.org/licenses/by/3.0), which permits unrestricted use, distribution, and reproduction in any medium, provided the original work is properly cited.

References

[1] United States Census Bureau. [Internet]. 2022. Available from: Census – Table Results [Accessed: April 23, 2022]

[2] Ortman JM, Velkoff VA, Hogan H. An Aging Nation: The Older Population in the United States. Washington, DC: US Census Bureau; 2014. pp. P25-P1140

[3] Senior Strong Organization. [Internet]. 2022. Available from: What Age Makes You A Senior Citizen? (seniorstrong.org) [Accessed: April 23, 2022]

[4] Bettelli G. Preoperative evaluation in geriatric surgery: Comorbidity, functional status and pharmacological history. Minerva Anestesiologica. 2011;**77**(6):637-646

[5] Inouye SK, Schlesinger MJ, Lydon TJ. Delirium: A symptom of how hospital care is failing older persons and a window to improve quality of hospital care. The American Journal of Medicine. 1999;**106**(5):565-573

[6] Cole MG, Primeau FJ. Prognosis of delirium in elderly hospital patients. Canadian Medial Association Journal. 1993;**149**(1):41-46

[7] Leslie DL, Inouye SK. The importance of delirium: Economic and societal costs. Journal of the American Geriatrics Society. 2011;**59**(Suppl 2):S241-S243

[8] Lee H, Lee E, Jang IY. Frailty and comprehensive geriatric assessment. Journal of Korean Medical Science. 2020;**35**(3):e16. DOI: 10.3346/jkm.2020.35.e16

[9] Xue DD, Cheng Y, Wu M, Zhang Y. Comprehensive geriatric assessment prediction of postoperative complications in gastrointestinal cancer patients: A meta-analysis. Clinical Interventions in Aging. 2018;**13**:723-736. DOI: 10.2147/CIA.S155409

[10] Kim KJ, Lee SB, Kim CO. How to Assess Frailty: Role of Comprehensive Geriatric Assessment. Journal of Korean Medical Science. 2020;**35**(3):e34. DOI: 10.3346/jkms.2020.35.3.e34

[11] Kong H, Xu LM, Wang DX. Perioperative neurocognitive disorders: A narrative review focusing on diagnosis, prevention, and treatment. CNS Neuroscience & therapeutics. 2022;**28**(8):P1147-P1167. DOI: 10.1111/cns.13873

[12] John Hopkins Medicine. [Internet]. 2022. Available from: Dementia and Delirium (hopkinsmedicine.org) [Accessed: July 29, 2022]

[13] Tatum Iii PE, Talebreza S, Ross JS. Geriatric assessment: An office-based approach. America Family Physician. 2018;**97**(12):P776-P784

[14] Inouye SK, Van Dyck CH, Alessi CA, Balkin S, Siegal AP, Horwitz RI. Clarifying confusion: The confusion assessment method. A new method for detection of delirium. Annals of Internal Medicine. 1990;**113**(12):P941-P948. DOI: 10.7326/0003-4819-113-12-941

[15] NSW Government. [Internet]. 2022. Available from: Screening and assessment tools for older people | Agency for Clinical Innovation (nsw.gov.au) [Accessed: July 29, 2022]

[16] World Health Organization. [Internet]. 2022. Available from: Malnutrition (who.int) [Accessed: July 29, 2022]

[17] Matsunaga T, Saito H, Osaki T, Takahashi S, Iwamoto A, Fukuda K, et al. Impact of geriatric nutritional risk index on outcomes after gastrectomy in elderly patients with gastric cancer: A retrospective multicenter study in Japan. BMC Cancer. 2022;**22**(1):540. DOI: 10.1186/s12885-022-09638-6

[18] Nutrition Care Systems. [Internet]. 2022. Available from: Malnutrition and the Elderly - Nutrition Care Systems [Accessed: July 29, 2022]

[19] Yu X, Chen L, Chen S, Qian W, Fang L. Application of care bundles in post anesthesia recovery for elderly patients with colorectal cancer. International Journal of. General Medicine. 2021;**14**:5949-5958

[20] Shahrokni A, Alexander K. What will perioperative geriatric assessment for older cancer patients look like in 2025? Advantages and limitations of new technologies in geriatric assessment. European Journal of Surgical Oncology: The Journal of the European Society of Surgical Oncology and the British Association of Surgical Oncology. 2020;**46**(3):305-309. DOI: 10.1016/j.ejso.2019.07.026

[21] Wieland D, Ferrucci L. Multidimensional geriatric assessment: Back to the future. The Journals of Gerontology, Series A, Biological Sciences and Medical Sciences. 2008;**63**(3):272-274. DOI: 10.1093/gerona/63.3.272

[22] Walston J, Buta B, Xue QL. Frailty Screening, and Interventions: Considerations for clinical practice. Clinics in Geriatric Medicine. 2018;**34**(1):P25-P38. DOI: 10.1016/j.cger.2017.09.004

[23] Chia CL, Tan KY. The era of geriatric surgery. Annals of the Academy of Medicine. 2019;**48**(11):P345-P346

[24] Gilardi F, Capanna A, Ferraro M, Scarcella P, Marazzi MC, Palombi L, et al. Frailty screening and assessment tools: A review of characteristics and use in Public Health. Annals of Surgery;**30**(2):128-139

[25] Carp L. Basic principles and geriatric surgery. Annals of Surgery. 1946;**123**(6):P1101-P1110

[26] Zhang J, Che J, Sun X, Ren W. Clinical application and perioperative anesthesia management based on enhanced recovery after surgery concept to elderly patients undergoing total knee replacement. Computational Intelligence and Neuroscience. 2022;**2022**:8039258. DOI: 10.1155/2022/8039358

[27] Paduraru M, Ponchietti L, Casas IM, Svenningsen P, Pereira J, Landaluce-Olavarria A, et al. Enhanced Recovery After Surgery (ERAS) the evidence in geriatric emergency surgery: A systematic review. Chirurgia. 2017;**112**(5):546-557

[28] Sharma R, Arora M, Garg R, Bansal P. A closer look at the 2019 Beers criteria. Drugs & Therapy Perspectives. 2020;**36**(3):116-122. DOI: 10.1007/s40267-019-00704-x

[29] By the 2019 American Geriatrics Society Beers Criteria® Update Expert Panel. American Geriatrics Society 2019 Updated AGS Beers Criteria® for Potentially Inappropriate Medication Use in Older Adults. Journal of the American Geriatrics Society. 2019;**67**(4):674-694. DOI: 10.1111/jgs.15767

[30] Williams K. Guidelines in practice: Moderate sedation and analgesia. Association of Perioperative Registered Nurses. 2022;**115**(6):P553-P564

[31] Liu M, Sun Y, Zhou L, Feng K, Wang T, Feng X. The median effective

dose and bispectral index of remimazolam tosilate for anesthesia induction in elderly patients: An up-and-down sequential allocation trial. Clinical Interventions in Aging. 2022;**17**:P837-P843

[32] Li X, Han C, Yu W. Comparison a femoral nerve block and fascia iliac block for proximal femoral fracture in the elderly patient: A meta- analysis. Geriatric Orthopedic Surgery and Rehabilitation. 2022;**13**:11647. DOI: 10.1177/21514593221111647